Shear Wave Elastography of Thyroid Nodules

Myung Hi Yoo • Hye Jeong Kim
In Ho Choi • Sumi Yun

Shear Wave Elastography of Thyroid Nodules

A Guide to Differential Diagnosis by Means of the Stiffness Map

Springer

Myung Hi Yoo
Department of Internal Medicine
Soonchunhyang University Hospital
Seoul
Korea (Republic of)

Hye Jeong Kim
Department of Internal Medicine
Soonchunhyang University Hospital
Seoul
Korea (Republic of)

In Ho Choi
Department of Pathology
Soonchunhyang University Hospital
Seoul
Korea (Republic of)

Sumi Yun
Department of Diagnostic Pathology
Samkwang Medical Laboratories
Seoul
Korea (Republic of)

ISBN 978-981-33-6872-9 ISBN 978-981-33-6873-6 (eBook)
https://doi.org/10.1007/978-981-33-6873-6

This Springer imprint is published by the registered company Springer Nature Singapore Pte Ltd.
The registered company address is: 152 Beach Road, #21-01/04 Gateway East, Singapore 189721, Singapore

Foreword

This is my Father's world.
All nature sings,
And God is the ruler. (Hymnal 478)
And so is the world of shear wave elastography.

Seoul, Korea (Republic of) Myung Hi Yoo

Preface

Fine needle aspiration cytology has been regarded as the gold standard in the differential diagnosis of thyroid nodules, but still the differential diagnosis of thyroid nodules with indeterminate cytology, especially follicular patterned lesions of thyroid nodules, needs further tools to aid the differential diagnosis which cannot be discriminated by fine needle aspiration cytology. Shear wave elastography may be helpful in the differentiation of follicular lesions which include nodular hyperplasia (NH) and follicular neoplasm (follicular adenoma and follicular carcinoma), because NH and follicular neoplasm show difference in the degree of fibrosis on histopathology, which can be detected on the stiffness map, i.e., shear wave elastography (SWE).

Also thyroid cancer, especially papillary carcinoma, is frequently accompanied by fibrosis which can be detected on shear wave elastography. So the evaluation of the degree and pattern of fibrosis can provide useful information about the pathology of the thyroid nodules, and we have reported several articles.

But for clinical application, demonstration of the representative clinical patient cases can help the readers figure out how stiffness map can be utilized for the differential diagnosis of the thyroid nodules. This book will give the readers clear concepts of the points of the differential diagnosis of thyroid nodules by SWE, through the presentation of clinical data of the patients even more effectively than by the articles published, especially for the practitioners and clinicians.

Shear wave elastography has been quite useful in the differential diagnosis of chronic liver disease by Fibroscan, which is another type of the stiffness map of the liver. Shear wave elastography has been recognized as a useful tool aiding the differential diagnosis of breast cancer. Now, it can be useful in the differential diagnosis of thyroid nodules leading to correct preoperative differential diagnosis. For the differentiation of benign and malignant nodules, SWE will provide additional information about the probability of possible histopathology and help the physician to decide the candidate nodule of FNA and further management.

This book presents the real data of the patients with thyroid nodules including conventional ultrasonogram (USG), shear wave elastography (SWE), fine needle aspiration cytology (FNA), and core needle biopsy (CNB) or surgical biopsy, giving the readers clear insight to guess the final histopathology by USG and SWE, so making correct differential diagnosis possible before FNA/CNB or surgical pathology. We hope this book will serve as a beginning reference for that purpose.

Seoul, Korea (Republic of)

Myung Hi Yoo
Hye Jeong Kim
In Ho Choi
Sumi Yun

Contents

1 Introduction

Thyroid nodule is a common disease found in up to 60% of the population on ultrasound (USG) examination [1, 2], and the malignancy rate is 5–15% of the thyroid nodules [3]. Fine-needle aspiration cytology (FNA) has been the gold standard in differentiating malignant thyroid nodules. Papillary carcinoma, which accounts for 80–90% of thyroid cancers, has several characteristic findings on USG and FNA [4–6], making accurate diagnosis is possible.

On the other hand, differential diagnosis of follicular patterned lesions including nodular hyperplasia (NH), follicular adenoma (FA), follicular carcinoma and follicular variant papillary carcinoma is not easy because there are no distinguishing and overlapping features on FNA [7–9] and USG [10, 11].

According to the Bethesda System for Reporting Thyroid Cytopathology (BSRTC) classification [3] and 2015 American Thyroid Association guidelines [12], for thyroid nodules in the indeterminate FNA including category III (atypia or follicular lesion of undetermined significance) and category IV (follicular neoplasm or suspicious for follicular neoplasm), diagnostic surgery (lobectomy) is recommended. The malignancy rate of the thyroid nodules of indeterminate category is reported as 20–50%, resulting in 50–80% of the patients ending up with unnecessary diagnostic surgery and leaving 20–50% of the patients with further completion thyroidectomy when further radioactive iodine treatment is needed [3, 7, 8, 13–18].

US elastography had been reported to be useful in the differentiation of benign and malignant thyroid nodules [19–23]. Strain elastography was initially developed with the operator using manual compression on the tissue to measure tissue displacement (strain) caused by the compression (stress) [24]. However, strain elastography had several disadvantages including high operator dependence in terms of compression and absence of sufficient quantitative information [25, 26].

Shear wave elastography (SWE) uses several focused ultrasonic pushing beams to generate shear waves and measures transversely propagated shear wave speed, and the subsequent ultrafast echographic imaging sequence generates a quantitative elastogram [27]. SWE has sufficient quantitative information and is operator independent in terms of compression; hence, it is expected to result in more reproducible findings than strain elastography, and two-dimensional SWE (2D-SWE) represents the focal tissue stiffness map [25, 27].

M. H. Yoo et al., *Shear Wave Elastography of Thyroid Nodules*,
https://doi.org/10.1007/978-981-33-6873-6_1

References

1. Bongiovanni M, Spitale A, Faquin WC, Mazzucchelli L, Baloch ZW. The Bethesda System for Reporting Thyroid Cytopathology: a meta-analysis. Acta Cytol. 2012;56:333–9.
2. Mazzaferri EL. Management of a solitary thyroid nodule. N Engl J Med. 1993;328:553–9.
3. Cibas ES, Ali SZ. The 2017 Bethesda System for Reporting Thyroid Cytopathology. Thyroid. 2017;27:1341–6.
4. Kumar V, Abbas AK, Aster JC. Robbins and Cotran pathologic basis of disease. 9th ed. Philadelphia, PA: Elsevier; 2015.
5. Lloyd RV, Osamura RY, Kloppel G, Rosai J. WHO classification of tumours of endocrine organs (medicine). 4th ed. Lyon: International Agency for Research on Cancer; 2017.
6. Ali SZ, Cibas ES. The Bethesda System for Reporting Thyroid Cytopathology: definitions, criteria and explanatory notes. New York, NY: Springer; 2010.
7. Alexander EK. Approach to the patient with a cytologically indeterminate thyroid nodule. J Clin Endocrinol Metab. 2008;93:4175–82.
8. Greaves TS, Olvera M, Florentine BD, Raza AS, Cobb CJ, Tsao-Wei DD, Groshen S, Singer P, Lopresti J, Martin SE. Follicular lesions of thyroid: a 5-year fine-needle aspiration experience. Cancer. 2000;90:335–41.
9. Maruta J, Hashimoto H, Suehisa Y, Yamashita H, Noguchi S, Aratake Y, Ohno E, Kobayashi TK. Improving the diagnostic accuracy of thyroid follicular neoplasms: cytological features in fine-needle aspiration cytology. Diagn Cytopathol. 2011;39:28–34.
10. Jeh SK, Jung SL, Kim BS, Lee YS. Evaluating the degree of conformity of papillary carcinoma and follicular carcinoma to the reported ultrasonographic findings of malignant thyroid tumor. Korean J Radiol. 2007;8:192–7.
11. Sillery JC, Reading CC, Charboneau JW, Henrichsen TL, Hay ID, Mandrekar JN. Thyroid follicular carcinoma: sonographic features of 50 cases. AJR Am J Roentgenol. 2010;194:44–54.
12. Haugen BR, Alexander EK, Bible KC, Doherty GM, Mandel SJ, Nikiforov YE, Pacini F, Randolph GW, Sawka AM, Schlumberger M, Schuff KG, Sherman SI, Sosa JA, Steward DL, Tuttle RM, Wartofsky L. 2015 American Thyroid Association Management Guidelines for Adult Patients with Thyroid Nodules and Differentiated Thyroid Cancer: The American Thyroid Association Guidelines Task Force on Thyroid Nodules and Differentiated Thyroid Cancer. Thyroid. 2016;26:1–133.
13. Marhefka GD, McDivitt JD, Shakir KM, Drake AJ 3rd. Diagnosis of follicular neoplasm in thyroid nodules by fine needle aspiration cytology: does the result, benign vs. suspicious for a malignant process, in these nodules make a difference? Acta Cytol. 2009;53:517–23.
14. Baloch ZW, Fleisher S, LiVolsi VA, Gupta PK. Diagnosis of "follicular neoplasm": a gray zone in thyroid fine-needle aspiration cytology. Diagn Cytopathol. 2002;26:41–4.
15. Yeh MW, Demircan O, Ituarte P, Clark OH. False-negative fine-needle aspiration cytology results delay treatment and adversely affect outcome in patients with thyroid carcinoma. Thyroid. 2004;14:207–15.
16. Bohacek L, Milas M, Mitchell J, Siperstein A, Berber E. Diagnostic accuracy of surgeon-performed ultrasound-guided fine-needle aspiration of thyroid nodules. Ann Surg Oncol. 2012;19:45–51.
17. Carling T, Udelsman R. Follicular neoplasms of the thyroid: what to recommend. Thyroid. 2005;15:583–7.
18. Yoon RG, Baek JH, Lee JH, Choi YJ, Hong MJ, Song DE, Kim JK, Yoon JH, Kim WB. Diagnosis of thyroid follicular neoplasm: fine-needle aspiration versus core-needle biopsy. Thyroid. 2014;24:1612–7.
19. Gregory A, Bayat M, Kumar V, Denis M, Kim BH, Webb J, Meixner DD, Ryder M, Knudsen JM, Chen S, Fatemi M, Alizad A. Differentiation of benign and malignant thyroid nodules by using comb-push ultrasound shear elastography: a preliminary two-plane view study. Acad Radiol. 2018;25:1388–97.
20. Veyrieres JB, Albarel F, Lombard JV, Berbis J, Sebag F, Oliver C, Petit P. A threshold value in Shear Wave elastography to rule out malignant thyroid nodules: a reality? Eur J Radiol. 2012;81:3965–72.
21. Kim H, Kim JA, Son EJ, Youk JH. Quantitative assessment of shear-wave ultrasound elastography in thyroid nodules: diagnostic performance for predicting malignancy. Eur Radiol. 2013;23:2532–7.
22. Park AY, Son EJ, Han K, Youk JH, Kim JA, Park CS. Shear wave elastography of thyroid nodules for the prediction of malignancy in a large scale study. Eur J Radiol. 2015;84:407–12.
23. Liu Z, Jing H, Han X, Shao H, Sun YX, Wang QC, Cheng W. Shear wave elastography combined with the thyroid imaging reporting and data system for malignancy risk stratification in thyroid nodules. Oncotarget. 2017;8:43406–16.
24. Chang N, Zhang X, Wan W, Zhang C, Zhang X. The preciseness in diagnosing thyroid malignant nodules using shear-wave elastography. Med Sci Monit. 2018;24:671–7.
25. Bardet S, Ciappuccini R, Pellot-Barakat C, Monpeyssen H, Michels JJ, Tissier F, Blanchard D, Menegaux F, de Raucourt D, Lefort M, Reznik Y, Rouxel A, Heutte N, Brenac F, Leconte A, Buffet C, Clarisse B, Leenhardt L. Shear wave elastography in thyroid nodules with indeterminate cytology: results of a prospective bicentric study. Thyroid. 2017;27:1441–9.
26. Bhatia KS, Tong CS, Cho CC, Yuen EH, Lee YY, Ahuja AT. Shear wave elastography of thyroid nodules in routine clinical practice: preliminary observations and utility for detecting malignancy. Eur Radiol. 2012;22:2397–406.
27. Swan KZ, Nielsen VE, Bibby BM, Bonnema SJ. Is the reproducibility of shear wave elastography of thyroid nodules high enough for clinical use? A methodological study. Clin Endocrinol (Oxf). 2017;86:606–13.

Elastography Physics

2

A detailed description of physics is out of the scope of this book, so a summary of the principles necessary for the clinical application will be provided. Basically, elasticity (stiffness) measures how a tissue will maintain its shape when force is applied. Elastography is the visual display of the stiffness of the tissue which can be obtained by measuring the displacement (strain) of the tissue in response to applied pressure.

In ultrasound elastography physics, the stiffness of the tissue is described by Young's elastic modulus E.

$$\sigma = E\varepsilon,$$

where $\sigma = \frac{F}{A}$, $\varepsilon = \frac{\Delta L}{L_0}$

Stress σ (F/A) is the applied force per unit area with units of pascals (Pa) and strain ε ($\Delta L/L_0$) is the deformation in length relative to its original length in response to the compression force (stress).

So Young's elastic modulus E is,

$$E = \frac{\sigma}{\varepsilon} = \left(\frac{F}{A}\right)\frac{L_0}{\Delta L}$$

So Young's elastic modulus E is inversely proportional to the amount of displacement ($\Delta L/L_0$) in response to stress, resulting less displacement (strain) in harder tissue [1, 2].

Initially, strain elastography was introduced and the operator applied compression on the tissue usually using the ultrasound transducer. Analyzing changes in the echo pattern before and after compression by measuring tissue displacement (strain) creates the strain elastogram. The strain elastogram is displayed adjacent to the B-mode image and color coded with scoring systems (4–5 scales) showing whether the lesion is hard or soft relative to the other tissues in the field of view. The lesion appears hard or soft depending on the stiffness of other tissues around, so the strain elastography produces a qualitative stiffness map [3]. And strain changes according to the compression pressure (stress) applied by the operator, so the strain elastography shows high operator-dependent variability in terms of compression. So strain elastography is limited by the wide interobserver variability and also by the qualitative data, which lacks quantitative information. To overcome these limitations, SWE was developed.

SWE uses several focused ultrasonic beams (pushing beams) at increasing depths, which are transmitted to generate shear waves. It uses constant acoustic pressure from the transducer, accomplishing the standardization of compression (stress) [2].

In shear waves particle motions are perpendicular to the direction of wave propagation and shear wave speed is approximately 1–10 m/s in soft tissues. The low wave speed in soft tissues allows high differences between tissues, giving suitable tissue contrast for elastography

M. H. Yoo et al., *Shear Wave Elastography of Thyroid Nodules*,
https://doi.org/10.1007/978-981-33-6873-6_2

measurements. On the other hand, in longitudinal ultrasonic waves where particle motions are parallel to the direction of wave propagation, the speed of the wave is approximately 1540 m/s in soft tissues. So it makes relatively small differences in wave speed between different soft tissues, which are not adequate for tissue contrast [4].

The transverse shear waves are rapidly attenuated, so immediately after generation of pushing beams, an ultrafast echographic imaging sequence (up to 20,000 frames/s) is performed to track the lateral movements of shear waves.

Young's modulus E can be approximated by

$$E = 3\rho c^2$$

Where ρ is the local density constant and equal to 1000 kg/m^3 in soft tissues and c is the shear wave speed (m/s). Based on Young's modulus formula, tissue elasticity can be calculated from shear wave propagation speed, resulting in quantitative data of the focal lesion in kPa or m/s.

Shear waves propagate faster through stiffer tissues, so the numerical value of the speed of shear wave propagation within a region of interest is a reasonable representation of tissue stiffness in the region [2]. A color-coded shear wave elastogram is displayed ranging from 0 to 240 kPa, which is superimposed on a B-mode scan, visualizing simultaneous anatomical and tissue stiffness information with the quantitative map of tissue stiffness. So, the shear wave elastogram has the advantage of being quantitative, reproducible and not operator dependent in terms of compression (stress) [5].

References

1. Kamaya A, Machtaler S, Safari Sanjani S, Nikoozadeh A, Graham Sommer F, Pierre Khuri-Yakub BT, Willmann JK, Desser TS. New technologies in clinical ultrasound. Semin Roentgenol. 2013;48:214–23.
2. Sigrist RMS, Liau J, Kaffas AE, Chammas MC, Willmann JK. Ultrasound elastography: review of techniques and clinical applications. Theranostics. 2017;7:1303–29.
3. Gennisson JL, Deffieux T, Fink M, Tanter M. Ultrasound elastography: principles and techniques. Diagn Interv Imaging. 2013;94:487–95.
4. Garra BS. Elastography: history, principles, and technique comparison. Abdom Imaging. 2015;40:680–97.
5. Evans A, Whelehan P, Thomson K, McLean D, Brauer K, Purdie C, Jordan L, Baker L, Thompson A. Quantitative shear wave ultrasound elastography: initial experience in solid breast masses. Breast Cancer Res. 2010;12:R104.

3 SWE of Thyroid Nodules

Studies using SWE to assess thyroid nodules have reported its usefulness in detecting malignant nodules. However, there was a wide range of cut-off values of the elasticity index (EI) in detecting malignant nodules ranging from 34 kPa to 90 kPa [1–11]. Thyroid nodules usually show heterogeneous images of EI within the nodule on 2D-SWE; thus, selecting different locations of region of interest (ROI) within the nodule displays different ROI even with the same operator [12, 13]. Difficulty in imaging and the subjective features of selecting representative location of ROI in thyroid nodules with heterogeneous EI contribute to variable EI profiles in SWE [14, 15]. Therefore, SWE is not operator dependent in terms of the added stress (compression) but operator dependent in the placement of ROI. To decrease this subjective variance in the placement of ROI in thyroid nodules, we let the total nodular area as the ROI by tracing the total nodular margin using the overlapping B-mode US.

Recently, we reported that the mean EI in the total nodular ROI showed higher reproducibility and better agreement in intra- and interrater assay than in the focal nodular ROI when evaluating the intraclass correlation coefficient, coefficient of variation, and Bland-Altman analysis. It may be due to the avoidance of the subjective variance of placement of ROI in the focal nodular ROI [16]. We suggested that the total nodular ROI method would be a valuable and standardized method in clinical practice. Also our report revealed that fibrosis increased SWE elasticity in the thyroid nodule, which might lead to the discrepancy of the cut-off values in detecting thyroid cancer. Our study showed that the percentage of high EI (>36 kPa) area of the nodule showed a correlation with the degree of fibrosis (percentage of fibrosis on surgical histopathology). Moreover, the EI of the thyroid nodule showed positive correlation with the degree of fibrosis on surgical pathology. Additionally, the location of the fibrosis on surgical pathology was concordant with the high EI area on SWE. Hence, the degree and location of fibrosis on histopathology were closely correlated with the high EI area of the thyroid nodule on SWE [16]. Diverse elasticities in papillary thyroid carcinoma (PTC) might reflect variable degrees of fibrosis in PTC. Because 80–90 % of the malignant nodules are composed of PTC, it may result in the discrepant cut-off values in the diagnosis of malignant thyroid nodules. A wide range of cut-off values of the EI in detecting malignancy from 34 kPa to 90 kPa have been reported [1–11]. It may be due to the various degrees of fibrosis in different patients and different types of tumors in the same study group and also in different study groups.

In the cytologic diagnosis of thyroid nodules, most difficult problem is the differential diagnosis of the follicular patterned lesions, It is the most frequently found entity comprising more than 50 % in FNA [17, 18]. Benign Follicular lesion (category II in Bethesda system) and

M. H. Yoo et al., *Shear Wave Elastography of Thyroid Nodules*,
https://doi.org/10.1007/978-981-33-6873-6_3

follicular neoplasm or suspicious for follicular neoplasm (category IV in Bethesda system) represent follicular patterned lesion, which histopathologically encompass nodular hyperplasia and follicular neoplasm including follicular adenoma and follicular carcinoma. Follicular thyroid carcinoma (FTC) has no reliable diagnostic cytologic findings on FNA [19–21] nor characteristic US findings [22, 23] showing similar or overlapping features with benign follicular lesions such as follicular adenoma (FA) and nodular hyperplasia (NH) both on FNA [24–26] and US. FTC is confirmed postoperatively by capsular invasion or angioinvasion, so preoperative distinction from FA is impossible by FNA. Postoperative evaluation of FTC revealed preoperative FNA was classified as benign follicular lesion (category II), atypia or follicular lesion of undetermined significance (AUS/FLUS, category III), follicular neoplasm or suspicious for follicular neoplasm (FN/SFN, category IV) or suspicious for malignancy (SM, category V) according to the Bethesda System [21, 27]. And diagnostic surgery of the thyroid nodules with FNA in category III or IV revealed malignancy rate was 20–50% [24, 25, 28–32]. So unnecessary diagnostic surgery for benign nodules was 50–80%, and about 30–50% of benign surgery was revealed as NH [25, 32].

In clinical management, if FNA of FTC showed category III or IV by showing microfollicular patterns, FTC may be detected by diagnostic surgery. But when it showed features of macrofollicular pattern compatible with category II on FNA, it is hard to select possible candidate of FTC in large numbers of benign nodules accounting for 65% of thyroid nodules [18], because FTC has no specific findings on FNA and US. And this infrequent case may make litigious episode, especially first diagnosed as benign on FNA and later clarified as malignant due to distant metastasis [26, 33, 34].

For decades, continuous efforts have been made to preoperatively differentiate malignant follicular lesions from benign lesions, including thyroxine suppression, analysis of clinical findings [35], US findings [36], core-needle biopsy (CNB) [37] and molecular tests [38–43]. CNB may help differentiate NH from FN [44–46], but it is not always possible and practical to perform CNB for the large numbers of benign thyroid nodules. Molecular tests help select malignant follicular lesion with high sensitivity but show low specificity of around 50% [38] and might show false positive results in benign follicular lesions. Also it is expensive to perform as routine screening tests.

Histopathologically, NH shows focal nonneoplastic hyperplasia and subsequent involutional changes accompanied by various degenerative changes including hemorrhage, infiltration of inflammatory cells and fibrotic change with incomplete capsule formation [47, 48], while FA is composed of neoplastic cells surrounded by complete capsulation and shows typically scanty amount of interstitial tissue [34], devoid of degenerative changes [49]. So, the degree and quantity of fibrosis is usually larger in NH than in FA.

Recent application of SWE showed it was useful in the evaluation of fibrosis, especially in the evaluation of chronic liver disease and liver cirrhosis. SWE of liver (Fibroscan), which measures the degree of fibrosis in chronic liver disease, has replaced CNB in the evaluation of the cirrhotic change of the chronic liver disease [50]. Besides, SWE of liver has the advantage of noninvasiveness; it can evaluate the whole hepatic parenchyma compared with the small pieces of tissue on CNB which sometimes does not represent the whole hepatic parenchymal change.

We evaluated SWE could detect the difference of fibrosis between NH and FA. We had studied the diagnostic performance of SWE to differentiate follicular neoplasm (FN) from NH in follicular lesions of thyroid nodules [51]. We analyzed the magnitude of EI and patterns of high EI area (EI > 36 kPa). The patterns of high EI area was classified as marginal pattern (high EI areas are restricted in the outer 1/3 of the nodule) and traversing pattern (high EI areas approaching further to the center of the nodule within inner 2/3 of the nodule). The EMax, EMean, ESD, and percent of high EI area were significantly lower in FN than NH ($p < 0.001$). The diagnostic performance to predict FN showed sensitivity, specificity, and accuracy of 95%, 90% and 92% by $E_{\mathrm{Max}} < 42.1$ kPa, and of 89%, 93% and 92% by marginal pattern of high EI area, respectively. We had reported the diagnostic criteria of E_{Max} less than 42.1 kPa and marginal pattern of high EI area on SWE can predict FN with high diagnostic accuracy. It might wave diagnostic surgery of NH in indeterminate cytology [51].

It is known that EI is different in magnitude in different tissues (fibrosis >carcinoma >glandular tissue >fat) [52]. We compared 2D-SWE of the thyroid nodules with the surgical histopathology specimens or CNB results. We investigated the relationship between the magnitude and patterns of elevated EI area on SWE and the fibrotic area on histopathology specimen stained with H & E stain and Masson's trichrome stain for visualizing collagen fiber. In the following chapter, we present cases of separate disease category with the data of SWE and surgical pathology or CNB. We will discuss the diagnostic performance of SWE in the differential diagnosis of thyroid nodules and try to figure out possible prediction of histopathology by 2D-SWE.

References

1. Wang F, Chang C, Chen M, Gao Y, Chen YL, Zhou SC, et al. Does lesion size affect the value of shear wave elastography for differentiating between benign and malignant thyroid nodules? J Ultrasound Med. 2018;37(3):601–9.
2. Azizi G, Keller JM, Mayo ML, Piper K, Puett D, Earp KM, et al. Shear wave elastography and Afirma gene expression classifier in thyroid nodules with indeterminate cytology: a comparison study. Endocrine. 2018;59(3):573–84.
3. Sebag F, Vaillant-Lombard J, Berbis J, Griset V, Henry JF, Petit P, et al. Shear wave elastography: a new ultrasound imaging mode for the differential diagnosis of benign and malignant thyroid nodules. J Clin Endocrinol Metab. 2010;95(12):5281–8.
4. Duan SB, Yu J, Li X, Han ZY, Zhai HY, Liang P. Diagnostic value of two-dimensional shear wave elastography in papillary thyroid microcarcinoma. OncoTargets Therapy. 2016;9:1311–7.
5. Gregory A, Bayat M, Kumar V, Denis M, Kim BH, Webb J, et al. Differentiation of benign and malignant thyroid nodules by using comb-push ultrasound shear elastography: a preliminary two-plane view study. Acad Radiol. 2018;25(11):1388–97.
6. Veyrieres JB, Albarel F, Lombard JV, Berbis J, Sebag F, Oliver C, et al. A threshold value in Shear Wave elastography to rule out malignant thyroid nodules: a reality? Eur J Radiol. 2012;81(12):3965–72.
7. Kim H, Kim JA, Son EJ, Youk JH. Quantitative assessment of shear-wave ultrasound elastography in thyroid nodules: diagnostic performance for predicting malignancy. Eur Radiol. 2013;23(9):2532–7.
8. Park AY, Son EJ, Han K, Youk JH, Kim JA, Park CS. Shear wave elastography of thyroid nodules for the prediction of malignancy in a large scale study. Eur J Radiol. 2015;84(3):407–12.
9. Liu Z, Jing H, Han X, Shao H, Sun YX, Wang QC, et al. Shear wave elastography combined with the thyroid imaging reporting and data system for malignancy risk stratification in thyroid nodules. Oncotarget. 2017;8(26):43406–16.
10. Chang N, Zhang X, Wan W, Zhang C, Zhang X. The preciseness in diagnosing thyroid malignant nodules using shear-wave elastography. Med Sci Monit. 2018;24:671–7.
11. Bhatia KS, Tong CS, Cho CC, Yuen EH, Lee YY, Ahuja AT. Shear wave elastography of thyroid nodules in routine clinical practice: preliminary observations and utility for detecting malignancy. Eur Radiol. 2012;22(11):2397–406.
12. Bardet S, Ciappuccini R, Pellot-Barakat C, Monpeyssen H, Michels JJ, Tissier F, et al. Shear wave elastography in thyroid nodules with indeterminate cytology: results of a prospective bicentric study. Thyroid. 2017;27(11):1441–9.
13. Garra BS. Imaging and estimation of tissue elasticity by ultrasound. Ultrasound Quart. 2007;23(4):255–68.
14. Swan KZ, Nielsen VE, Bibby BM, Bonnema SJ. Is the reproducibility of shear wave elastography of thyroid nodules high enough for clinical use? A methodological study. Clin Endocrinol. 2017;86(4):606–13.
15. Anvari A, Dhyani M, Stephen AE, Samir AE. Reliability of shear-wave elastography estimates of the Young Modulus of tissue in follicular thyroid neoplasms. AJR Am J Roentgenol. 2016;206(3):609–16.
16. Yoo MH, Kim HJ, Choi IH, Park S, Kim SJ, Park HK, et al. Shear wave elasticity by tracing total nodule showed high reproducibility and concordance with fibrosis in thyroid cancer. BMC Cancer. 2020;20(1):118.
17. Bongiovanni M, Spitale A, Faquin WC, Mazzucchelli L, Baloch ZW. The Bethesda System for Reporting Thyroid Cytopathology: a meta-analysis. Acta Cytol. 2012;56(4):333–9.
18. Ali SZ, Cibas ES. The Bethesda System for Reporting Thyroid Cytopathology: definitions, criteria and explanatory notes, vol. 2010. New York, NY: Springer; 2010.

19. Alexander EK. Approach to the patient with a cytologically indeterminate thyroid nodule. J Clin Endocrinol Metab. 2008;93(11):4175–82.
20. Greaves TS, Olvera M, Florentine BD, Raza AS, Cobb CJ, Tsao-Wei DD, et al. Follicular lesions of thyroid: a 5-year fine-needle aspiration experience. Cancer. 2000;90(6):335–41.
21. Maruta J, Hashimoto H, Suehisa Y, Yamashita H, Noguchi S, Aratake Y, et al. Improving the diagnostic accuracy of thyroid follicular neoplasms: cytological features in fine-needle aspiration cytology. Diagn Cytopathol. 2011;39(1):28–34.
22. Jeh SK, Jung SL, Kim BS, Lee YS. Evaluating the degree of conformity of papillary carcinoma and follicular carcinoma to the reported ultrasonographic findings of malignant thyroid tumor. Korean J Radiol. 2007;8(3):192–7.
23. Sillery JC, Reading CC, Charboneau JW, Henrichsen TL, Hay ID, Mandrekar JN. Thyroid follicular carcinoma: sonographic features of 50 cases. AJR Am J Roentgenol. 2010;194(1):44–54.
24. Marhefka GD, McDivitt JD, Shakir KM, Drake AJ 3rd. Diagnosis of follicular neoplasm in thyroid nodules by fine needle aspiration cytology: does the result, benign vs. suspicious for a malignant process, in these nodules make a difference? Acta Cytol. 2009;53(5):517–23.
25. Baloch ZW, Fleisher S, LiVolsi VA, Gupta PK. Diagnosis of "follicular neoplasm": a gray zone in thyroid fine-needle aspiration cytology. Diagn Cytopathol. 2002;26(1):41–4.
26. Yeh MW, Demircan O, Ituarte P, Clark OH. False-negative fine-needle aspiration cytology results delay treatment and adversely affect outcome in patients with thyroid carcinoma. Thyroid. 2004;14(3):207–15.
27. Bohacek L, Milas M, Mitchell J, Siperstein A, Berber E. Diagnostic accuracy of surgeon-performed ultrasound-guided fine-needle aspiration of thyroid nodules. Ann Surg Oncol. 2012;19(1):45–51.
28. Bahar G, Braslavsky D, Shpitzer T, Feinmesser R, Avidan S, Popovtzer A, et al. The cytological and clinical value of the thyroid "follicular lesion". Am J Otolaryngol. 2003;24(4):217–20.
29. Carling T, Udelsman R. Follicular neoplasms of the thyroid: what to recommend. Thyroid. 2005;15(6):583–7.
30. Yoon RG, Baek JH, Lee JH, Choi YJ, Hong MJ, Song DE, et al. Diagnosis of thyroid follicular neoplasm: fine-needle aspiration versus core-needle biopsy. Thyroid. 2014;24(11):1612–7.
31. Cibas ES, Ali SZ. The 2017 Bethesda System for Reporting Thyroid Cytopathology. Thyroid. 2017;27(11):1341–6.
32. Jo VY, Stelow EB, Dustin SM, Hanley KZ. Malignancy risk for fine-needle aspiration of thyroid lesions according to the Bethesda System for Reporting Thyroid Cytopathology. Am J Clin Pathol. 2010;134(3):450–6.
33. Zeiger MA, Dackiw AP. Follicular thyroid lesions, elements that affect both diagnosis and prognosis. J Surg Oncol. 2005;89(3):108–13.
34. Lloyd RV, Osamura RY, Kloppel G, Rosai J. WHO classification of tumours of endocrine organs (Medicine). 4th ed. Lyon: International Agency for Research on Cancer; 2017.
35. Gulcelik NE, Gulcelik MA, Kuru B. Risk of malignancy in patients with follicular neoplasm: predictive value of clinical and ultrasonographic features. Archiv Otolaryngol Head Neck Surg. 2008;134(12):1312–5.
36. Yoon JH, Kim EK, Youk JH, Moon HJ, Kwak JY. Better understanding in the differentiation of thyroid follicular adenoma, follicular carcinoma, and follicular variant of papillary carcinoma: a retrospective study. Int J Endocrinol. 2014;2014:321595.
37. Nasrollah N, Trimboli P, Guidobaldi L, Cicciarella Modica DD, Ventura C, Ramacciato G, et al. Thin core biopsy should help to discriminate thyroid nodules cytologically classified as indeterminate. A new sampling technique. Endocrine. 2013;43(3):659–65.
38. Alexander EK, Kennedy GC, Baloch ZW, Cibas ES, Chudova D, Diggans J, et al. Preoperative diagnosis of benign thyroid nodules with indeterminate cytology. N Engl J Med. 2012;367(8):705–15.
39. Nikiforov YE. Role of molecular markers in thyroid nodule management: then and now. Endocr Pract. 2017;23(8):979–88.
40. Taye A, Gurciullo D, Miles BA, Gupta A, Owen RP, Inabnet WB III, et al. Clinical performance of a next-generation sequencing assay (ThyroSeq v2) in the evaluation of indeterminate thyroid nodules. Surgery. 2018;163(1):97–103.
41. Valderrabano P, Khazai L, Thompson ZJ, Leon ME, Otto KJ, Hallanger-Johnson JE, et al. Impact of oncogene panel results on surgical management of cytologically indeterminate thyroid nodules. Head Neck. 2018;40(8):1812–23.
42. Yang SE, Sullivan PS, Zhang J, Govind R, Levin MR, Rao JY, et al. Has Afirma gene expression classifier testing refined the indeterminate thyroid category in cytology? Cancer Cytopathol. 2016;124(2):100–9.
43. Nikiforova MN, Mercurio S, Wald AI, Barbi de Moura M, Callenberg K, Santana-Santos L, et al. Analytical performance of the ThyroSeq v3 genomic classifier for cancer diagnosis in thyroid nodules. Cancer. 2018;124(8):1682–90.
44. Min HS, Kim JH, Ryoo I, Jung SL, Jung CK. The role of core needle biopsy in the preoperative diagnosis of follicular neoplasm of the thyroid. APMIS. 2014;122(10):993–1000.
45. Chen BT, Jain AB, Dagis A, Chu P, Vora L, Maghami E, et al. Comparison of the efficacy and safety of ultrasound-guided core needle biopsy versus fine-needle aspiration for evaluating thyroid nodules. Endocr Pract. 2015;21(2):128–35.

46. Trimboli P, Crescenzi A. Thyroid core needle biopsy: taking stock of the situation. Endocrine. 2015;48(3):779–85.
47. Kumar V, Abbas AK, Aster JC. Robbins and Cotran pathologic basis of disease. 9th ed. Philadelphia, PA: Elsevier; 2015.
48. DeMay RM. Follicular lesions of the thyroid. W(h) ither follicular carcinoma? Am J Clin Pathol. 2000;114(5):681–3.
49. Baloch ZW, Livolsi VA. Follicular-patterned lesions of the thyroid: the bane of the pathologist. Am J Clin Pathol. 2002;117(1):143–50.
50. Barr RG, Ferraioli G, Palmeri ML, Goodman ZD, Garcia-Tsao G, Rubin J, et al. Elastography assessment of liver fibrosis: Society of Radiologists in Ultrasound Consensus Conference Statement. Radiology. 2015;276(3):845–61.
51. Yoo MH, Kim HJ, Choi IH, Mok J, Park HK, Byun DW, et al. Differential diagnosis of thyroid follicular neoplasm from nodular hyperplasia by shear wave elastography. Soonchunhyang Med Sci. 2019;25(1):10–9.
52. Hedrick W. Technology for diagnostic sonography. St Louis: Elsevier Mosby; 2013.

Differential Diagnosis of Thyroid Nodules

4

4.1 Nodular Hyperplasia (Adenomatous Goiter)

Nodular hyperplasia (NH) occurs as unifocal or multifocal thyroid nodules and recurrent episodes of hyperplasia and involution produce irregular enlargement of the thyroid [1]. Uneven follicular hyperplasia with formation of new follicles appears and is subsequently followed by the involutional change with accumulation of colloid which leads to the rupture of the follicles and vessels accompanied by the hemorrhage, fibrosis with calcification and cystic change [1]. Microscopically, histological variabilities showing areas of hyperplastic follicles along with neighboring degenerative colloid rich follicles lined by flattened epithelial cells with interstitial inflammatory change, hemorrhage and fibrosis are observed [2].

According to the Bethesda system, about 65% of thyroid nodules are categorized as category II, benign. Category II benign nodules are subclassified as benign follicular nodules, thyroiditis and other less common entities [3]. And the benign follicular nodule (BFN) is the most commonly sampled lesion by FNA and encompasses cytologic features of the nodules classified histologically as nodular goiter, adenomatous hyperplasic nodules and follicular neoplasm with macrofollicular type.

Follicular neoplasm (adenoma and carcinoma) with microfollicles and sometimes NH with hyperplastic follicles also show cellular FNA and numerous follicular celles forming clusters of microfollicules with little or thick colloid and may be classified as category III (atypia) or IV (suspicious follicular neoplasm). On the other hand, follicular neoplasm (follicular adenoma or follicular carcinoma) with macrofollicular architecture shows abundant colloid with follicular cells arranged in monolayer sheets, similar to category II benign nodules by FNA [4]. So the distinction between malignant and benign follicular neoplasm is not possible by FNA [5–7], and especially category III and IV nodules often need diagnostic surgery to exclude malignancy.

Histopathologically NH shows focal nonneoplastic hyperplasia and subsequent involutional changes accompanied by various degenerative changes including hemorrhage, infiltration of inflammatory cells and fibrotic change with incomplete capsule formation [1, 8]. In contrast, FA is mainly composed of neoplastic cells and surrounded by the complete capsulation, and shows typically scanty amount of interstitial tissue [9] and devoid of degenerative change [2]. So the degree and quantity of fibrosis is larger in NH than FA.

Recent application of SWE showed it was useful in the evaluation of fibrosis, especially in the evaluation of chronic liver disease and liver cirrhosis. SWE of liver (Fibroscan) which

M. H. Yoo et al., *Shear Wave Elastography of Thyroid Nodules*,
https://doi.org/10.1007/978-981-33-6873-6_4

measures the degree of fibrosis in chronic liver disease has replaced CNB in the evaluation of cirrhotic change of the chronic liver disease [10]. Besides the SWE of liver has the advantage of noninvasiveness, it can evaluate the whole hepatic parenchyma compared with the small pieces of tissue on CNB.

We tried to apply SWE in thyroid nodules and evaluate whether SWE can differentiate the degree and patterns of fibrosis of NH from those of follicular neoplasm in thyroid nodules so that preoperative exclusion of NH from diagnostic surgery may avoid unnecessary thyroidectomy due to NH. We tried to evaluate the magnitude of SWE EI and pattern of elevated elasticity in the follicular patterned lesions of thyroid nodules. Diagnosis was confirmed by the surgically resected specimen or CNB results. We found difference in the magnitude (EI) and pattern of elevated elasticity on 2D-SWE between follicular neoplasm and NH.

Follicular patterned thyroid nodules with NH show a higher EI ($E_{Max} > 42.1$ kPa) in 90% of the nodules, while thyroid nodules with follicular neoplasm show a lower EI ($E_{Max} \leq 42.1$ kPa) in 90% of the nodules. And the patterns of high elasticity on 2D-SWE show difference between NH and follicular neoplasm. Thyroid nodules with NH show traversing patterns of increased elasticity traversing further than 1/3 of the transverse diameter toward the center from the margin of the nodule and more than 90% of the nodules with NH showed traversing patterns on SWE. Thyroid nodules with follicular neoplasm show no or marginal patterns of increased elasticity residing less than 1/3 of the transverse diameter toward the center from the margin of the nodules, usually expressing no or encircling or spotty increased elasticity around the margin of the nodules. More than 90% of the nodules with follicular neoplasm showed marginal patterns on SWE.

4.1.1 Case 1

60-year old woman was referred for a growing thyroid nodule during regular follow up. B-mode ultrasonogram showed isoechoic partially cystic 4.74 cm right nodule with round margin (Figs. 4.1, 4.2, and 4.3). Shear wave elastogram showed traversing pattern of high elasticity and E_{Max} was 76.6 kPa (Fig. 4.4). Core needle biopsy result was nodular hyperplasia with thick fibrous interstitial tissue showing similar patterned follicles in both sides of the fibrous tissue (arrows, Figs. 4.5 and 4.6). She underwent total thyroidectomy and histopathology was nodular hyperplasia (Fig. 4.7) showing thick interstitial fibrosis (arrows).

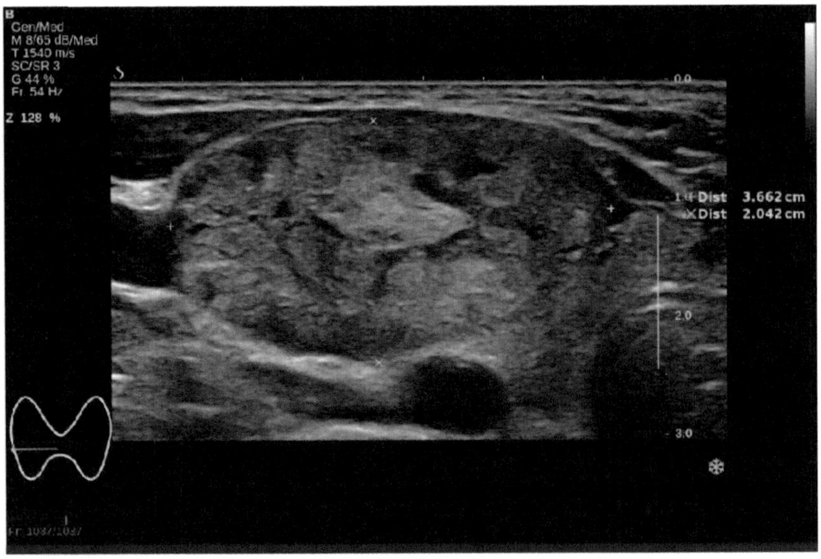

Fig. 4.1 B-mode ultrasonogram showing isoechoic partially cystic 4.74 cm right nodule with round margin

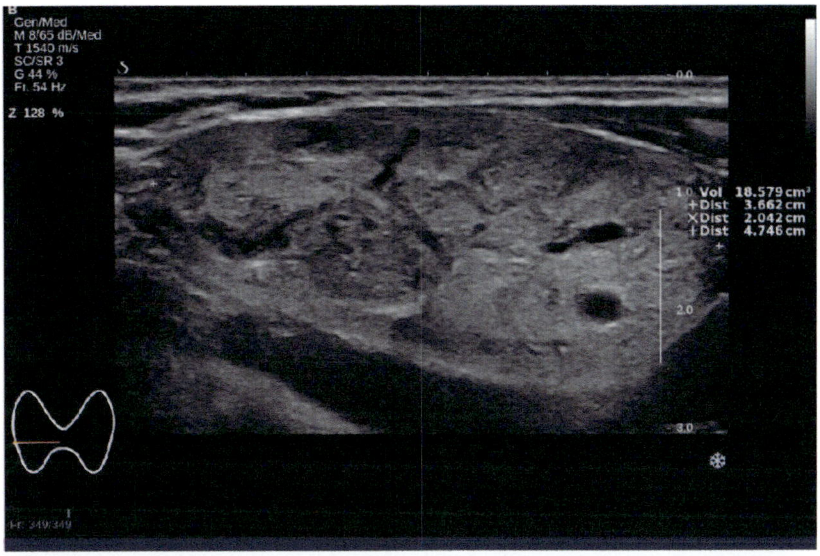

Fig. 4.2 B-mode ultrasonogram showing isoechoic partially cystic 4.74 cm right nodule with round margin

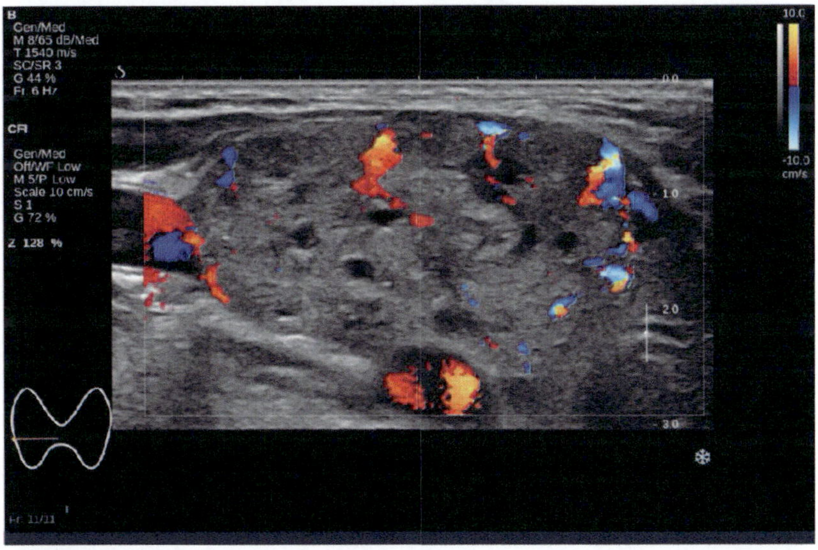

Fig. 4.3 Color Doppler showed moderately increased internal blood flow within the nodule

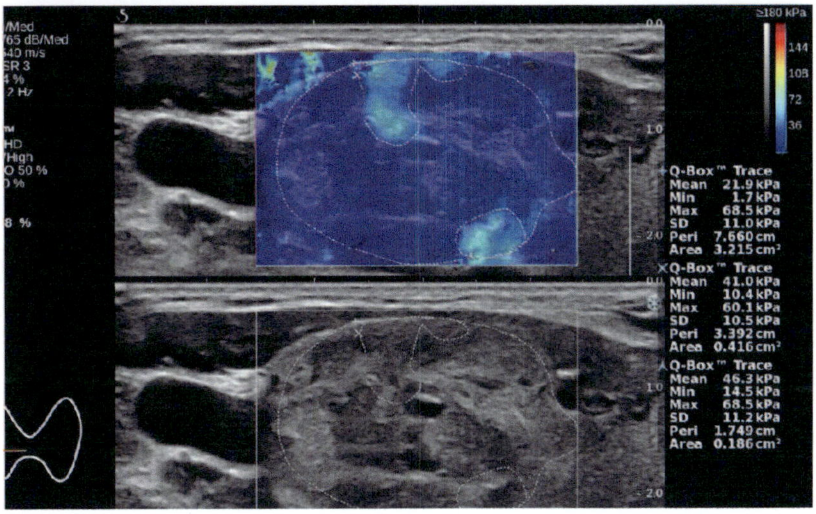

Fig. 4.4 Shear wave elastogram showing traversing pattern of high elasticity and E_{Max} 76.6 kPa

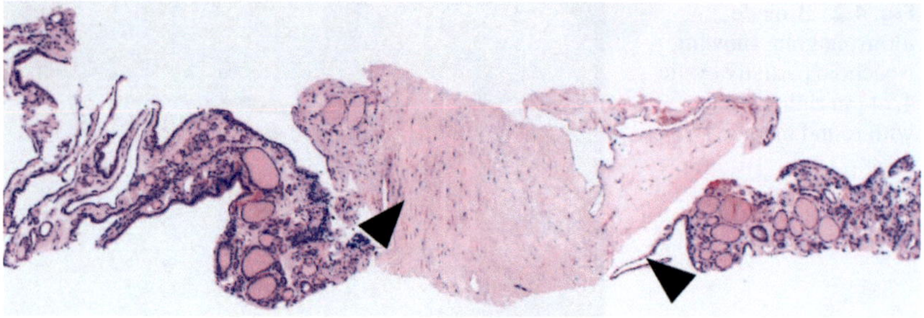

Fig. 4.5 Core needle biopsy suggested nodular hyperplasia with thick fibrous tissue (arrows)

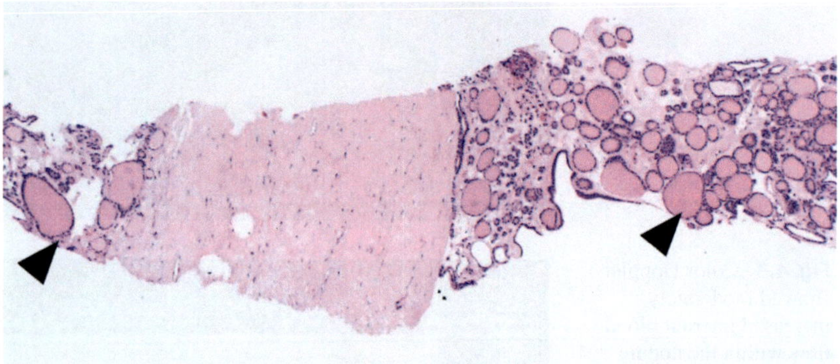

Fig. 4.6 Core needle biopsy suggested nodular hyperplasia with thick fibrous tissue showing similar patterned follicles in both sides (arrows)

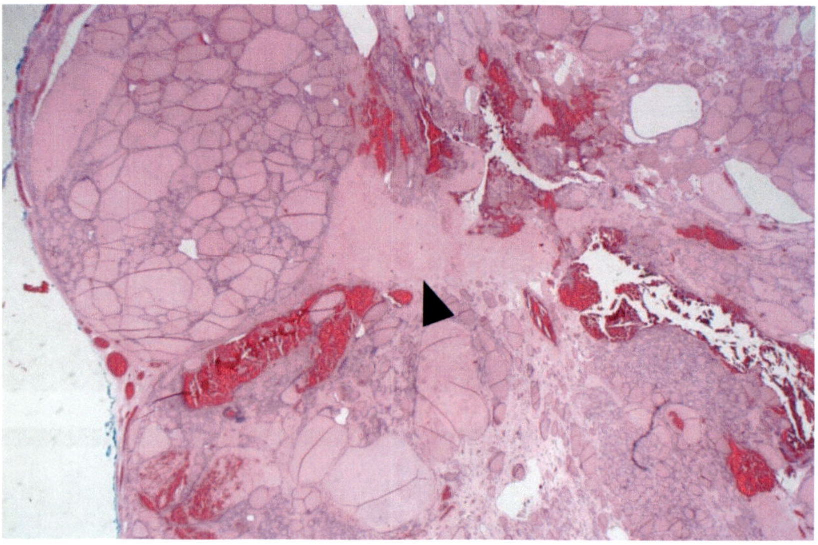

Fig. 4.7 Surgical histopathology was nodular hyperplasia showing thick interstitial fibrosis (arrow)

4.1.2 Case 2

65-year-old man was found to have a 1.39 cm right nodule on routine check. B-mode ultrasonogram showed a hypoechoic nodule with round margin (Figs. 4.8, 4.9 and 4.10).

Shear wave elastogram showed a traversing pattern of high elasticity and E_{Max} was 74.0 kPa (Fig. 4.11). FNA showed a benign follicular nodule (Figs. 4.12 and 4.13) and CNB showed nodular hyperplasia (Figs. 4.14 and 4.15).

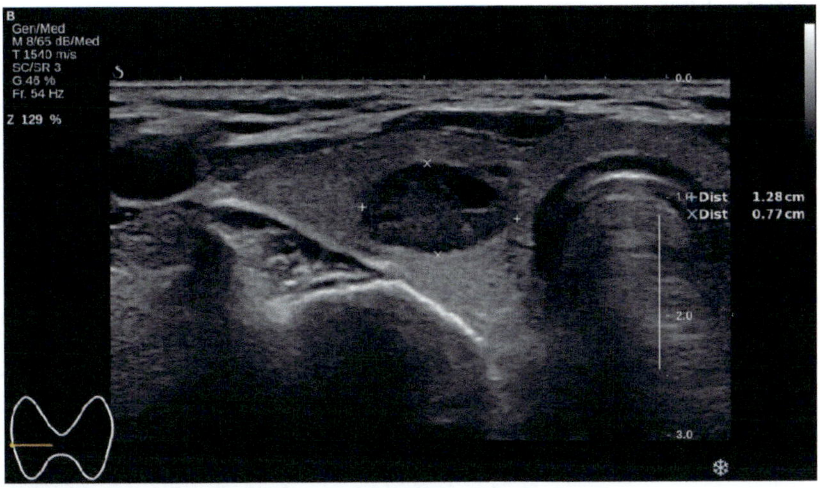

Fig. 4.8 B-mode ultrasonogram showed hypoechoic nodule with round margin

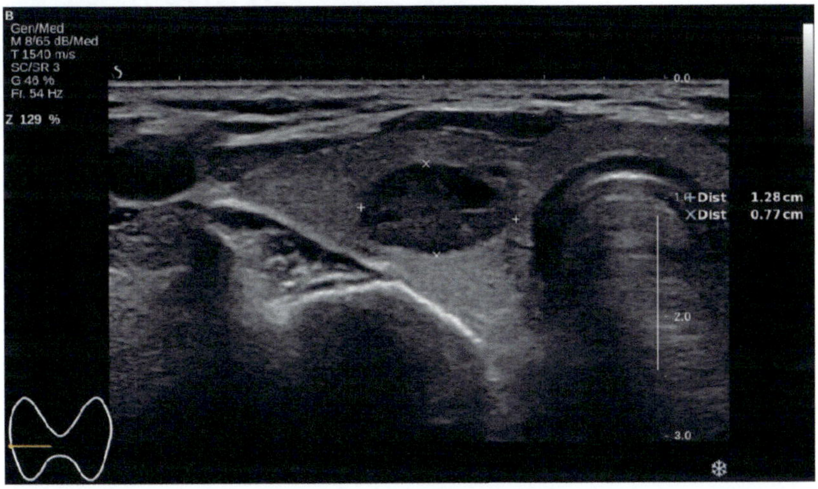

Fig. 4.9 B-mode ultrasonogram showed hypoechoic nodule with round margin

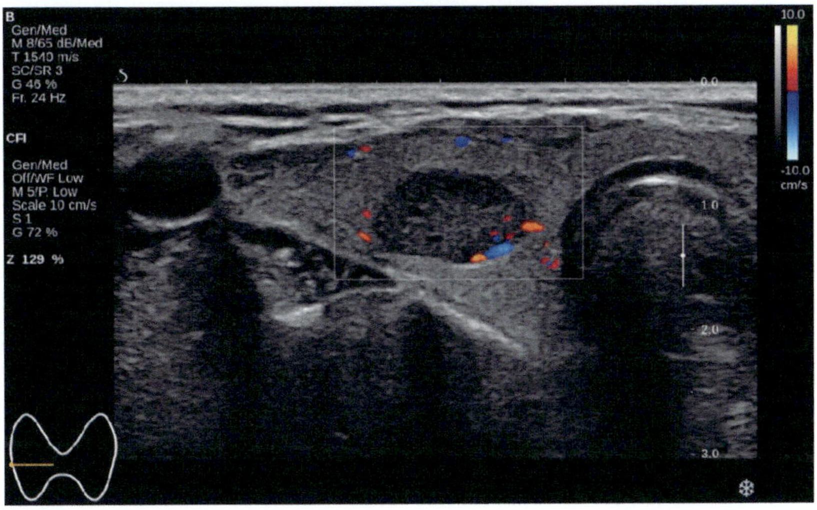

Fig. 4.10 Color Doppler showed little internal blood flow within the nodule

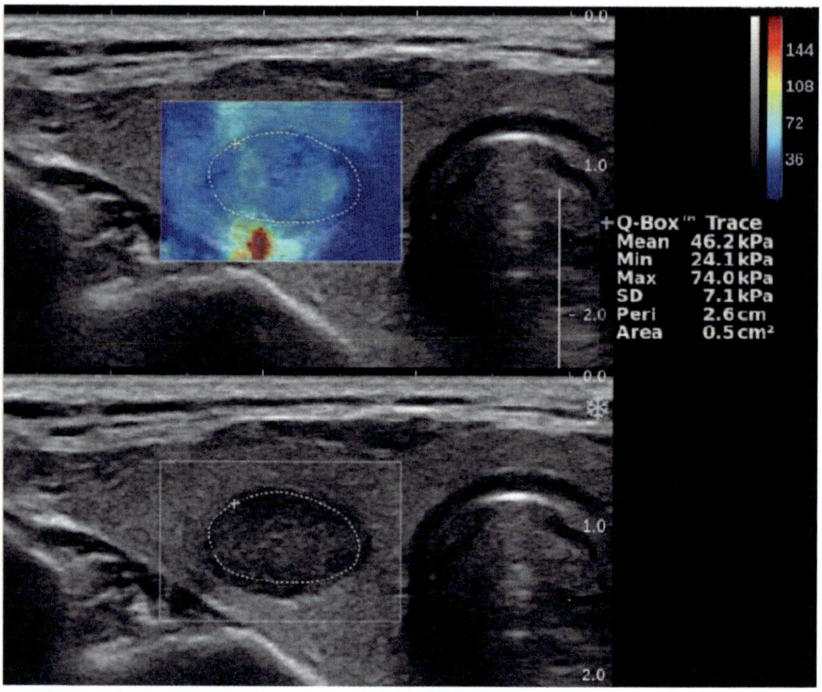

Fig. 4.11 Shear wave elastogram showed traversing pattern of high elasticity and E_{Max} was 74.0 kPa

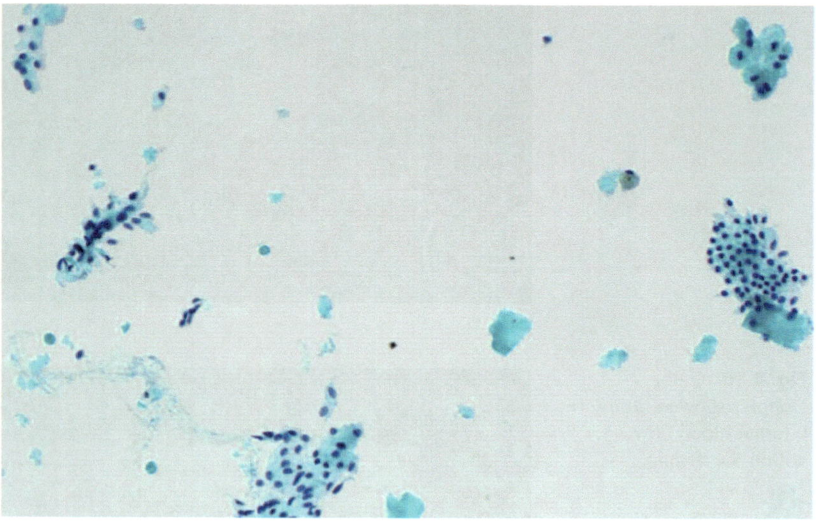

Fig. 4.12 FNA showed benign follicular nodule

4.1.3 Case 3

A 37-year-old woman was referred to have a thyroid nodule on routine check. B-mode ultrasonogram showed a 3.55 cm isoechoic right nodule with round margin with little internal vascularity (Figs. 4.16, 4.17, and 4.18). Shear wave elastogram showed a traversing pattern of high elasticity and E_{Max} was 60.1 kPa (Fig. 4.19). Core needle biopsy suggested nodular hyperplasia (Fig. 4.20) showing dilated involutional follicles.

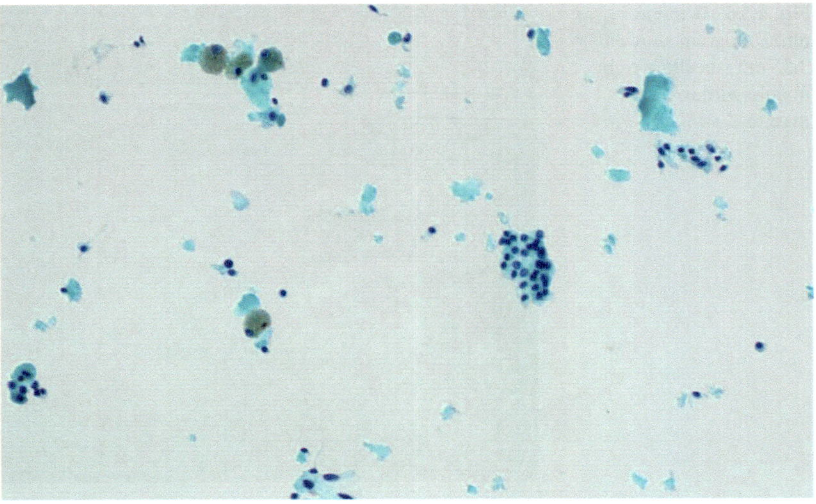

Fig. 4.13 FNA showed benign follicular nodule

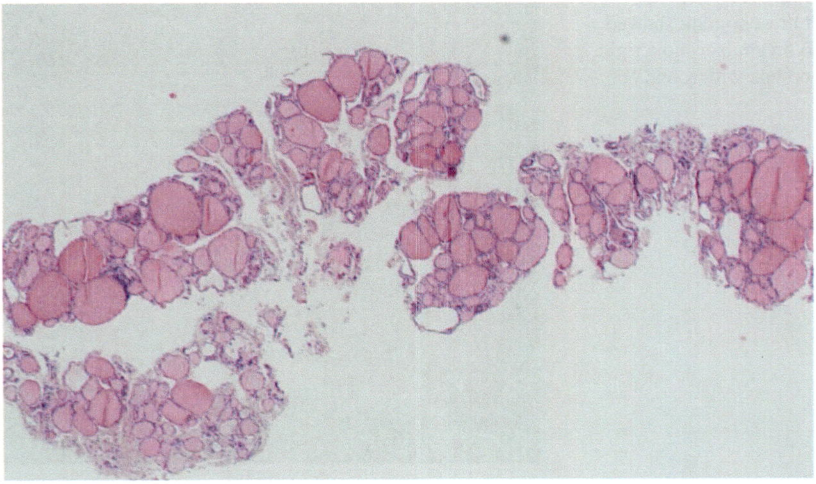

Fig. 4.14 CNB result was nodular hyperplasia

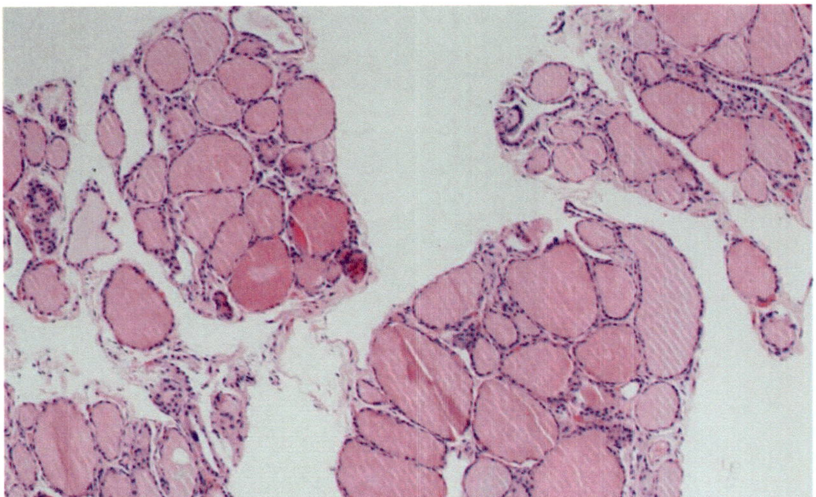

Fig. 4.15 CNB result was nodular hyperplasia

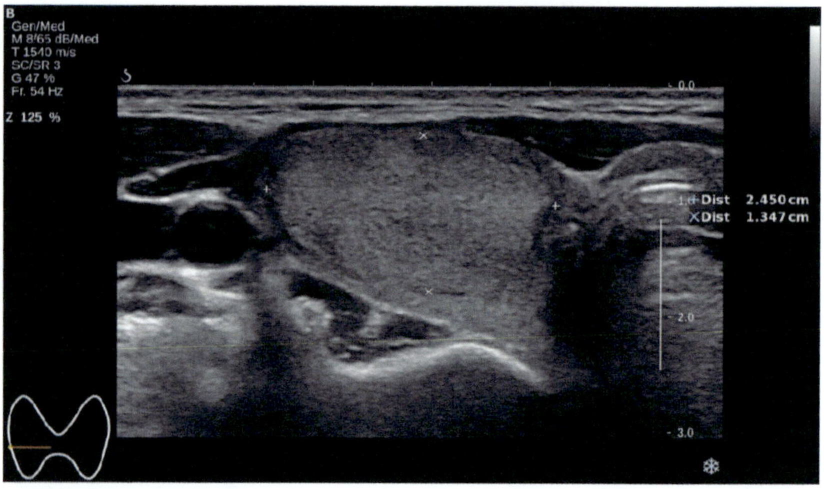

Fig. 4.16 B-mode ultrasonogram showed 3.55 cm isoechoic right nodule with round margin

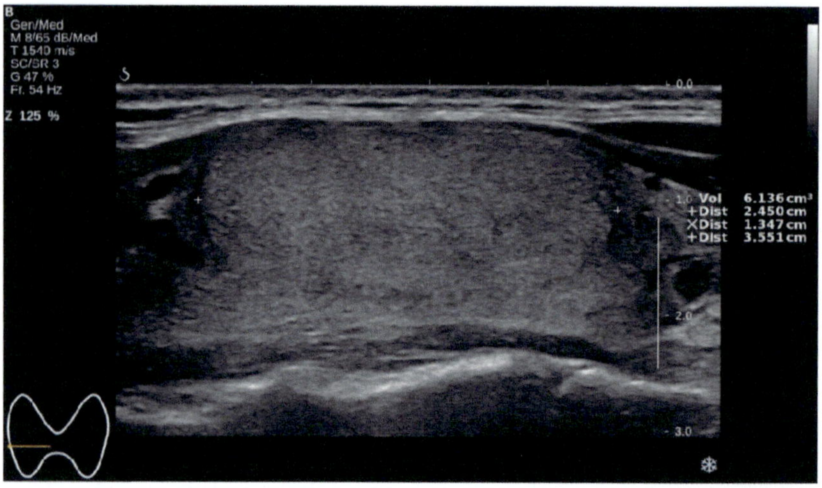

Fig. 4.17 B-mode ultrasonogram showed 3.55 cm isoechoic right nodule with round

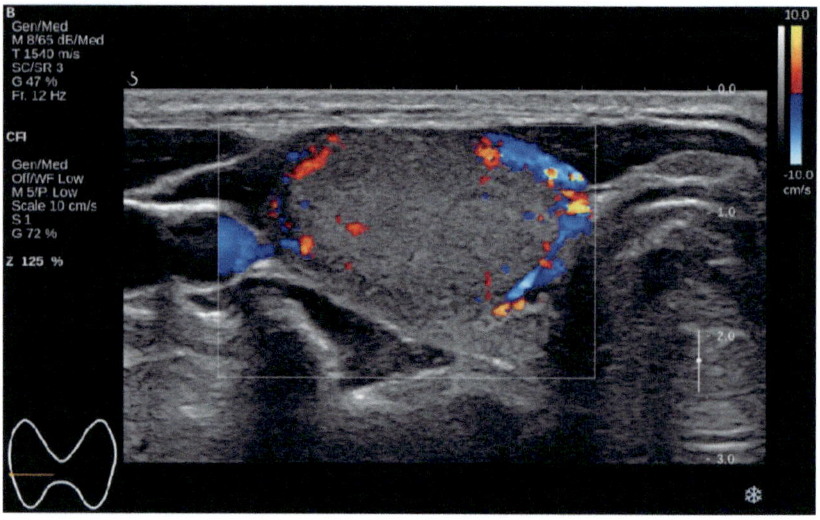

Fig. 4.18 Color Doppler showed little internal blood flow within the nodule

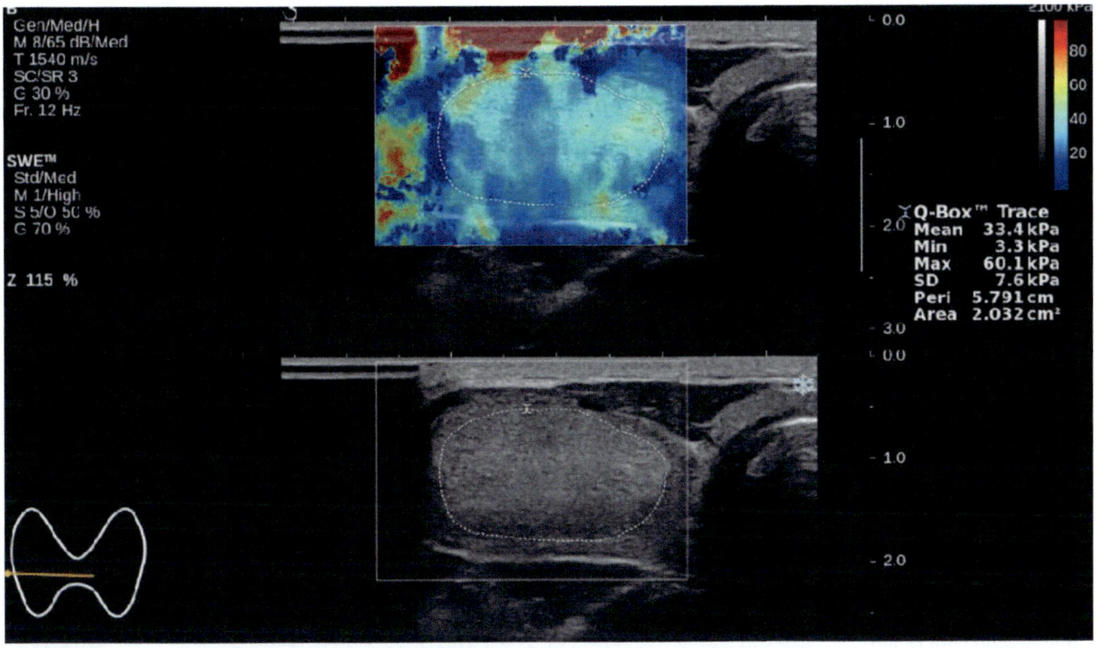

Fig. 4.19 Shear wave elastogram showed traversing pattern of high elasticity and E_{Max} was 60.1 kPa

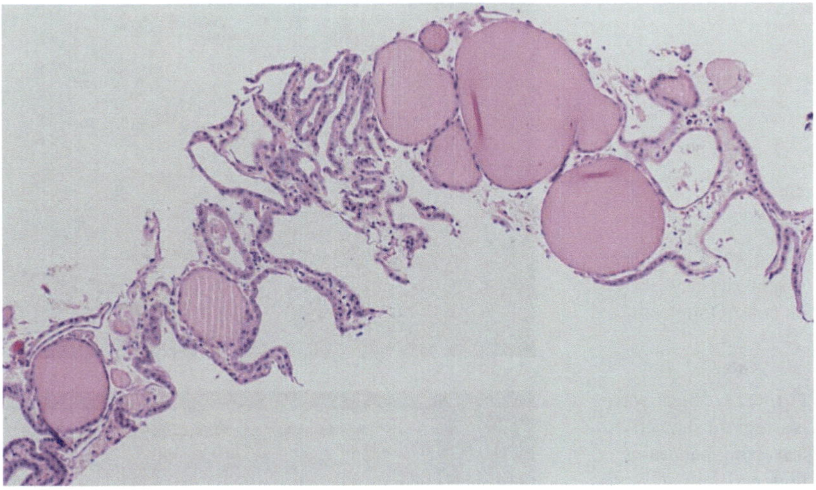

Fig. 4.20 Core needle biopsy suggested nodular hyperplasia showing dilated involutional follicles

4.1.4 Case 4

A 51-year-old woman was found to have a 1.03 cm left nodule that was growing to 1.58 cm during regular follow-up. B-mode ultrasonogram showed a partially cystic 1.58 cm solid nodule with round margin (Figs. 4.21 and 4.22), and FNA showed a benign follicular nodule. Shear wave elastogram showed a traversing pattern of high elasticity (E_{Max} 50.1 kPa, Figs. 4.23 and 4.24). She underwent thyroidectomy and histopathology revealed nodular hyperplasia (Figs. 4.25 and 4.26) showing incomplete formation of the surrounding capsule and interstitial fibrosis (arrow, Figs. 4.25, 4.26 and 4.27).

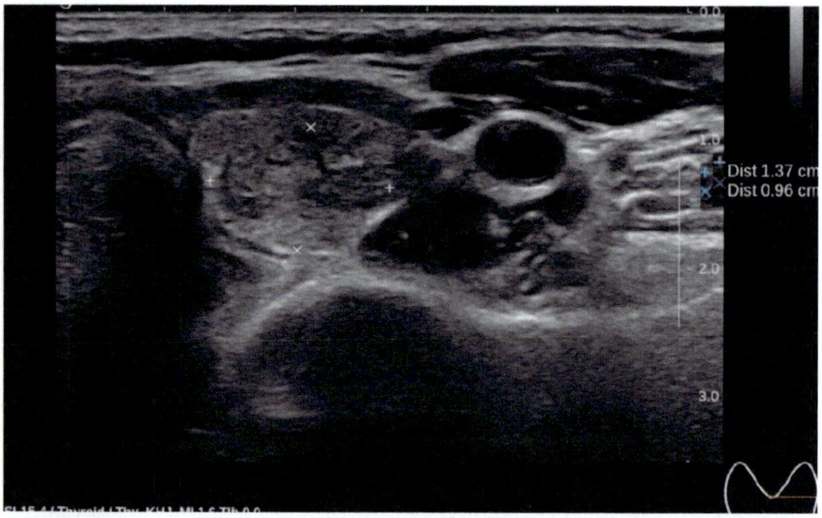

Fig. 4.21 B-mode ultrasonogram showed partially cystic 1.58 cm solid nodule with round margin in the left middle lobe

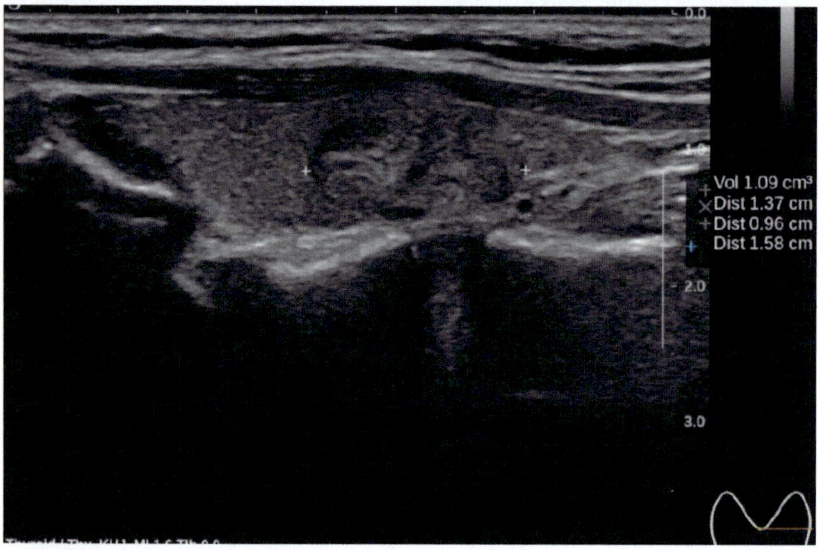

Fig. 4.22 B-mode ultrasonogram showed partially cystic 1.58 cm solid nodule with round margin in the left middle lobe

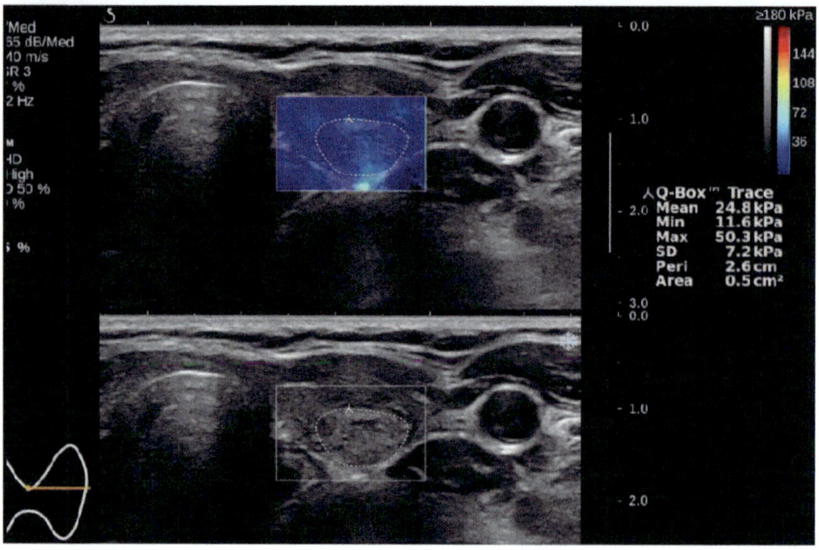

Fig. 4.23 Shear wave elastogram showed traversing pattern of high elasticity. E_{Max} was 50.1 kPa

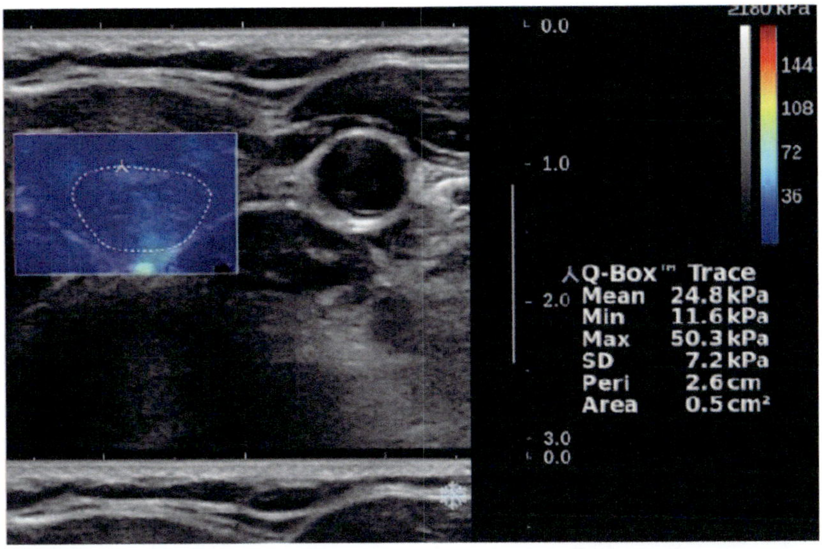

Fig. 4.24 Shear wave elastogram showed traversing pattern of high elasticity. E_{Max} was 50.1 kPa

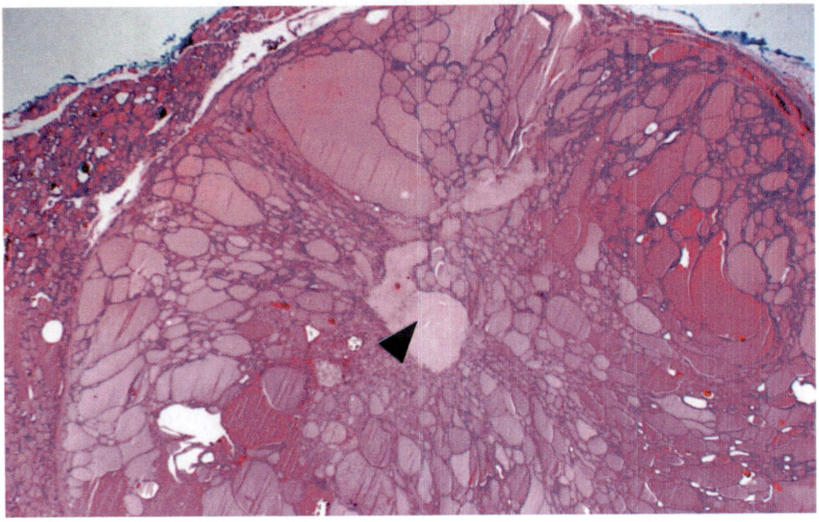

Fig. 4.25 Surgical histopathology revealed nodular hyperplasia. showing incomplete formation of surrounding capsule and interstitial fibrosis (arrow)

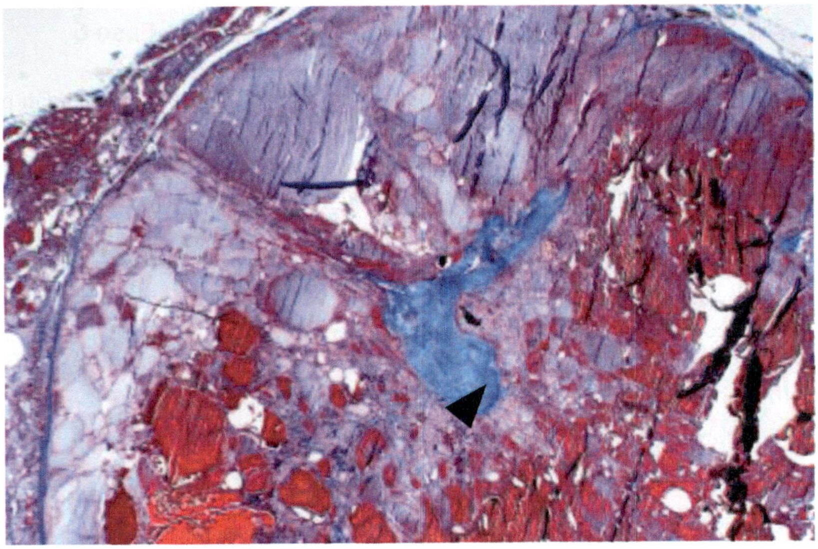

Fig. 4.26 Surgical histopathology revealed nodular hyperplasia.showing incomplete formation of surrounding capsule and interstitial fibrosis (arrow)

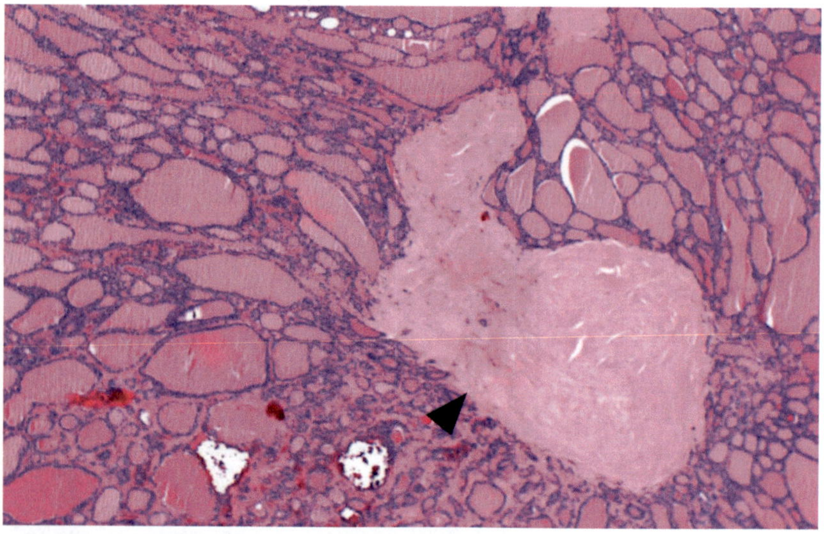

Fig. 4.27 Surgical histopathology revealed nodular hyperplasia. showing interstitial fibrosis (arrow)

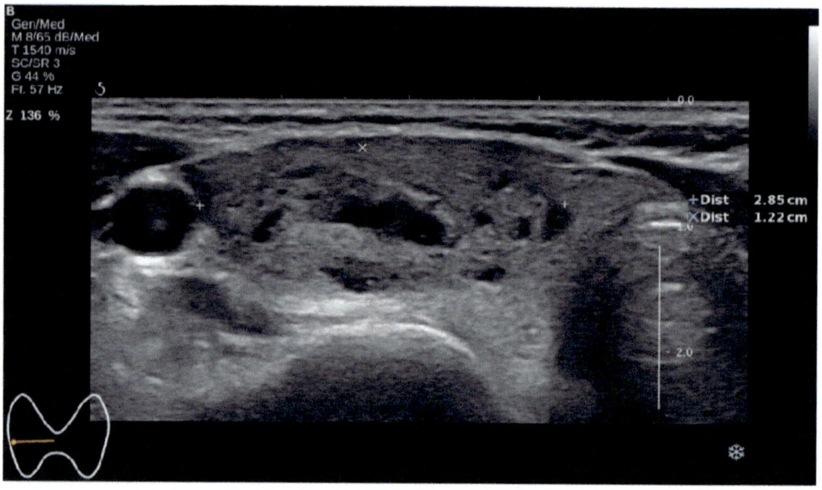

Fig. 4.28 B-mode ultrasonogram showed partially cystic 4.31 cm nodule in the left lobe

4.1.5 Case 5

33-year-old woman was referred to have a growing thyroid nodule during regular follow-up. B-mode ultrasonogram showed a partially cystic 4.31 cm left nodule with moderate internal vascularity (Figs. 4.28, 4.29, and 4.30). Shear wave elastogram showed a traversing pattern of high elasticity and E_{Max} was 150.8 kPa (Fig. 4.31). Core needle biopsy suggested nodular hyperplasia showing dilated follicles and interstitial infiltration of inflammatory cells (arrow, Fig. 4.32) and fibrotic change.

4.1.6 Case 6

A 48-year-old woman presented a right neck mass found recently. She had been diagnosed as a thyroid nodule (right, 0.8 cm) nine years ago and FNA at that time had revealed follicular lesion, but follow-up evaluation was lost. B-mode USG revealed a 5.25 cm mixed solid and cystic nodule with little internal vascularity in the right lobe (Figs. 4.33, 4.34 and 4.35). SWE showed scattered increased elasticity along the solid portions of the nodule (E_{Max} 140.4 kPa, Fig. 4.36). CNB was performed in the solid portion of the nodule and showed thick

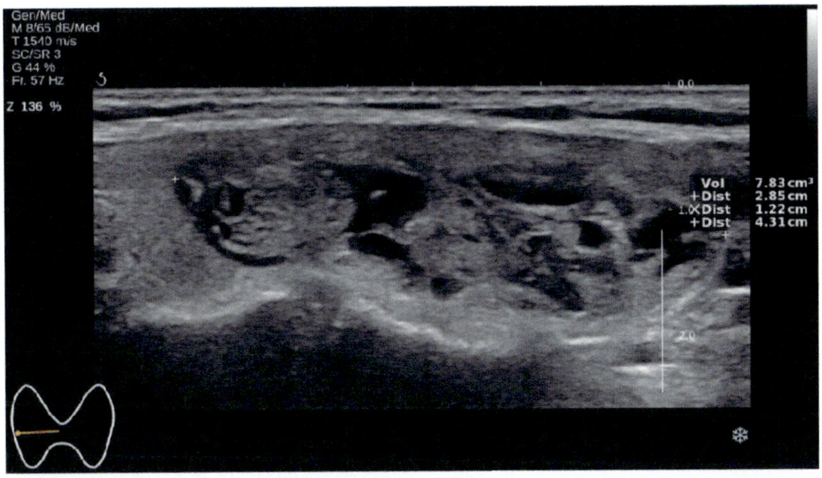

Fig. 4.29 B-mode ultrasonogram showed partially cystic 4.31 cm nodule inthe left lobe

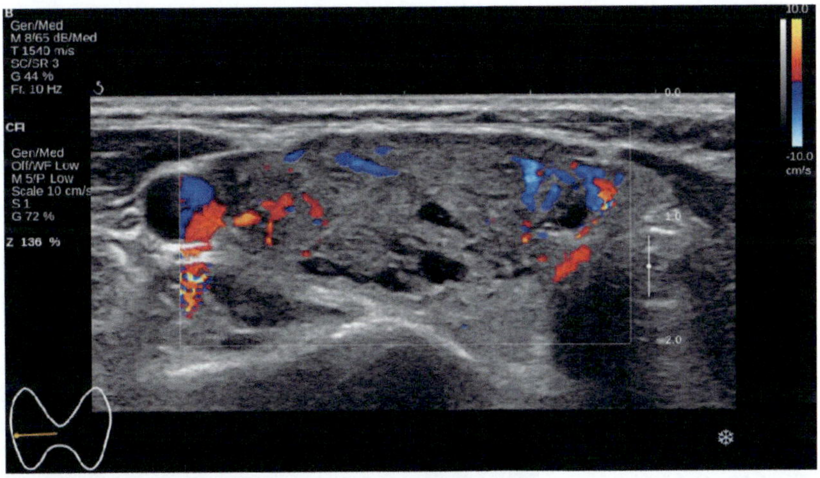

Fig. 4.30 Color Doppler showed moderately increased internal vascularity within the nodule

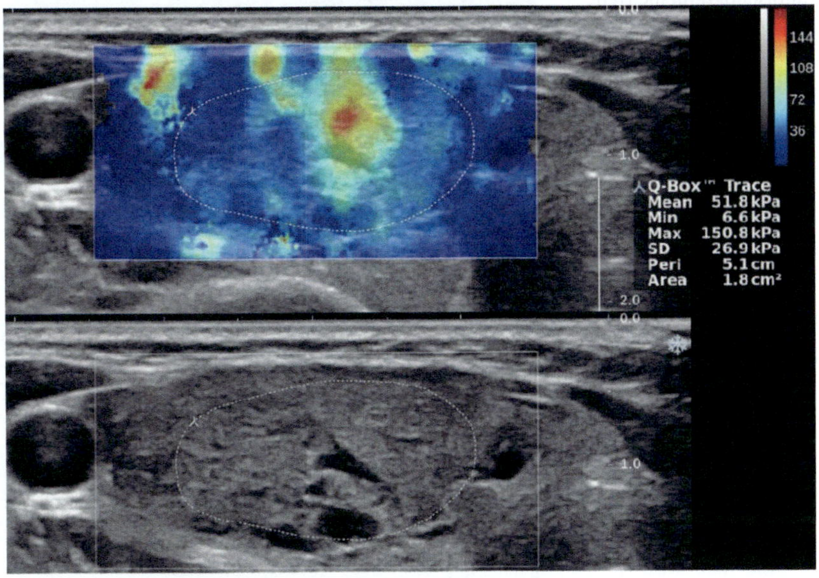

Fig. 4.31 Shear wave elastogram showed traversing pattern of high elasticity and E_{Max} was 150.8 kPa

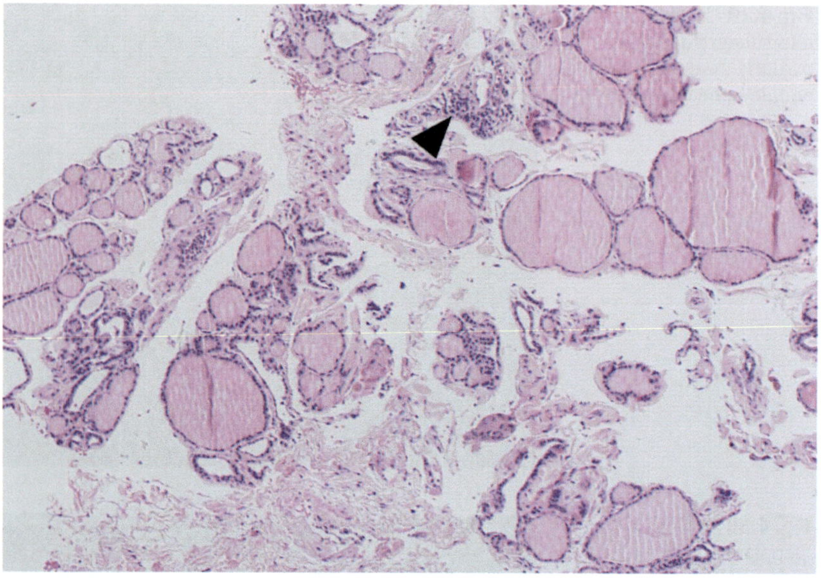

Fig. 4.32 Core needle biopsy suggested nodular hyperplasia showing dilated follicles and interstitial infiltration of inflammatory cells (arrow) and fibrotic change

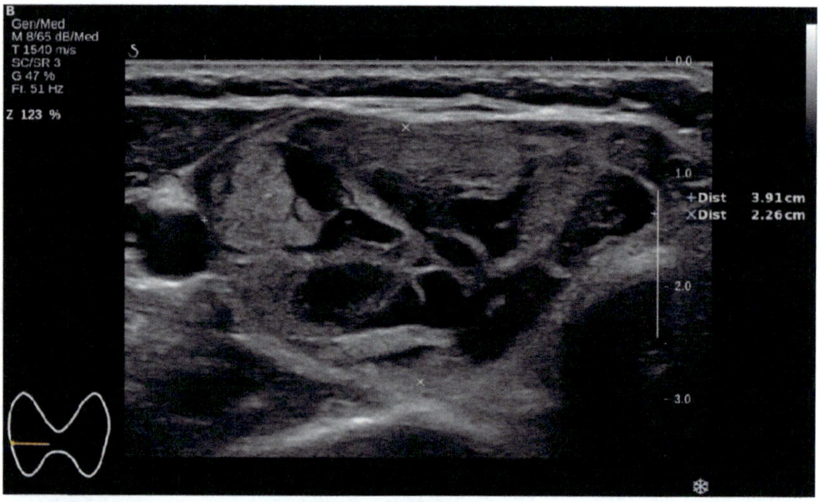

Fig. 4.33 B mode USG revealed 5.25 cm mixed solid and cystic nodule in the right middle lobe

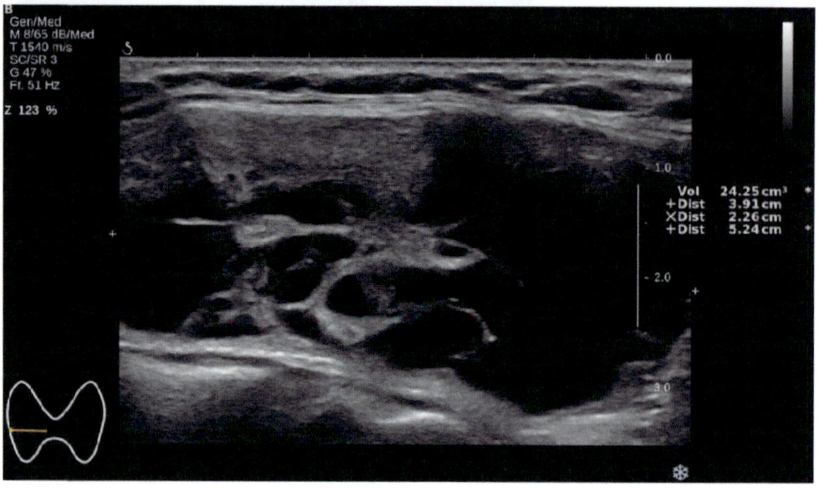

Fig. 4.34 B mode USG revealed 5.25 cm mixed solid and cystic nodule in the right middle lobe

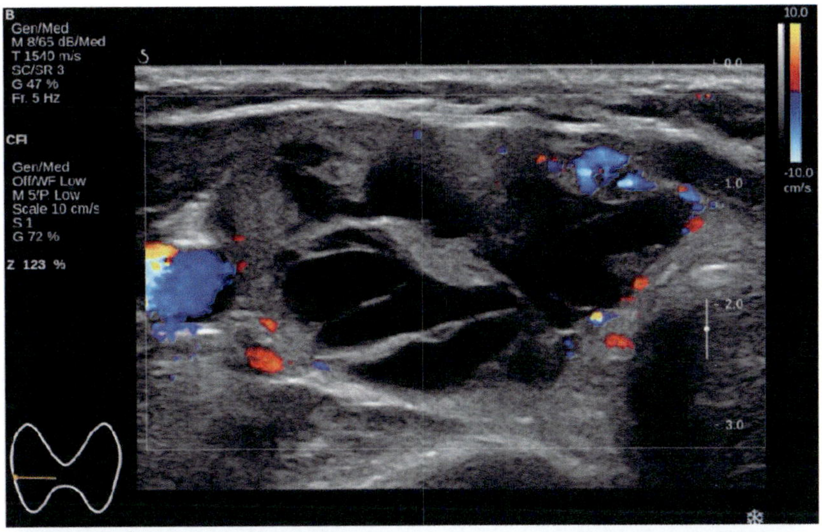

Fig. 4.35 Color Doppler showed little internal vascularity within the nodule

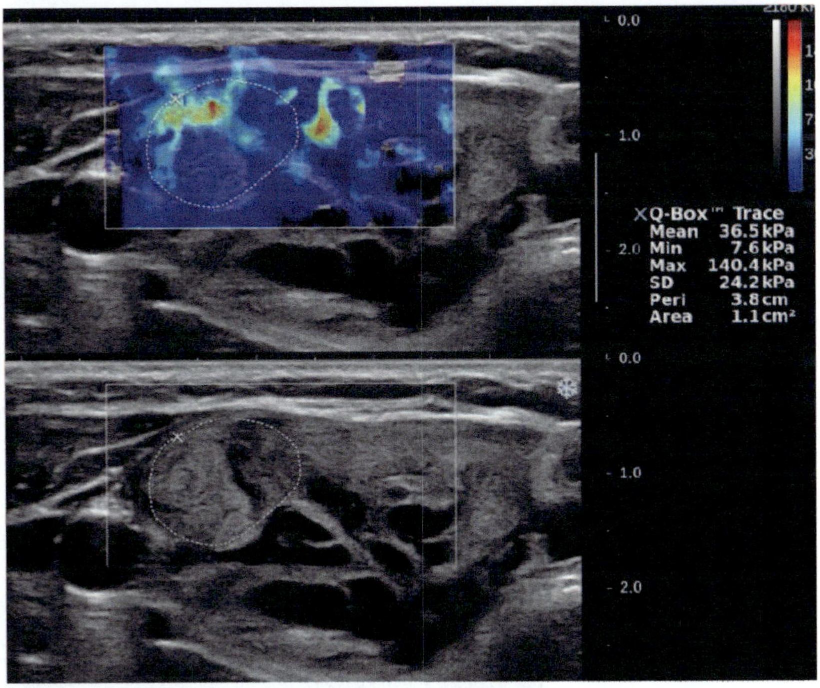

Fig. 4.36 SWE showed scattered increasd elasticity along the solid portions of the nodule (E_{Max} 140.4 kPa)

fibrous areas accompanied by the involutional change in flattened thyroid follicular cells (arrow) suggesting nodular hyperplasia (Fig. 4.37), which is compatible with SWE, the stiffness map.

4.1.7 Case 7

A 49-year-old woman was found to have a thyroid nodule in the right lobe on routine check. On ultrasonogram, a 1.9 cm hypoechoic nodule was observed in the right lower lobe (Figs. 4.38 and 4.39). On SWE elevated EI area traversing the nodule was observed (E_{Max} 69.3 kPa, Fig. 4.40). FNA showed normal follicular cells (Benign follicular nodule, Fig. 4.41) and CNB suggested NH showing variable-sized follicles (Fig. 4.42).

4.1.8 Case 8

46-year-old woman presented a palpable mass on the right side of the neck. B-mode ultrasonogram showed a predominantly solid 3.6 cm

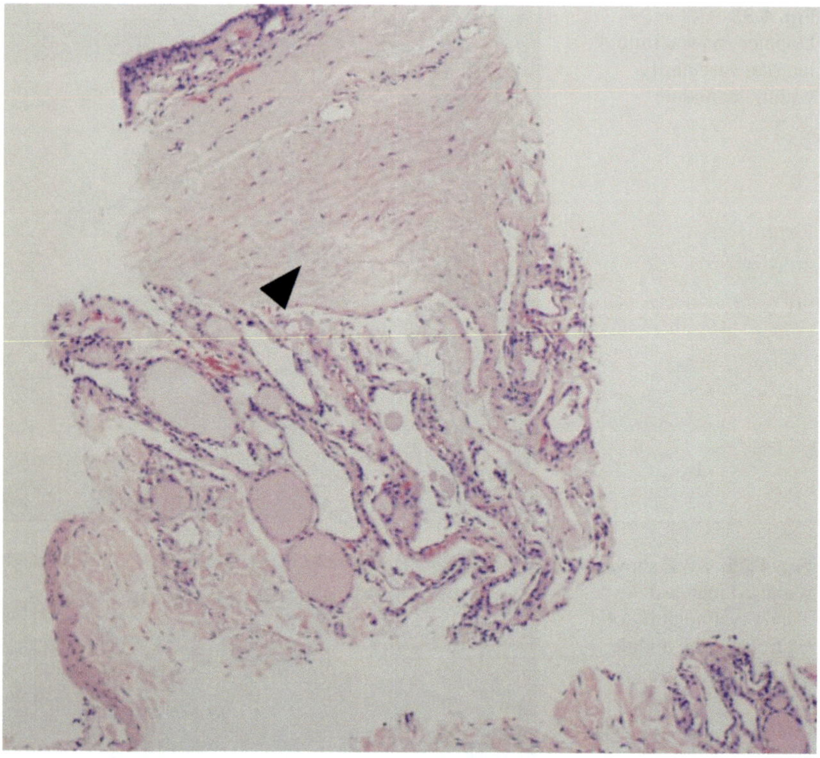

Fig. 4.37 CNB showed thick fibrous areas (arrow) accompanied by the involutional change of flattened thyroid follicular cells suggesting nodular hyperplasia

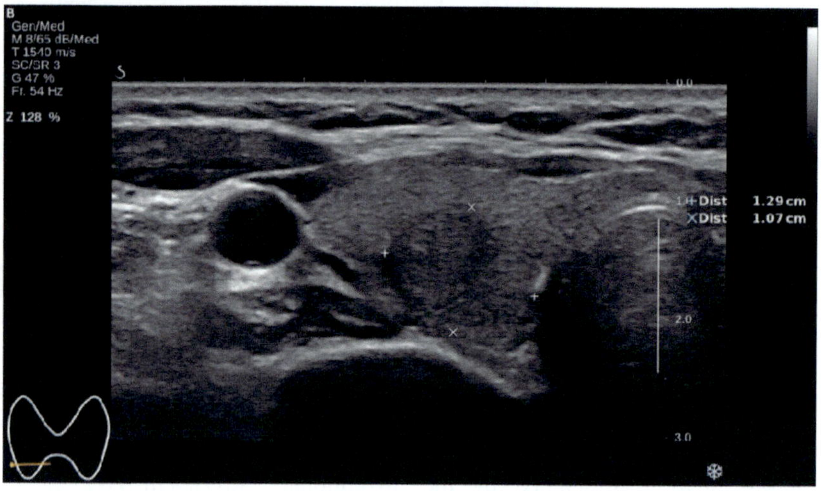

Fig. 4.38 On ultrasonogram, 1.9 cm hypoechoic nodule was observed in the right lower lobe

round nodule with little internal vascularity in the right lower lobe (Figs. 4.43, 4.44, and 4.45) and also a hypoechoic 0.8 cm nodule with irregular margin in the left middle lobe. Shear wave elastogram of the right nodule showed increased with traversing pattern, E_{Max} was 134.9 kPa (Figs. 4.46 and 4.47). Core needle biopsy of the right nodule revealed nodular hyperplasia and FNA of the left nodule showed papillary carcinoma. She underwent total thyroidectomy and surgical histopathology was nodular hyperplasia in the right nodule (Figs. 4.48 and 4.49) showing incomplete capsulation of the right nodule (arrow, Fig. 4.48) and fibrosis (arrow, Fig. 4.49). The left nodule was diagnosed as papillary carcinoma.

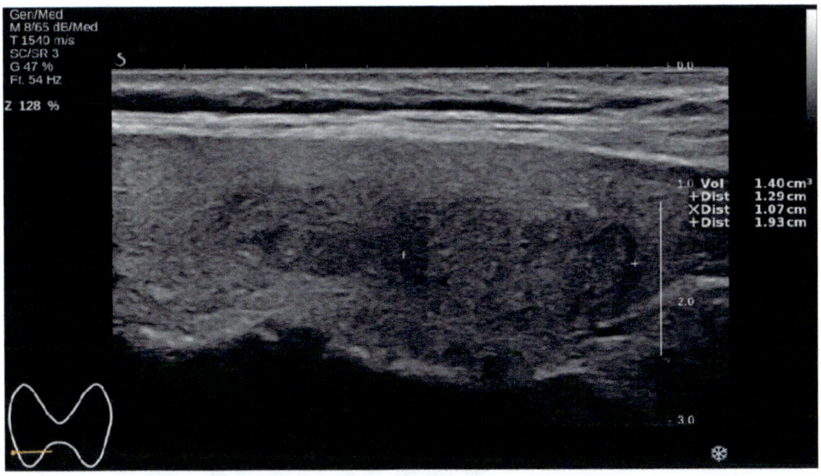

Fig. 4.39 On ultrasonogram, 1.9 cm hypoechoic nodule was observed in the right lower lobe

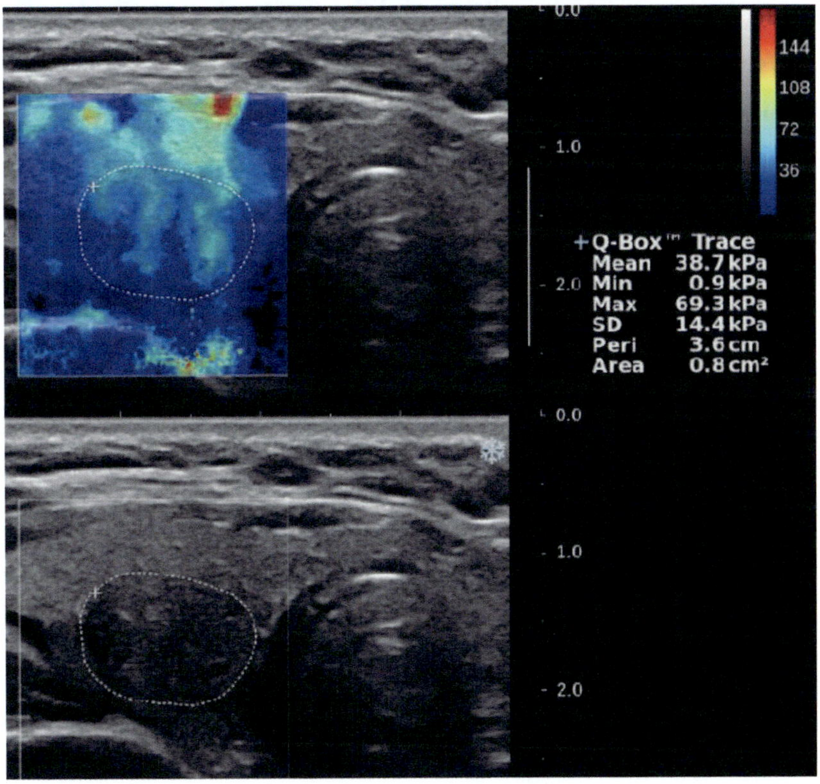

Fig. 4.40 On SWE elevated EI area traversing the nodule was observed. E_{Max} was 69.3 kPa

4.1.9 Case 9

A 33-year-old woman was referred for thyroid nodule. USG showed a 2.07 cm mixed nodule with moderate internal vascularity in the right lower lobe (Figs. 4.50, 4.51, and 4.52). Shear wave elastogram showed scattered traversing patterns of high elasticity (E_{Max} 54.9 kPa, Fig. 4.53), and CNB showed dilated follicles suggesting nodular hyperplasia (Fig. 4.54).

4.1.10 Case 10

45-year-old woman was referred for the evaluation of a growing thyroid nodule during regular

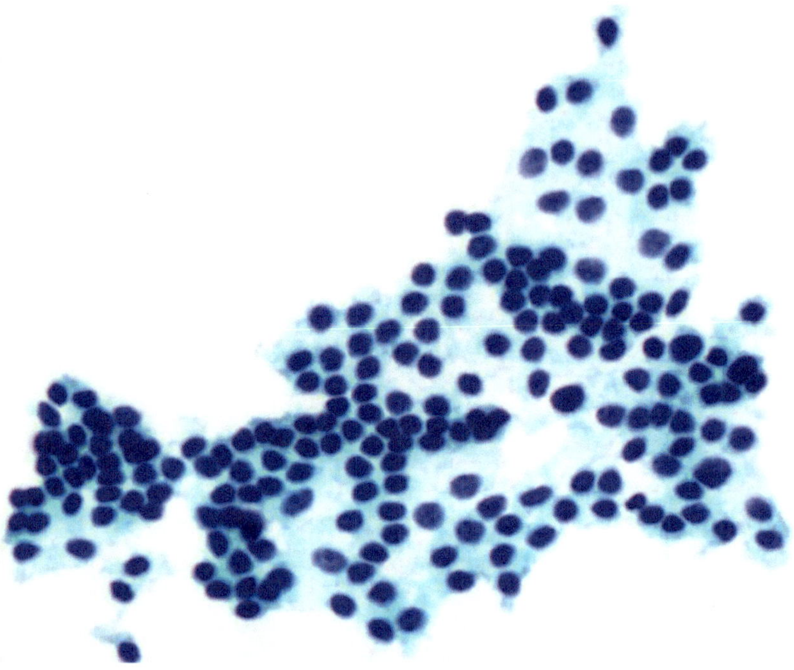

Fig. 4.41 FNA showed sheets of the normal follicular cells (Benign follicular nodule)

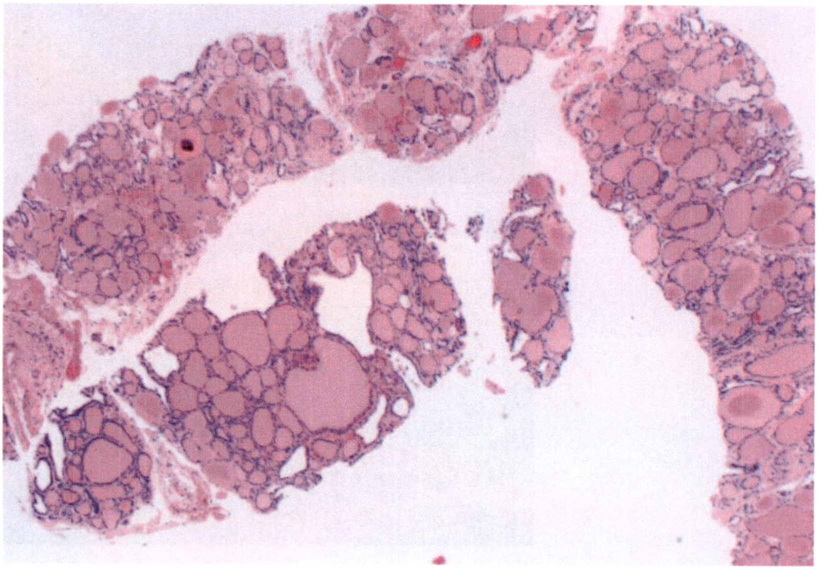

Fig. 4.42 CNB suggested nodular hyperplasia with variable sized follicles, showing small hyperplastic follicles and large involutional follicles together

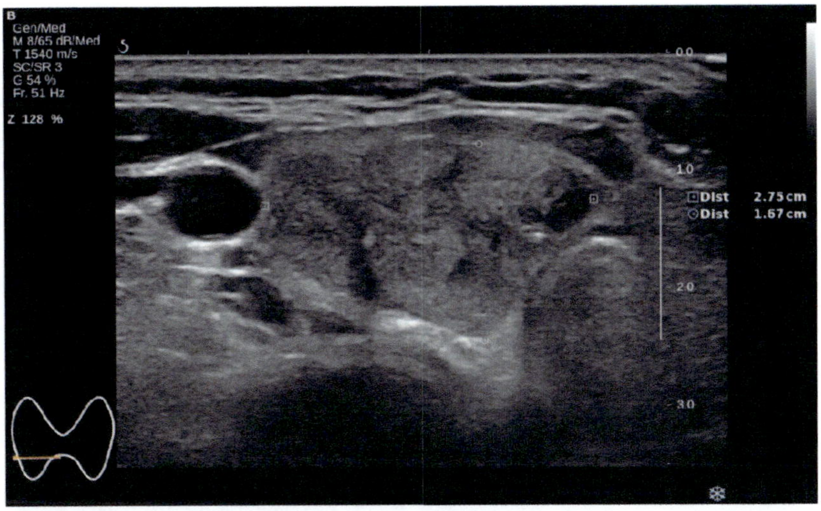

Fig. 4.43 Ultrasonogram showed predominantly solid 3.6 cm round nodule in the right lower lobe

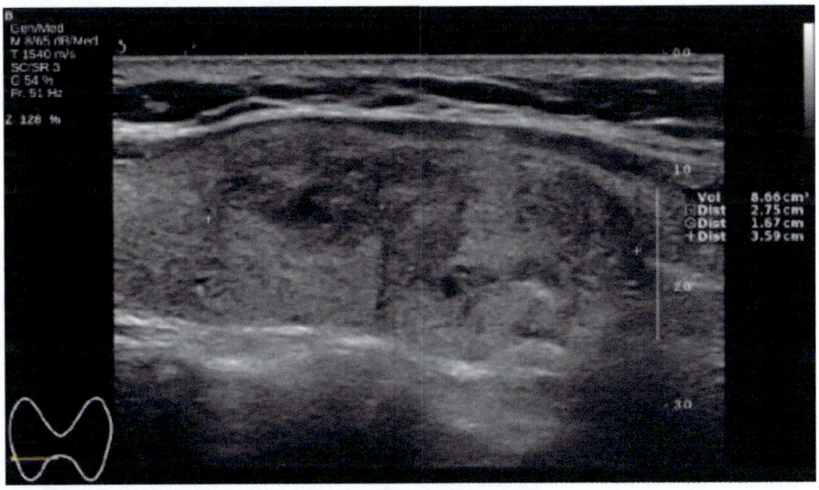

Fig. 4.44 Ultrasonogram showed predominantly solid 3.6 cm round nodule

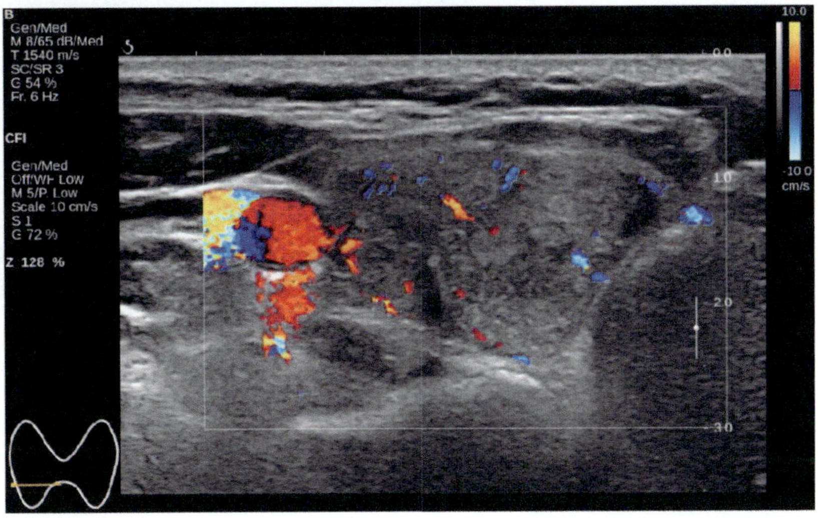

Fig. 4.45 Color Doppler showed little internal vascularity within the nodule

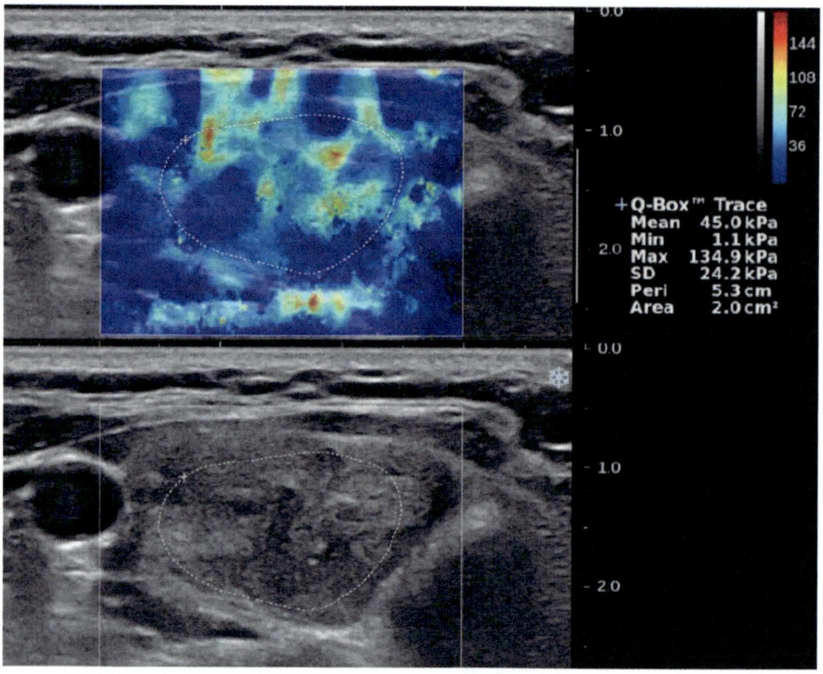

Fig. 4.46 Shear wave elastogram of the right nodule showed traversing pattern of increased EI and E_{Max} was 134.9 kPa

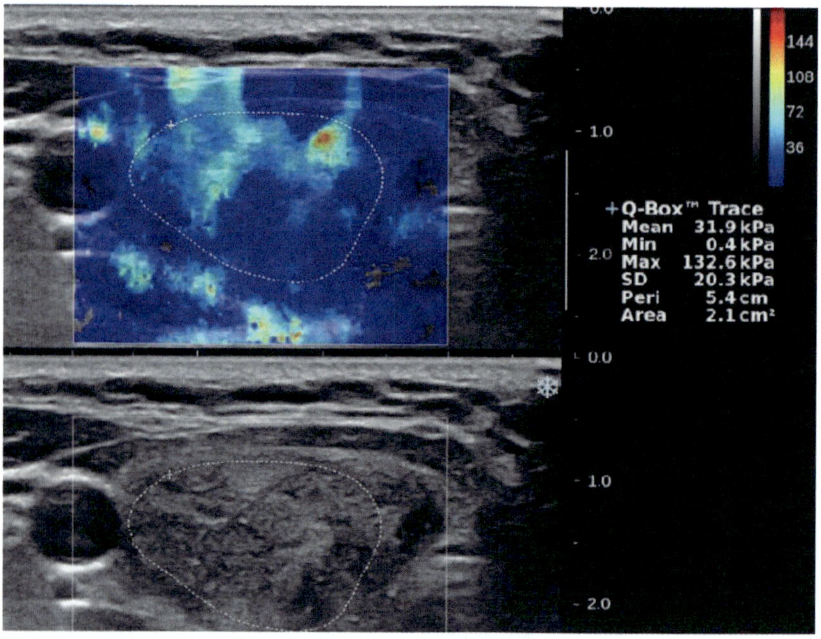

Fig. 4.47 Shear wave elastogram of the right nodule showed traversing pattern of increased EI and E_{Max} was 132.6 kPa

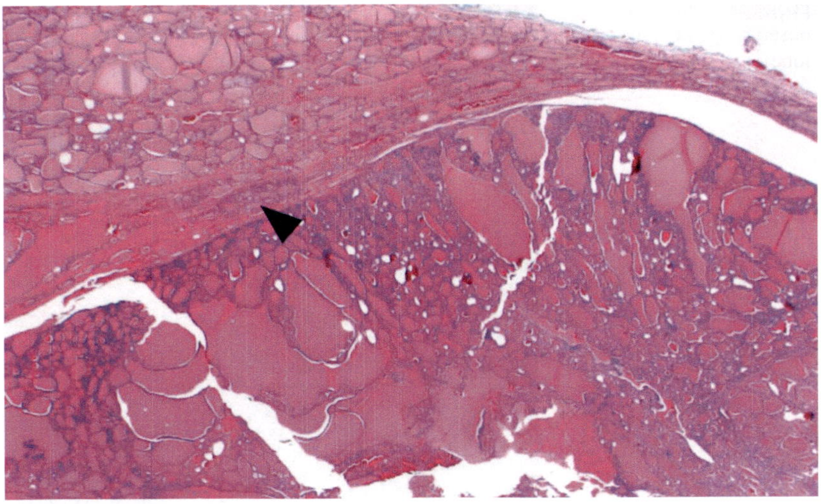

Fig. 4.48 Surgical histopathology revealed nodular hyperplasia in the right nodule showing incomplete capsulation (arrow)

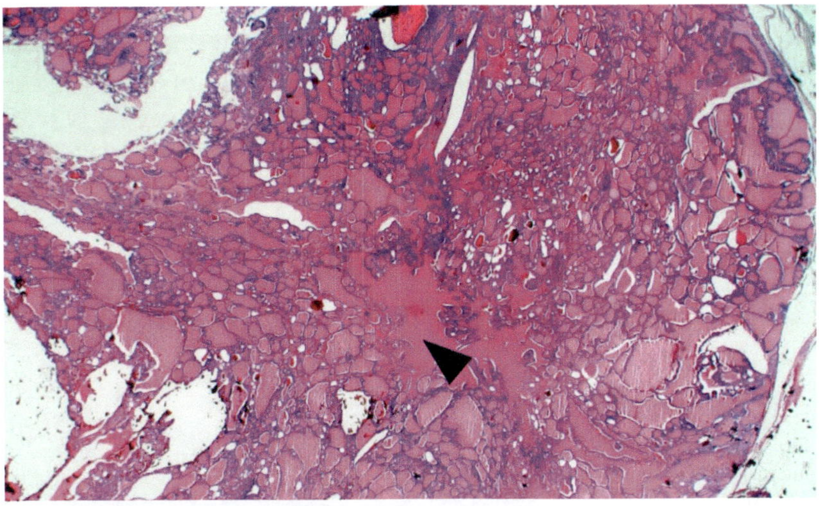

Fig. 4.49 Surgical histopathology revealed nodular hyperplasia showing fibrosis (arrow)

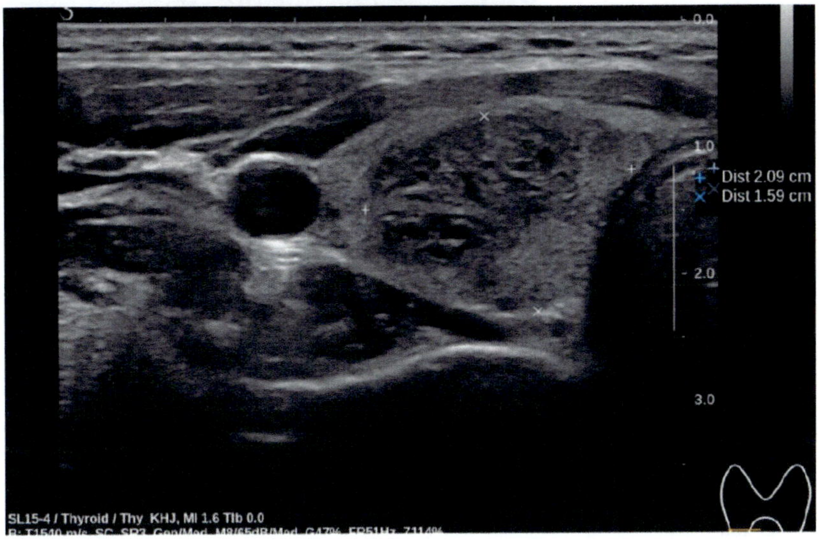

Fig. 4.50 USG showed 2.07 cm mixed nodule in the right lower lobe

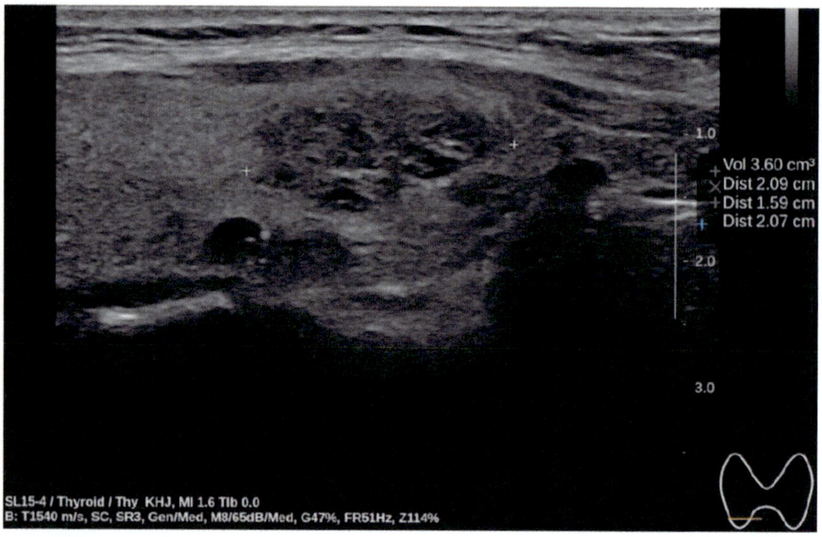

Fig. 4.51 USG showed 2.07 cm mixed nodule in the right lower lobe

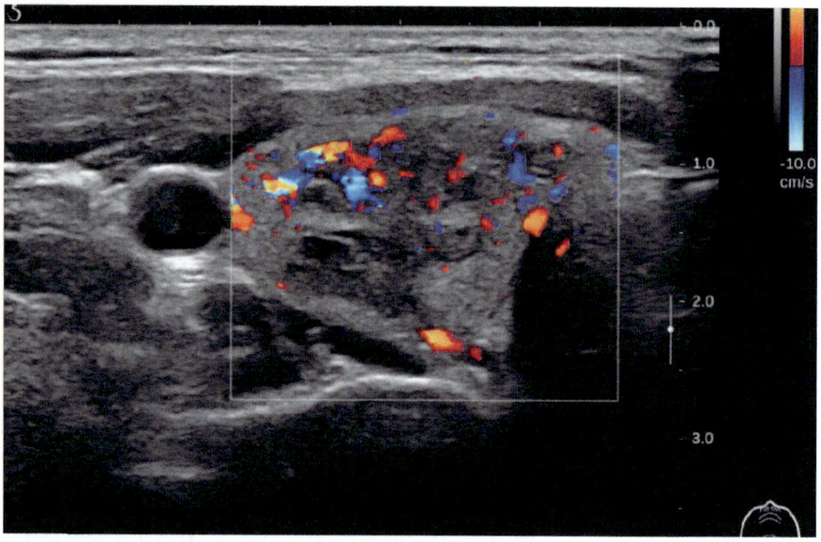

Fig. 4.52 Color Doppler showed moderately increased internal blood flow within the nodule

follow-up. B-mode ultrasonogram showed a solid 2.25 cm isoechoic round nodule with a halo in the left upper lobe (Figs. 4.55, 4.56, and 4.57). SWE showed diffuse increased elasticity (E_{Max} 141.2 kPa, Fig. 4.58). Core needle biopsy showed involutional follicles with interstitial fibrosis (arrow, Fig. 4.59) suggesting nodular hyperplasia.

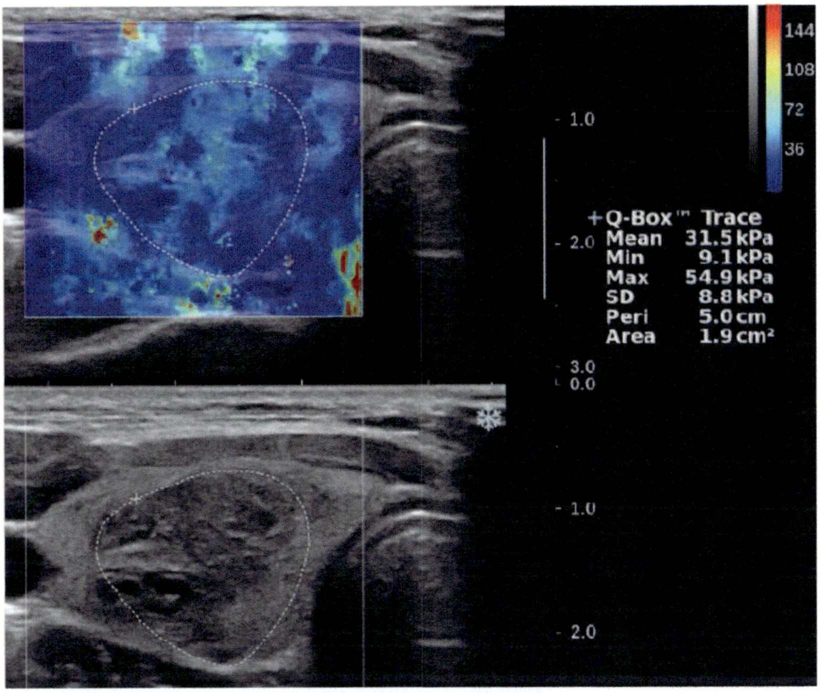

Fig. 4.53 Shear wave elastogram showed scattered traversing patterns of high elasticity and E_{Max} was 54.9 kPa

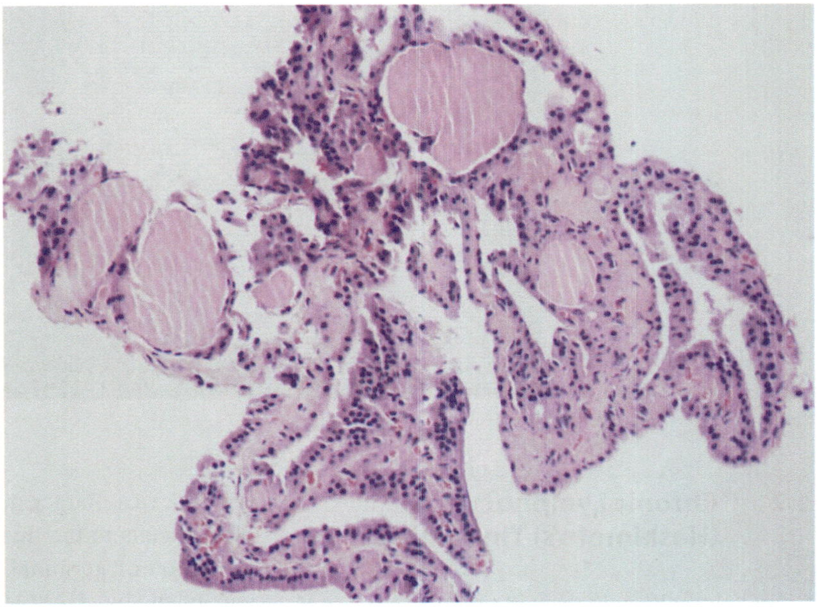

Fig. 4.54 CNB showed dilated involutional follicles suggesting nodular hyperplasia

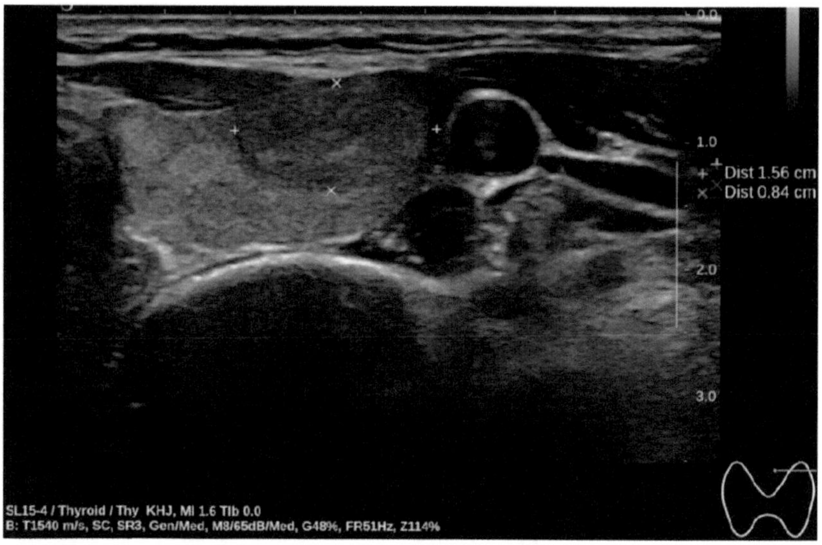

Fig. 4.55 B-mode ultrasonogram showed solid 2.25 cm round isoechoic nodule with halo in the left upper lobe

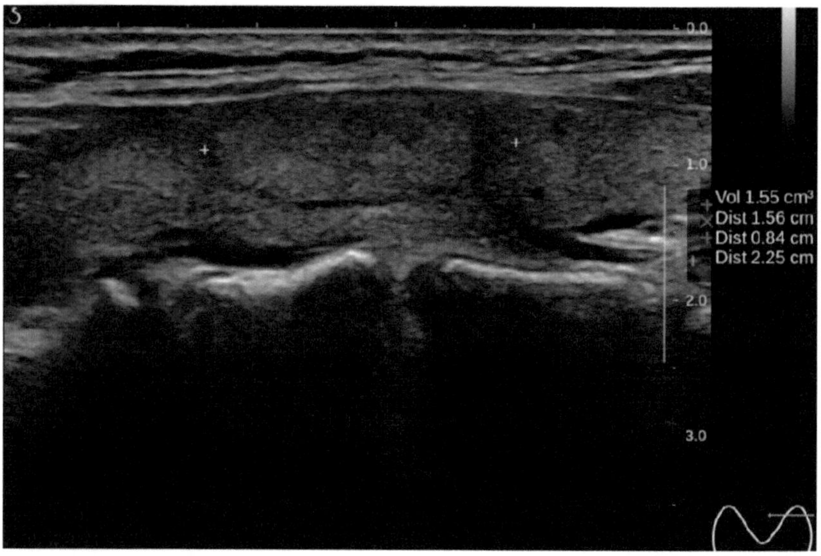

Fig. 4.56 B-mode ultrasonogram showed solid 2.25 cm round isoechoic nodule with halo in the left upper lobe

4.2 Chronic Lymphocytic (Hashimoto's) Thyroiditis

Chronic lymphocytic thyroiditis is the most common cause of hypothyroidism and is usually associated with the high titers of autoantibodies to thyroid peroxidase (TPO) and thyroglobulin. Progressive autoimmune destructions of thyroid epithelial cells are associated with infiltration of polymorphic lymphoid cells including small lymphocytes, larger reactive lymphocytes and plasma cells to the thyroid parenchyma with the formation of germinal centers. Thyroid follicles are lined by Hürthle cells (oncocytes) with abundant eosinophilic granular cytoplasm and a large nuclei, and interstitial connective tissue is increased with fibrosis [1]. The inflammatory process causes a diffused enlargement of thyroid but sometimes localized enlargement may be seen as focal thyroid nodules.

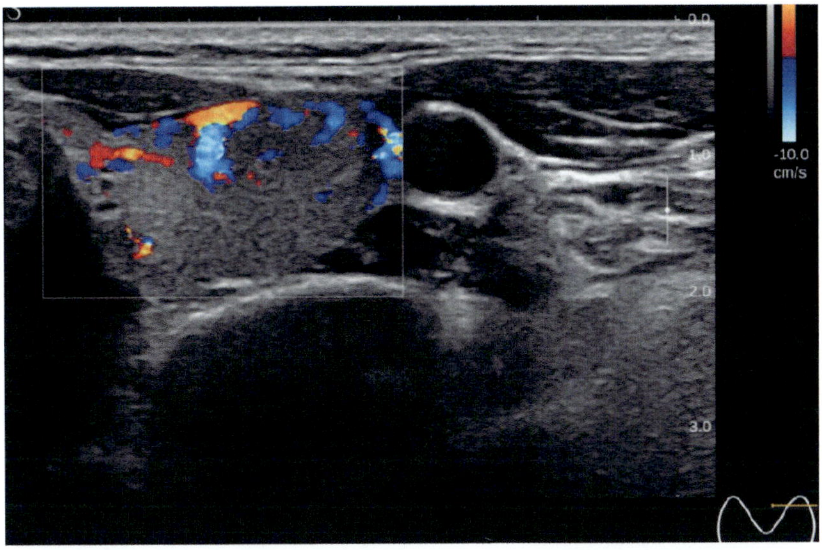

Fig. 4.57 Color Doppler showed moderately increased internal blood flow within the nodule

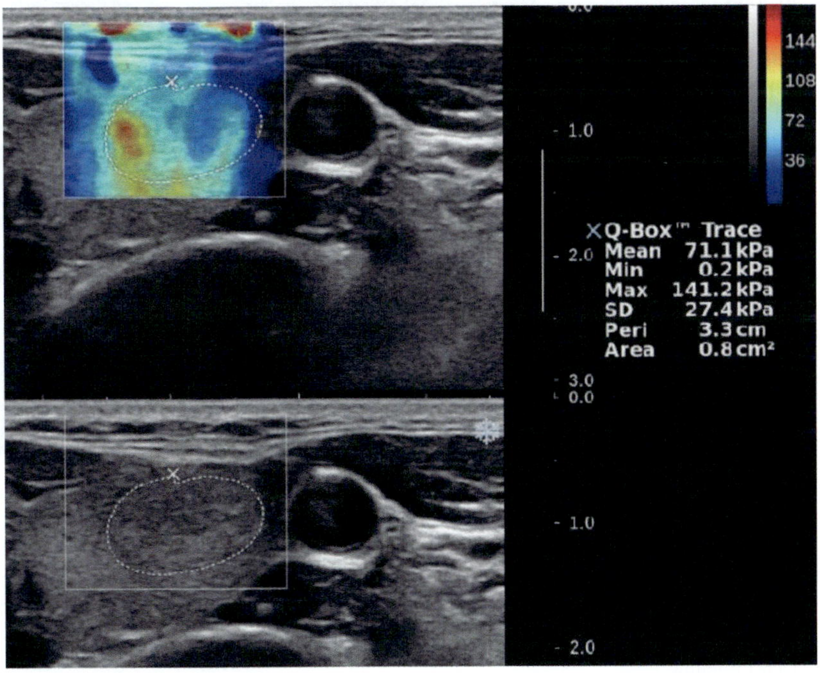

Fig. 4.58 SWE showed diffuse increased elasticity and E_{Max} was 141.2 kPa

On B-mode ultrasound of chronic lymphocytic thyroiditis, the parenchyma is heterogeneous and coarse with multiple hypoechoic solid nodules, sometimes surrounded by fibrosis. SWE showed increased elasticity depending the degree of fibrosis [11].

4.2.1 Case 1

A 54-year-old woman was found to have a nodule on routine check and was referred for the evaluation. Ultrasonogram showed a 1.77 cm isoechoic round nodule in the left lobe (Figs. 4.60

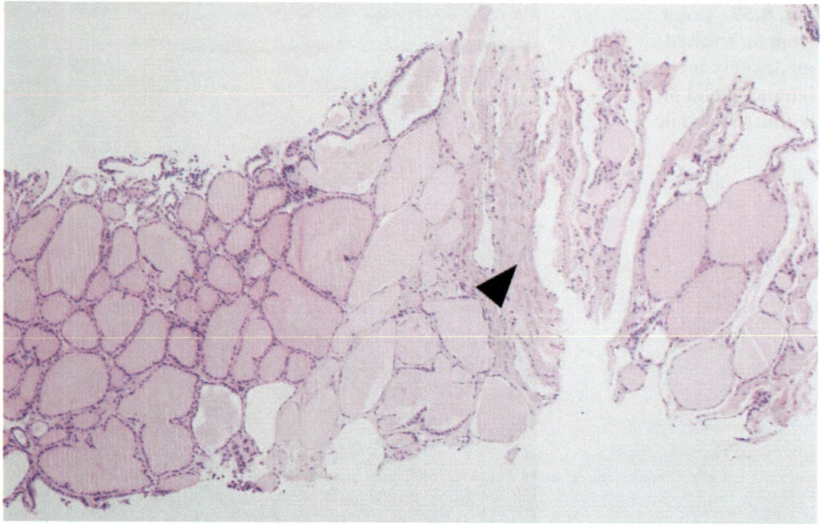

Fig. 4.59 Core needle biopsy showed involutional follicles with interstitial fibrosis (arrow) suggesting nodular hyperplasia

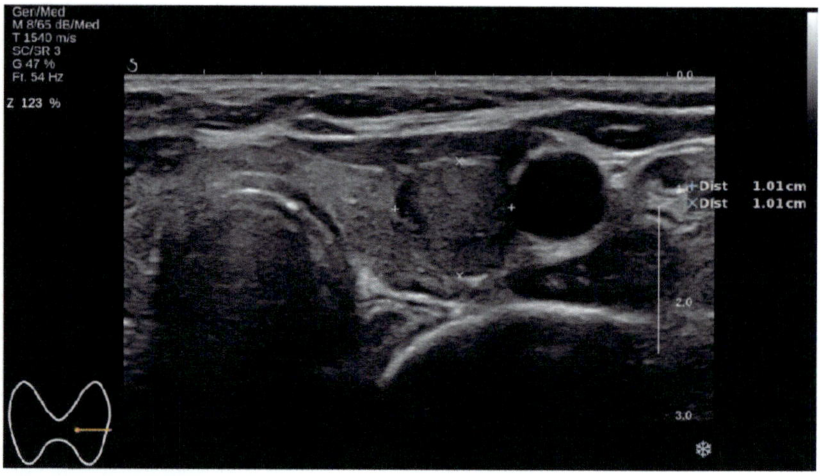

Fig. 4.60 Ultrasonogram showed 1.77 cm isoechoic round nodule in the left lower lobe

and 4.61) with moderate internal blood flow on color Doppler (Fig. 4.62). Shear wave elastogram showed scattered increased elasticity within the nodule (E_{Max} 50.3 kPa, Fig. 4.63). FNA showed many oxyphilic cells (Fig. 4.64), and the CNB result was chronic lymphocytic thyroiditis showing lymphocytic infiltration (arrow, Fig. 4.65) and interstitial fibrosis (thin arrow, Fig. 4.65) causing increased elasticity on SWE (Fig. 4.63).

4.2.2 Case 2

A 68-year-old woman presented with right neck mass. On ultrasonogram, an isoechoic solid 4.09 cm nodule was found in the right lower lobe (Figs. 4.66 and 4.67) with markedly increased blood flow on color Doppler (Fig. 4.68). Shear wave elastogram showed diffusely increased elasticity with E_{Max}

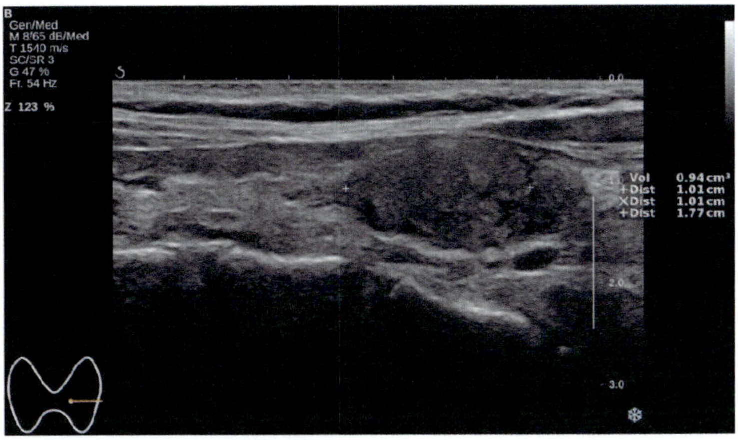

Fig. 4.61 Ultrasonogram showed 1.77 cm isoechoic round nodule in the left lower lobe

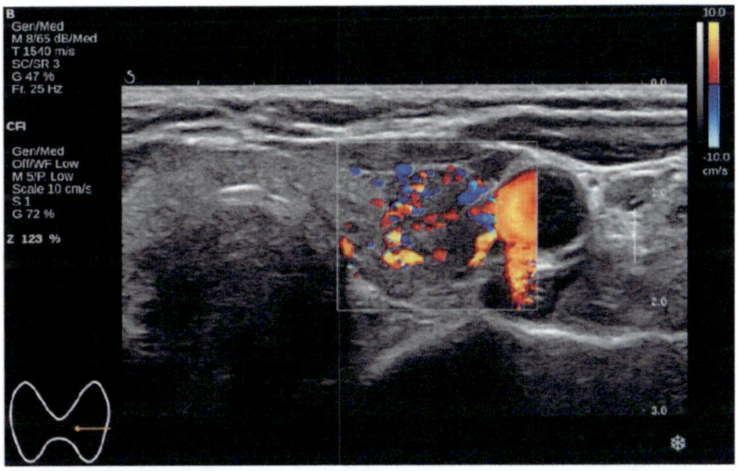

Fig. 4.62 Color Doppler showed moderately increased internal blood flow within the nodule

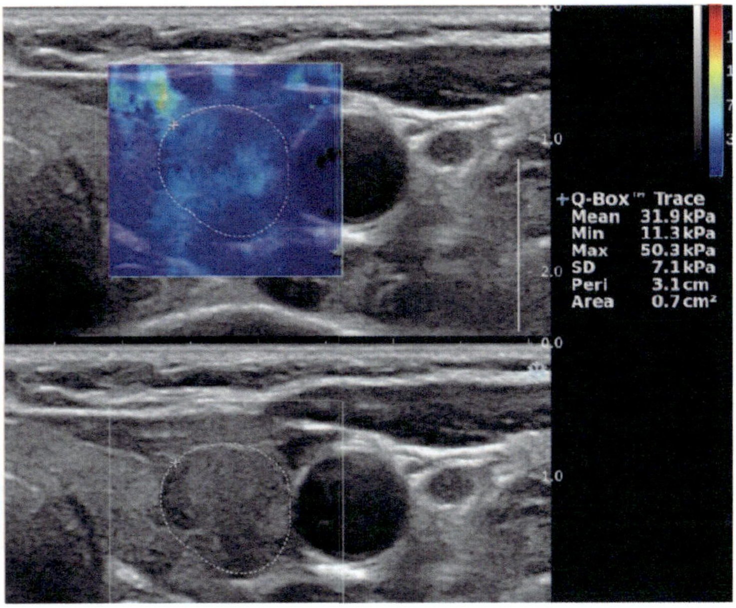

Fig. 4.63 Shear wave elastogram showed scattered increased elasticity within the nodule and E_{Max} was 50.3 kPa

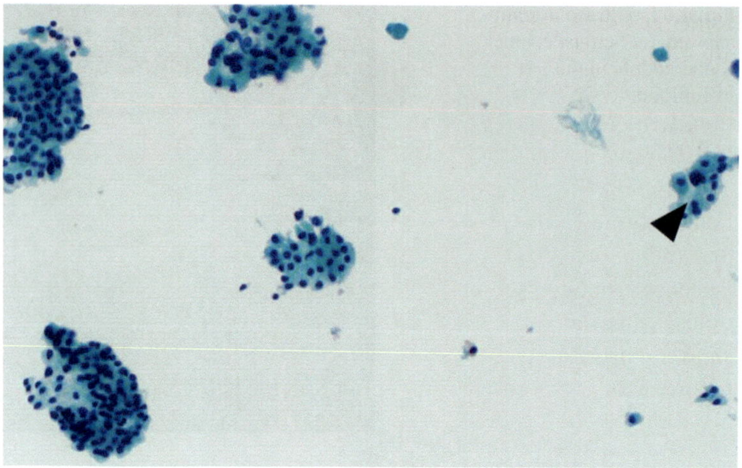

Fig. 4.64 FNA showed many oxyphilic cells (arrow)

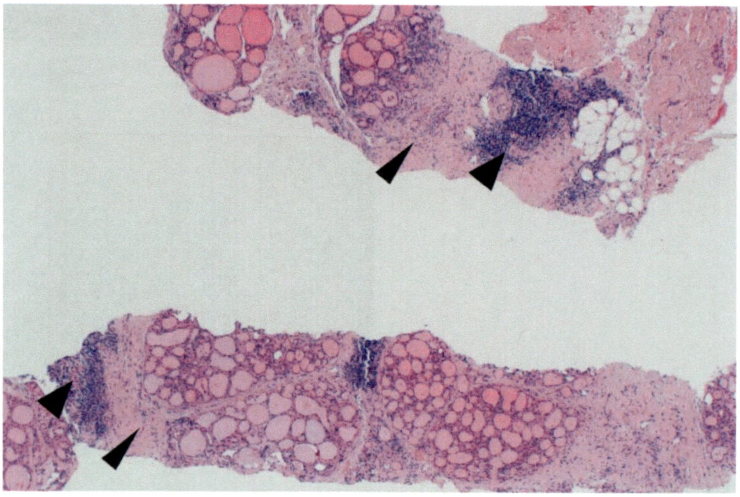

Fig. 4.65 CNB result was chronic lymphocytic thyroiditis showing lymphocytic infiltration (arrows), and interstitial fibrosis (thin arrows)

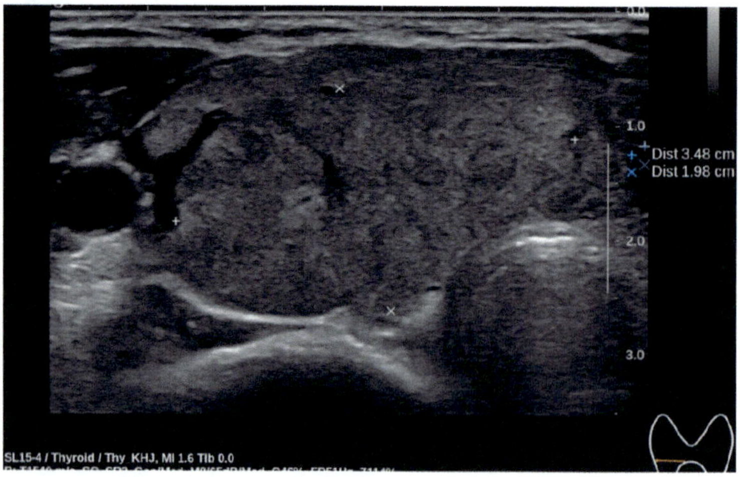

Fig. 4.66 On ultrasonogram, isoechoic solid 4.09 cm nodule was found in the right lower lobe

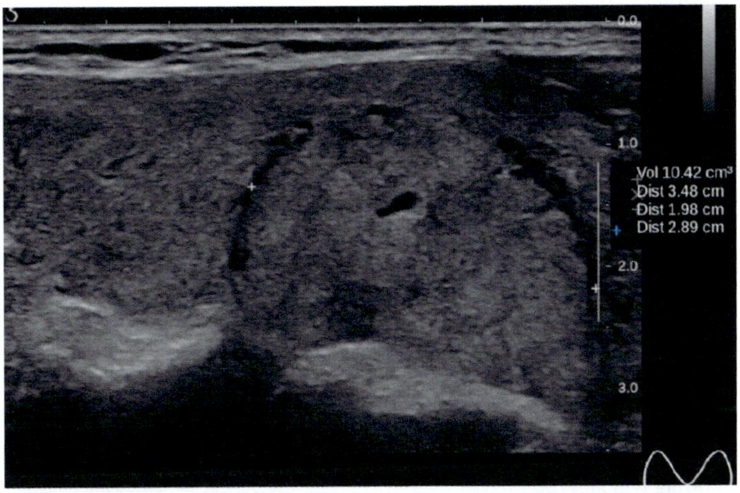

Fig. 4.67 On ultrasonogram, isoechoic solid 4.09 cm nodule was found in the right lower lobe

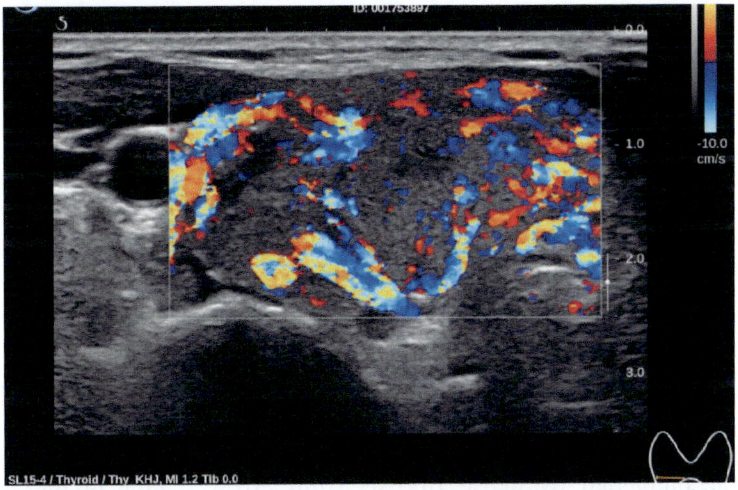

Fig. 4.68 Markedly increased internal vascularity was observed on color Doppler

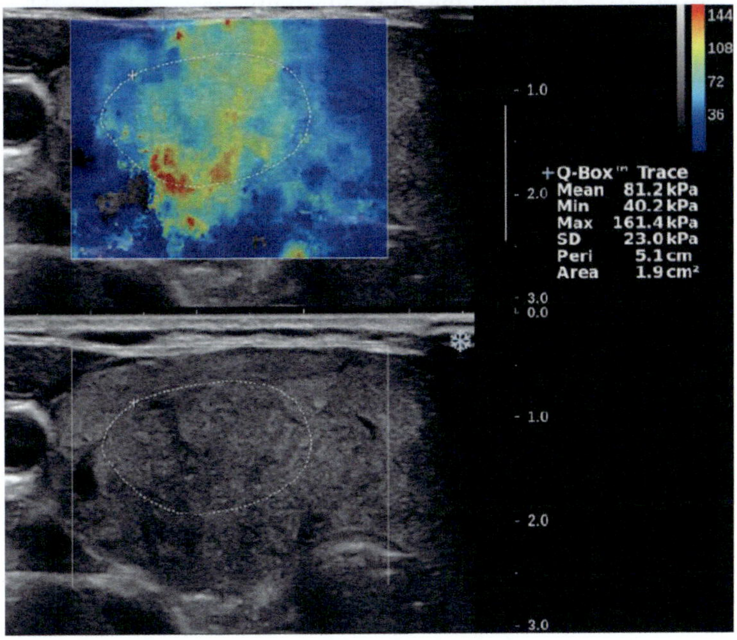

Fig. 4.69 Shear wave elastogram showed diffusely increased elasticity with E_{Max} 161.4 kPa

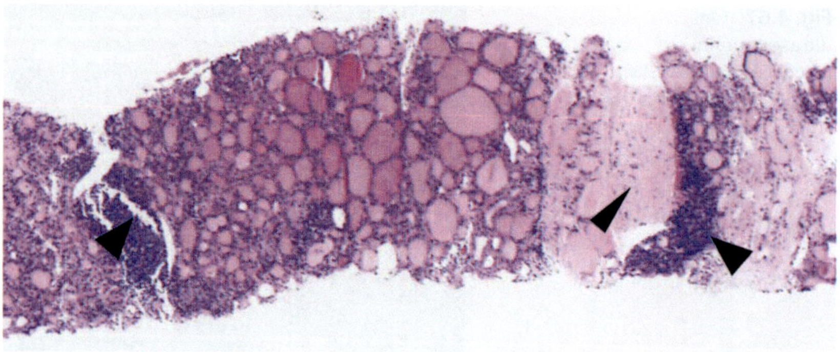

Fig. 4.70 CNB revealed chronic lymphocytic thyroiditis showing lymphocytic infiltration (arrows) accompanied by dense fibrosis (thin arrow)

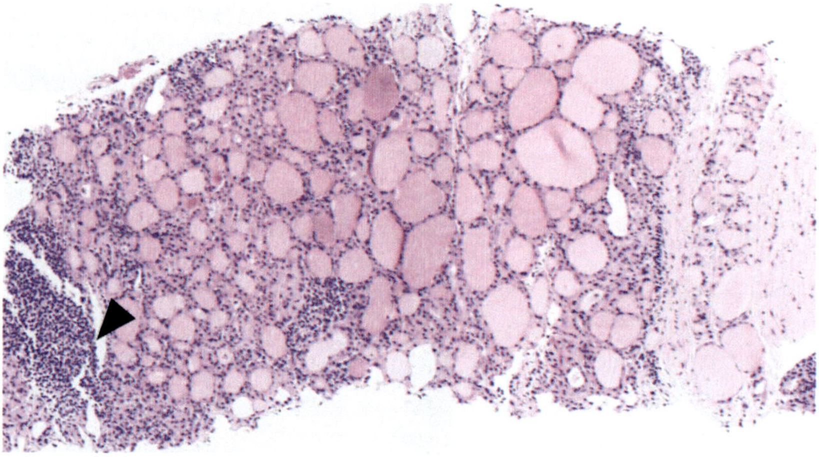

Fig. 4.71 CNB revealed. chronic lymphocytic thyroiditis showing lymphocytic infiltration (arrow)

161.4 kPa (Fig. 4.69). CNB revealed chronic lymphocytic thyroiditis showing lymphocytic infiltration (arrow, Figs. 4.70 and 4.71), accompanied by dense fibrosis (thin arrow, Fig. 4.70) explaining the high elasticity on SWE (Fig. 4.69).

4.2.3 Case 3

A 71-year-old woman was found to have a nodule on routine check and was referred for evaluation. Ultrasonogram showed a 3.22 cm isoechoic nodule with moderate internal vascularity in the left middle lobe (Figs. 4.72, 4.73, and 4.74). Shear wave elastogram showed diffusely increased elasticity within the nodule with E_{Max} 145.7 kPa (Fig. 4.75). The CNB result was chronic lymphocytic thyroiditis (Fig. 4.76) showing oxyphilic follicular cells (arrow, Fig. 4.77) and lymphocytic infiltration.

4.2.4 Case 4

A 62-year-old woman was referred for the evaluation of thyroid nodule. She had been treated with thyroid hormone for 10 years under the diagnosis of hypothyroidism. On B-mode ultrasonogram, a hypoechoic 1 cm nodule was found in the right middle lobe (Figs. 4.78 and 4.79). Shear wave elastogram showed diffusely high elasticity and E_{Max} was 132.7 kPa (Fig. 4.80). CNB revealed chronic lymphocytic thyroiditis showing infiltration of lymphocytic cells (thin arrow, Fig. 4.81) and oxyphilic change of follicular epithelial cells (arrow Fig. 4.82).

4.2.5 Case 5

A 60-year-old woman presented with left thyroid nodule. On B-mode USG, a 1.43 cm predominantly solid nodule with central cystic change

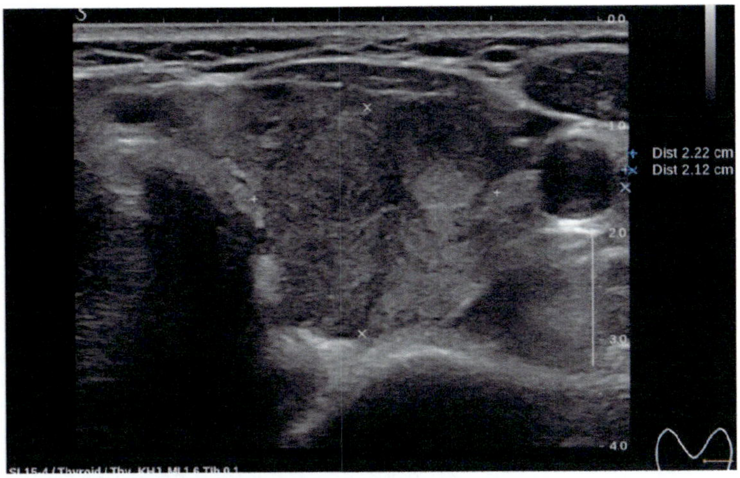

Fig. 4.72 Ultrasonogram showed 3.22 cm isoechoic nodule in the left lobe

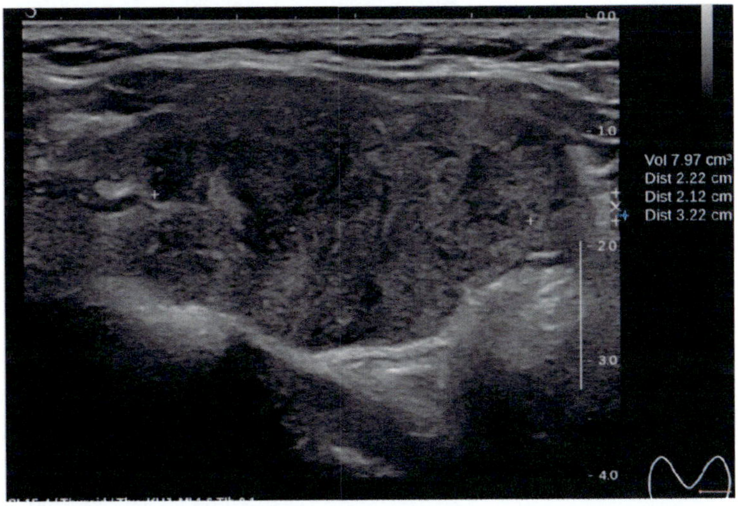

Fig. 4.73 Ultrasonogram showed 3.22 cm isoechoic nodule in the left lobe

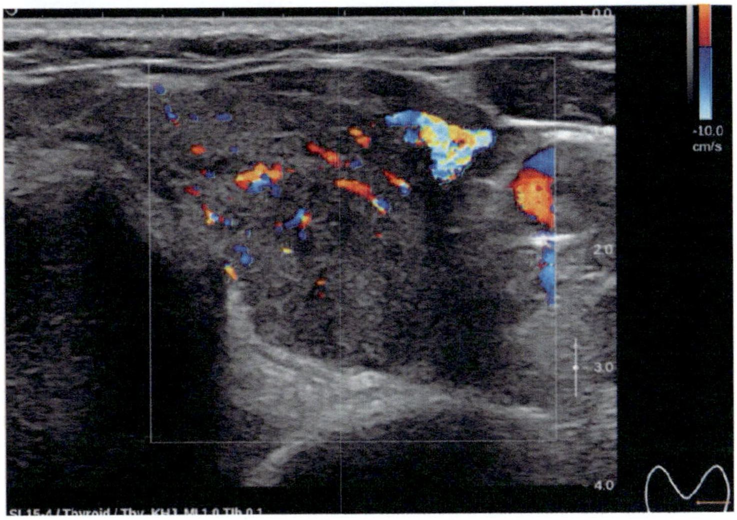

Fig. 4.74 Moderately increased internal vascularity was observed on color doppler

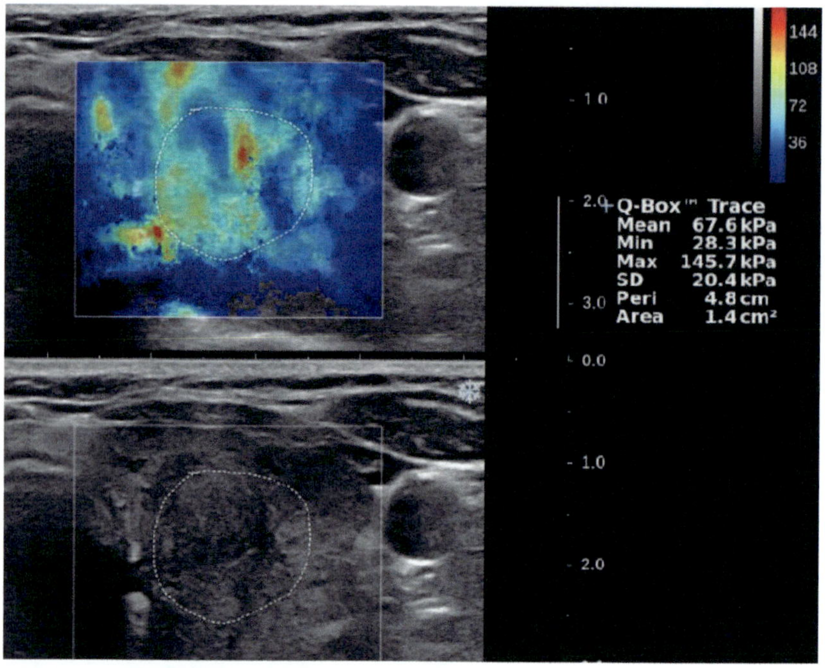

Fig. 4.75 Shear wave elastogram showed diffusely increased elasticity within the nodule with E_{Max} 145.7 kPa

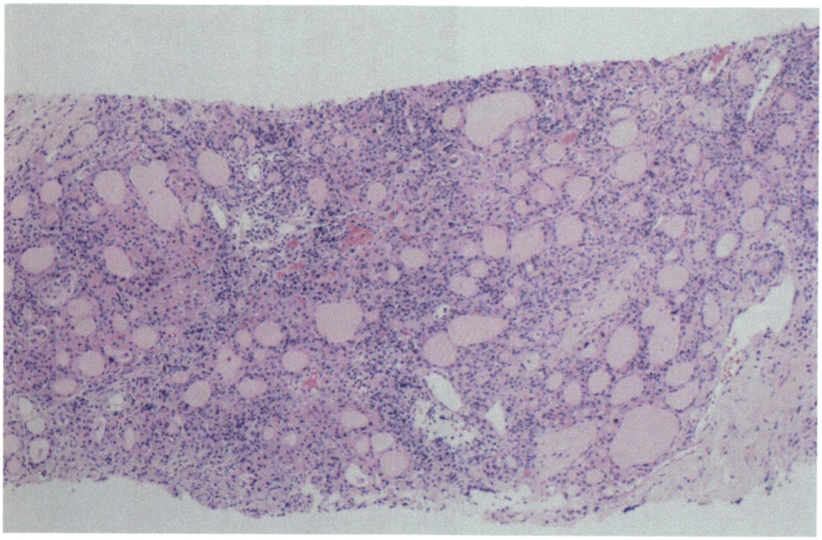

Fig. 4.76 CNB result was chronic lymphocytic thyroiditis showing lymphocytic infiltration

and moderate internal vascularity was observed in the left lobe (Figs. 4.83, 4.84 and 4.85). SWE showed low elasticity (E_{Max} 32.2 kPa, Fig. 4.86). CNB showed chronic lymphocytic thyroiditis with heavy infiltration of lymphoid cells (thin arrow, Fig. 4.87) and oxyphilic cells (arrow, Fig. 4.87).

4.2.6 Case 6

A 71-year-old woman was found to have a nodule on routine check and was referred for evaluation. Ultrasonogram showed a 1.54 cm isoechoic round nodule in the right lower lobe (Figs. 4.88 and 4.89) with little internal blood flow on color

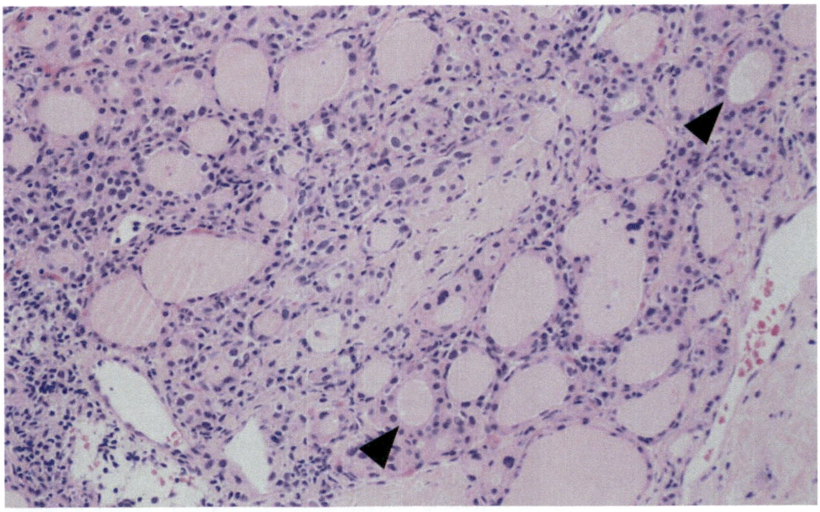

Fig. 4.77 CNB result was chronic lymphocytic thyroiditis showing oxyphilic follicular cells (arrow)

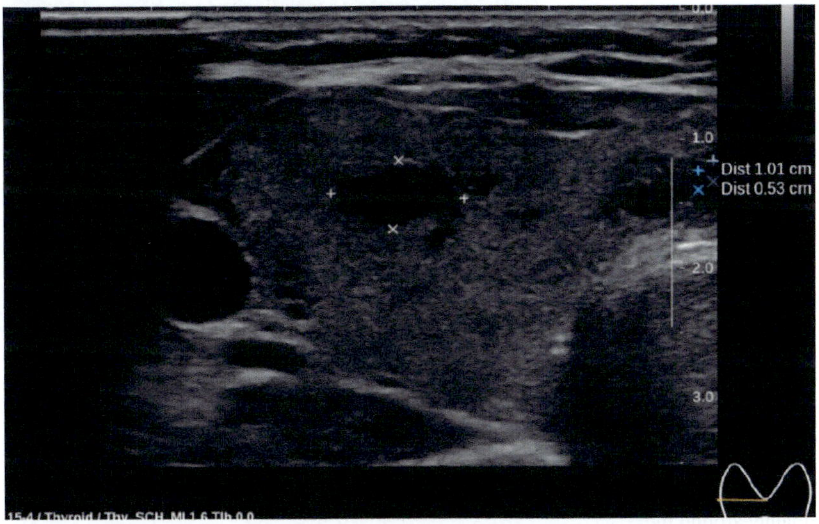

Fig. 4.78 On B-mode ultrasonogram, hypoechoic 1 cm nodule was found in the right middle lobe

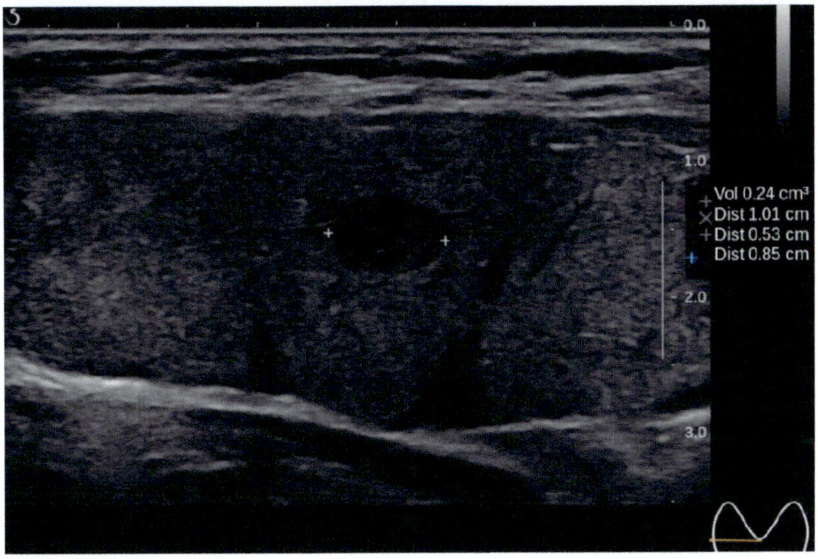

Fig. 4.79 On B-mode ultrasonogram, hypoechoic 1 cm nodule was found in the right middle lobe

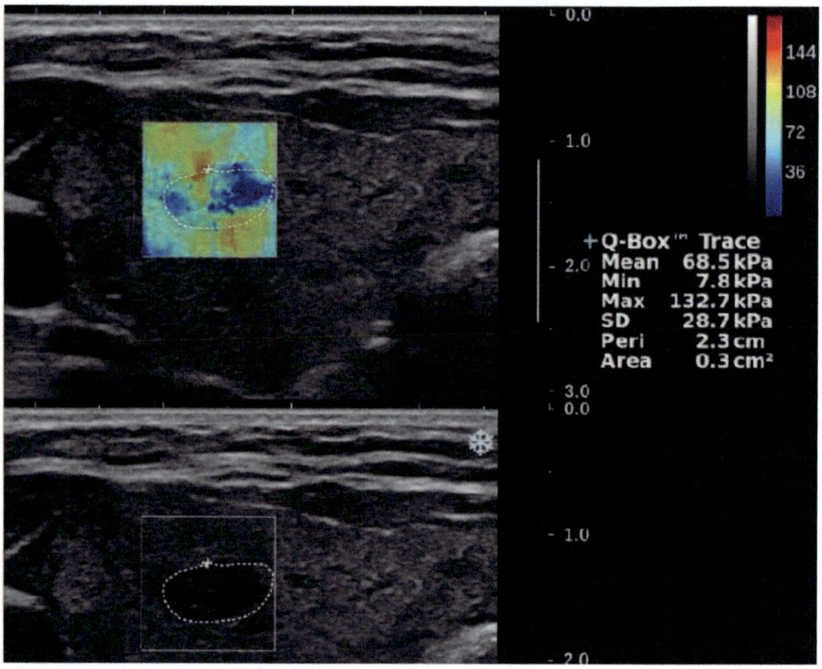

Fig. 4.80 Shear wave elastogram showed diffuse high elasticity and E_{Max} was 132.7 kPa

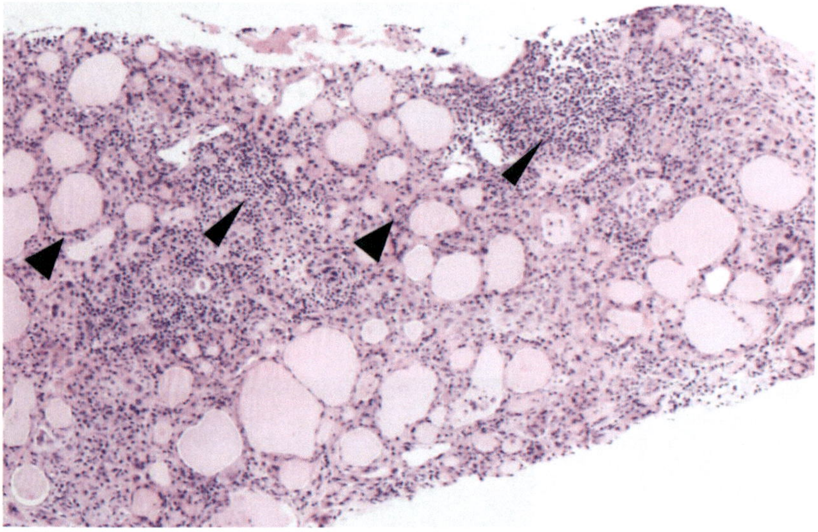

Fig. 4.81 CNB revealed chronic lymphocytic thyroiditis showing infiltration of lymphocytic cells (thin arrow) and oxyphilic change of follicular epithelial cells (arrow)

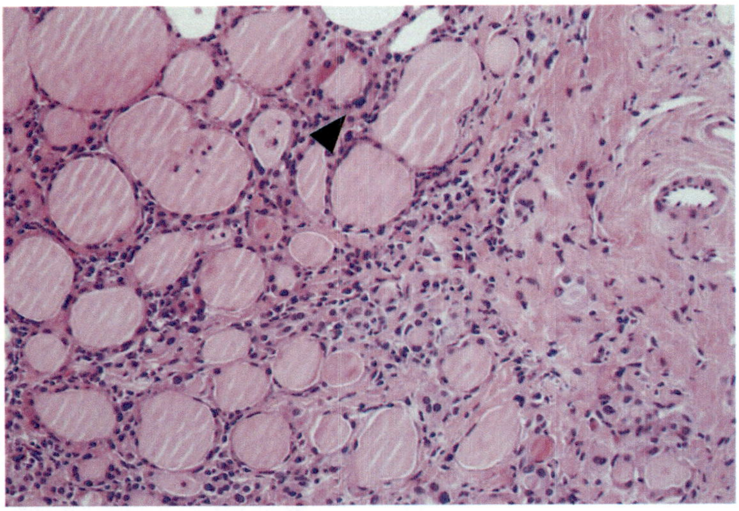

Fig. 4.82 CNB revealed chronic lymphocytic thyroiditis showing oxyphilic change of follicular epithelial cells (arrow)

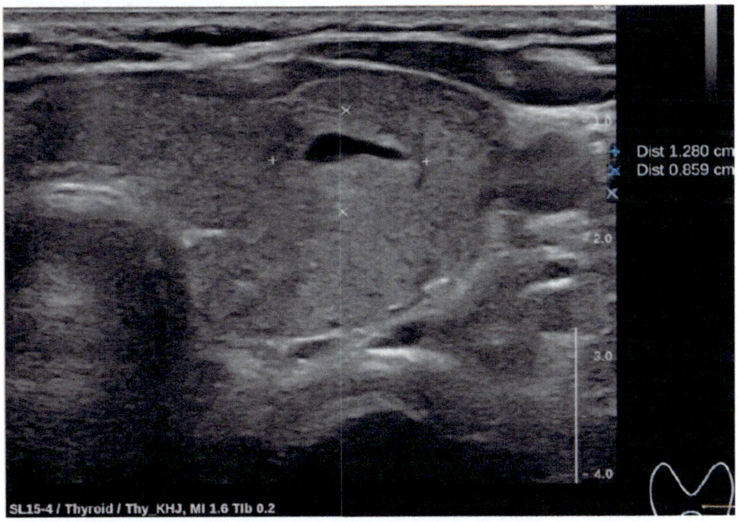

Fig. 4.83 On B mode USG, 1.43 cm predominantly solid nodule with central cystic change was observed in the left middle lobe

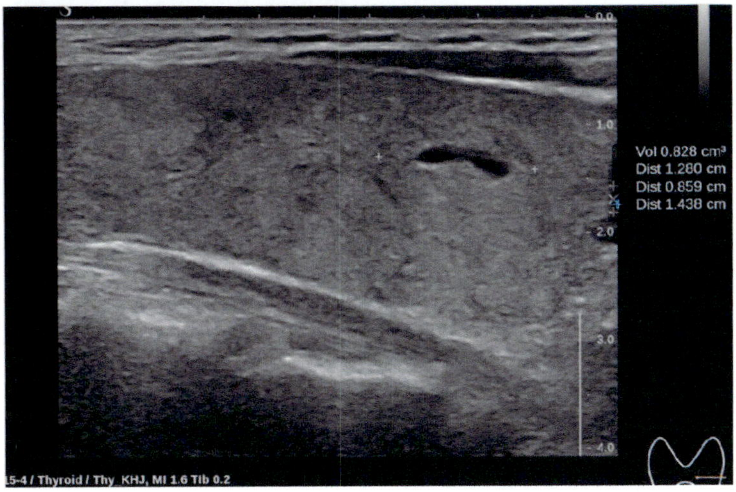

Fig. 4.84 On B mode USG, 1.43 cm predominantly solid nodule with central cystic change was observed in the left lobe

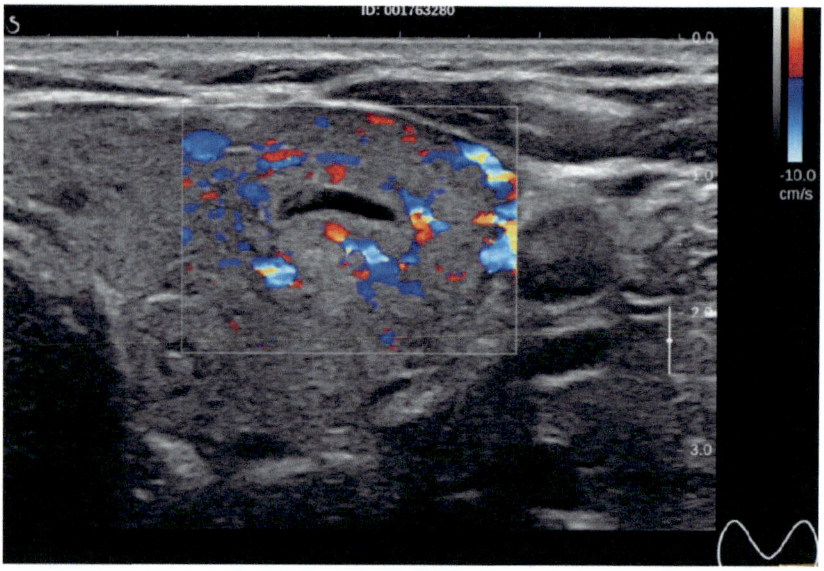

Fig. 4.85 Moderate internal vascularity was observed on color Doppler

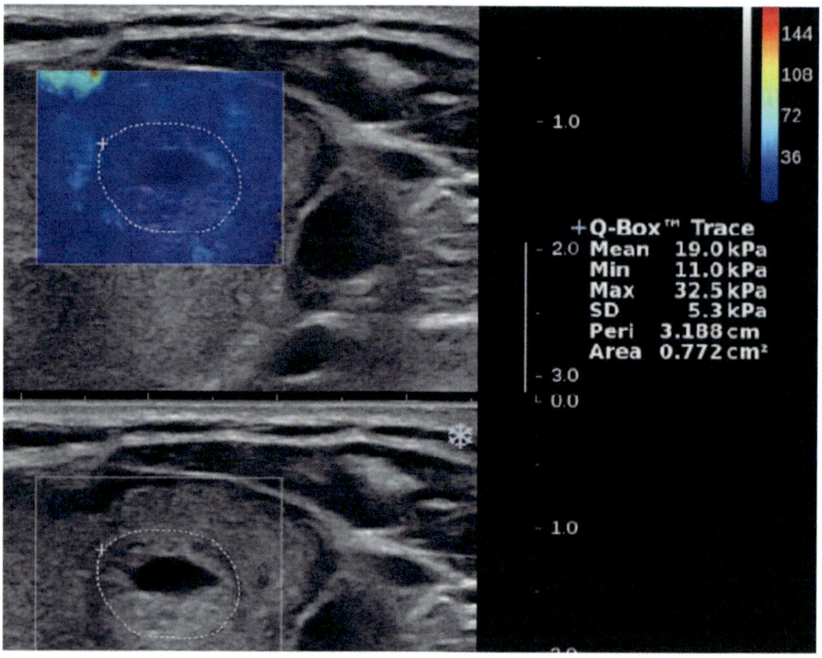

Fig. 4.86 Moderate internal vascularity was observed on color Doppler

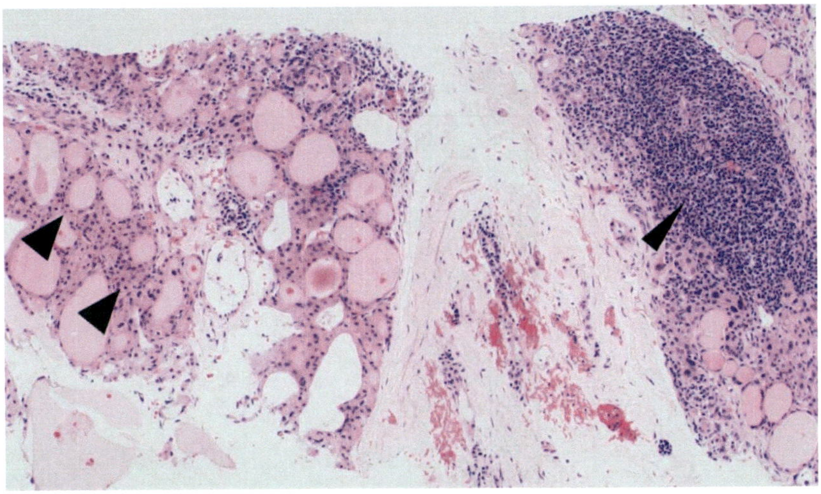

Fig. 4.87 CNB showed chronic lymphocytic thyroiditis with heavy infiltration of lymphoid cells (thin arrow) and oxyphilic cells (arrows)

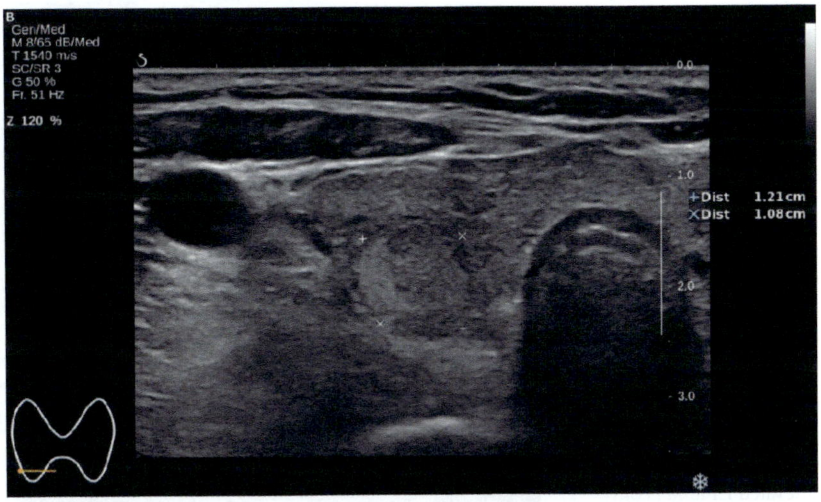

Fig. 4.88 Ultrasonogram showed 1.54 cm isoechoic round nodule in the right lower lobe

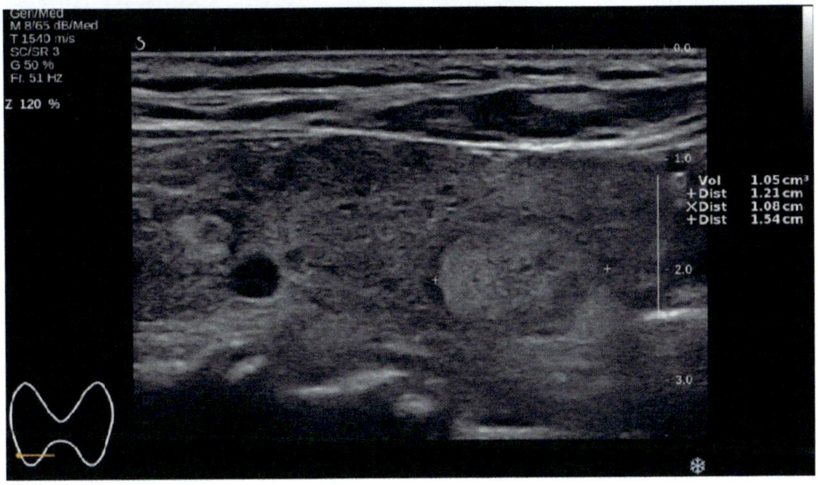

Fig. 4.89 Ultrasonogram showed 1.54 cm isoechoic round nodule in the right lower lobe

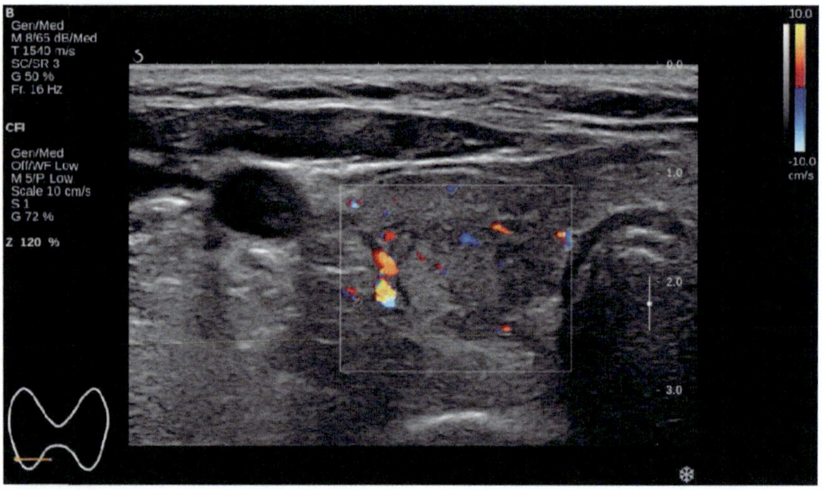

Fig. 4.90 Little internal vascularity was observed on color Doppler

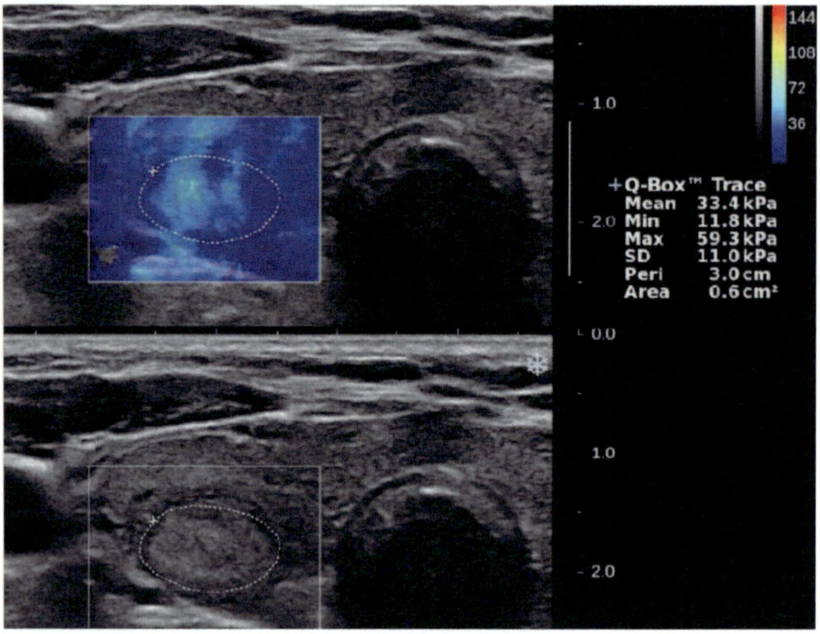

Fig. 4.91 Shear wave elastogram showed diffusely increased elasticity within the nodule and E_{Max} was 59.3 kPa

Doppler (Fig. 4.90). Shear wave elastogram showed diffusely increased elasticity within the nodule (E_{Max} 59.3 kPa, Fig. 4.91). CNB showed chronic lymphocytic thyroiditis showing heavy lymphocytic infiltration (Figs. 4.92 and 4.93).

4.2.7 Case 7

A 61-year-old woman was found to have a nodule on routine check and was referred for evaluation. She had been treated for hypothyroidism for 10

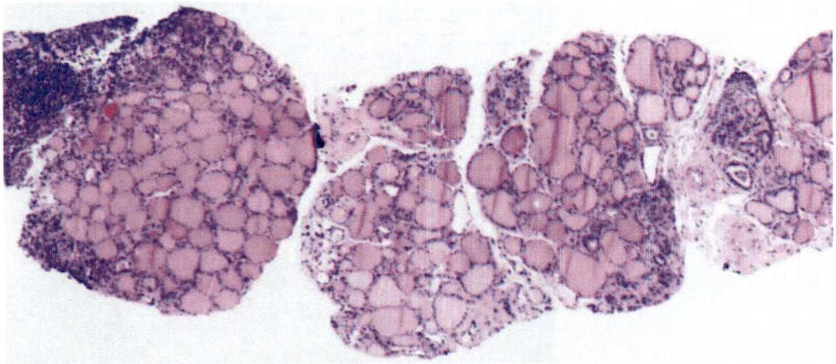

Fig. 4.92 CNB showed chronic lymphocytic thyroiditis showing heavy lymphocytic infitration

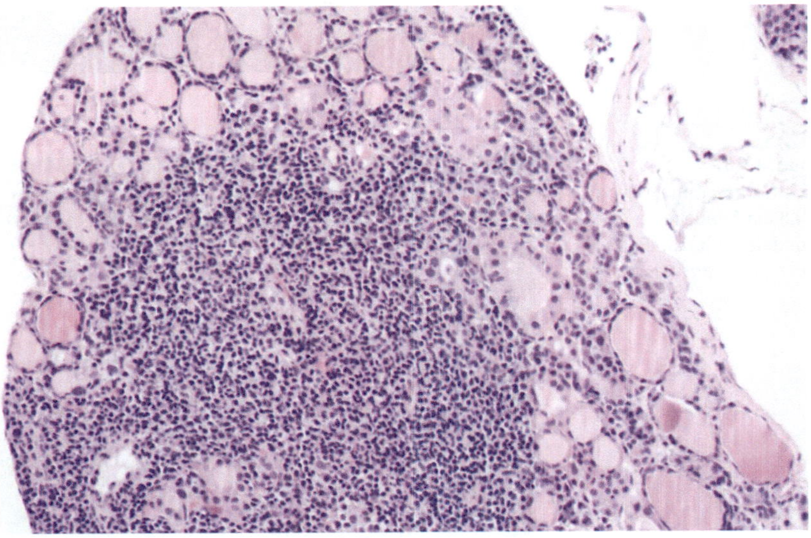

Fig. 4.93 CNB showed chronic lymphocytic thyroiditis showing heavy lymphocytic infitration

years. Ultrasonogram showed a 0.8 cm hypoechoic nodule with a calcified rim in the left lobe (Figs. 4.94 and 4.95) with little internal vascularity on color Doppler (Fig. 4.96). Shear wave elastogram showed increased elasticity under the calcified rim within the nodule (Fig. 4.97). CNB showed chronic lymphocytic thyroiditis (Fig. 4.98).

4.3 Granulomatous (Subacute, de Quervain's) Thyroiditis

Granulomatous (Subacute) thyroiditis is associated with proceeding viral infection and usually appears after a viral upper respiratory tract infection, and occurrences with coxachievirus, mumps, measles and adenovirus have also been reported. The thyroid glands show painful diffused enlargement, firm to hard in consistency and usually with severe tenderness. Initially hyperthyroidism appears, followed by hypothyroidism, which shows self-limited recovery to an euthyroid state in 6 to 8 wks.

Histopathology granulomatous thyroiditis showed infiltration of epitheloid histiocytes, lymphocytes, macrophages and multinucleated giant cells encircling colloid follicles. Later chronic inflammatory infiltrate and fibrosis replaces and regeneration of thyroid follicles results self-limited resolution [1].

On B-mode ultrasound of subacute thyroiditis ill-defined patchy hypoechoic areas with geographic patterns area observed which usually show resolution after remission of the disease. SWE showed much more elevated elasticity than chronic lymphocytic thyroiditis [12, 13].

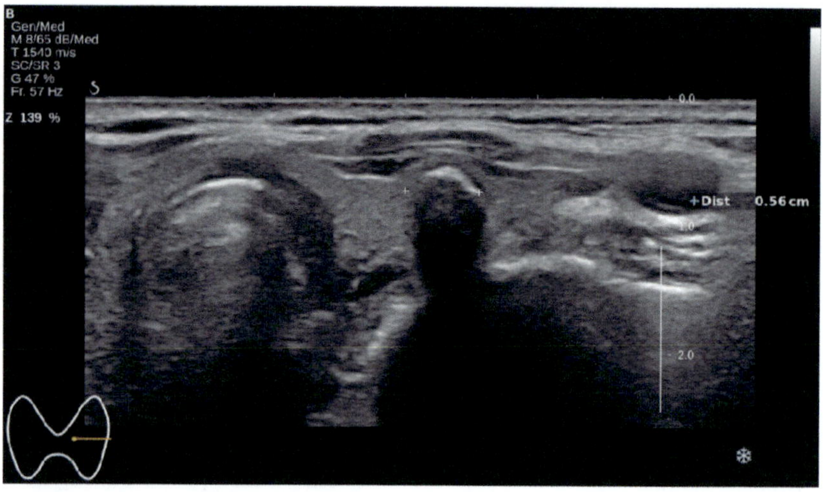

Fig. 4.94 Ultrasonogram showed 0.8 cm hypoechoic nodule with calcified rim in the left lobe

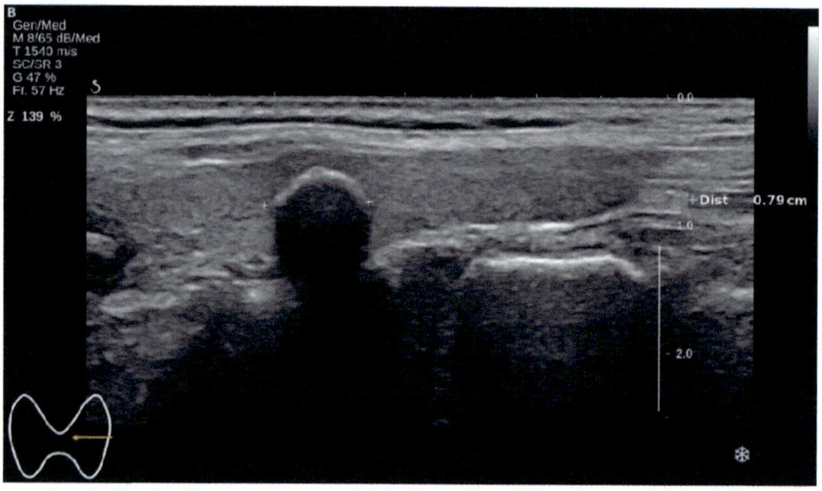

Fig. 4.95 Ultrasonogram showed 0.8 cm hypoechoic nodule with calcified rim in the left lobe

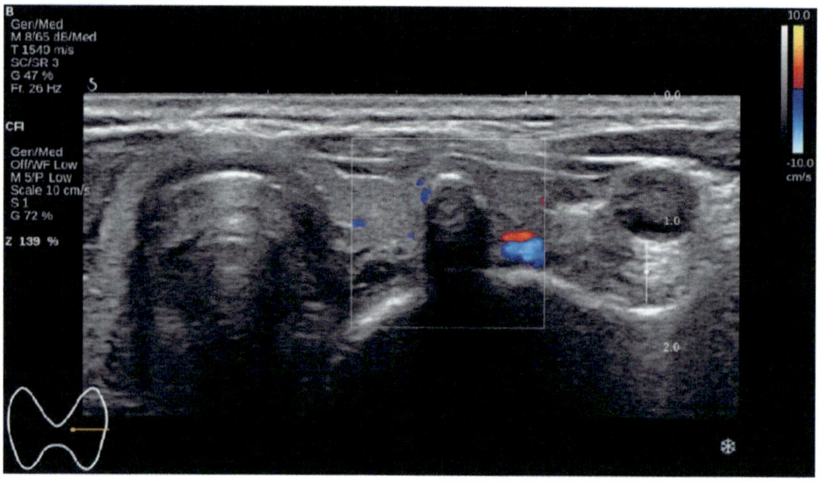

Fig. 4.96 Little internal vascularity was observed on color Doppler

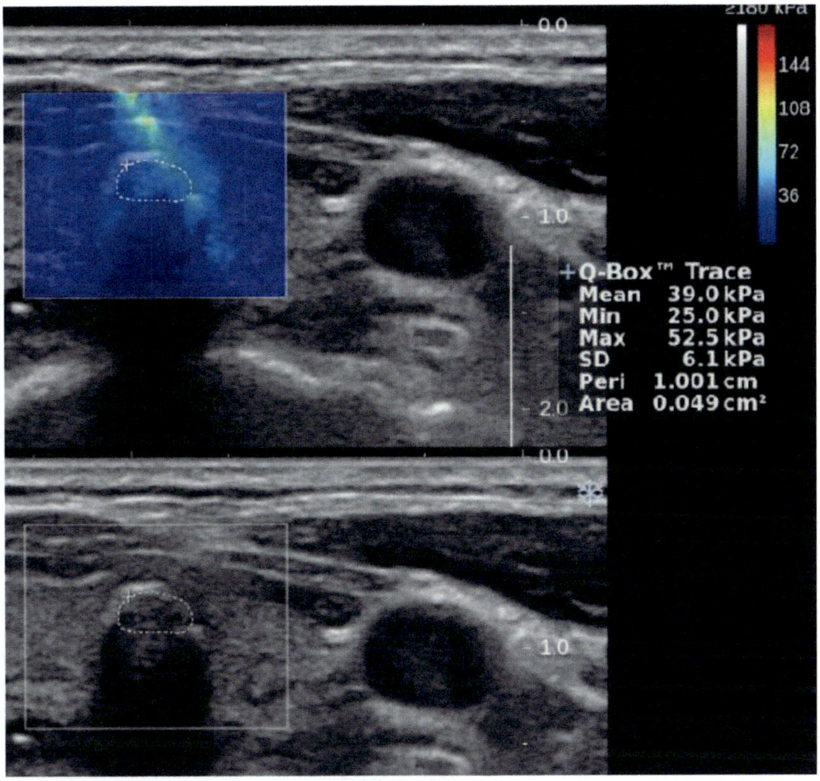

Fig. 4.97 Shear wave elastogram showed increased elasticity under the calcified rim within the nodule and E_{Max} was 52.5 kPa

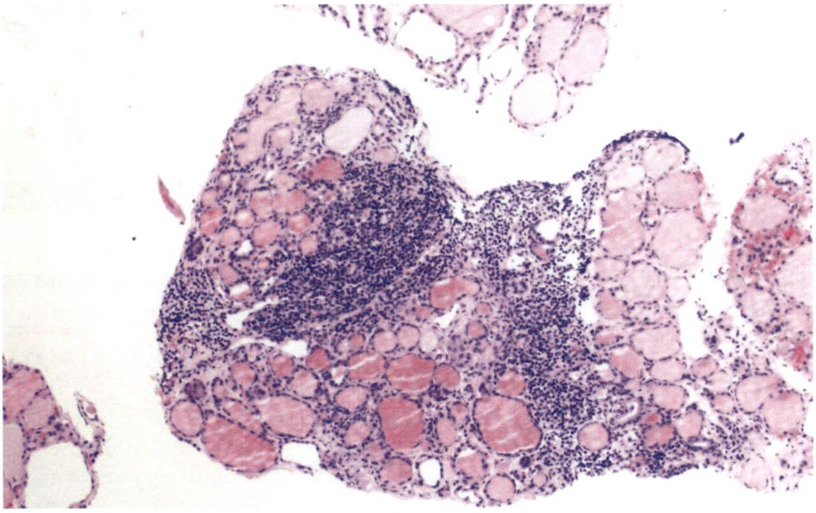

Fig. 4.98 CNB result was chronic lymphocytic thyroiditis

4.3.1 Case 1

A 50-year-old woman was found to have a painful right neck mass. She denied recent upper respiratory infection. On ultrasonogram, the right thyroid gland was diffusely enlarged and showed hypoechogenic irregular bordered lesion (Figs. 4.99 and 4.100) and little blood flow on color Doppler (Fig. 4.101). Shear wave elastogram showed markedly increased elasticity with E_{Max} 265.8 kPa (Fig. 4.102). The CNB result was subacute granulomatous thyroiditis showing diffuse infiltration of inflammatory cells and giant cells (arrow, Figs. 4.103 and 4.104).

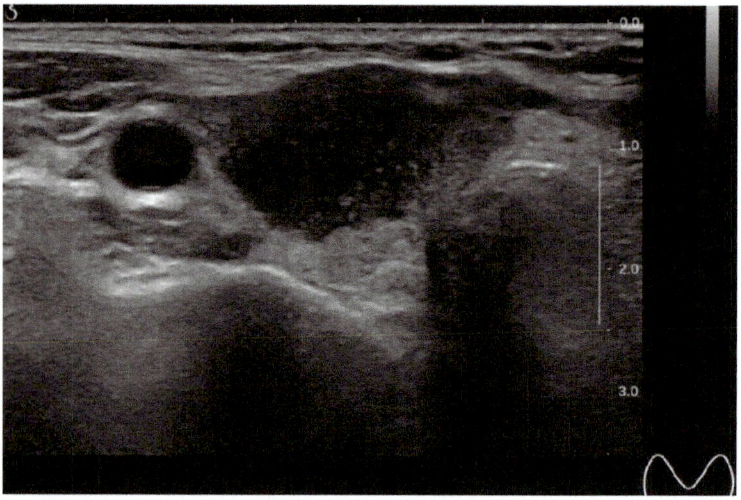

Fig. 4.99 On ultrasonogram, the right thyroid gland was diffusely enlarged and showed hypoechogenic irregular bordered lesion

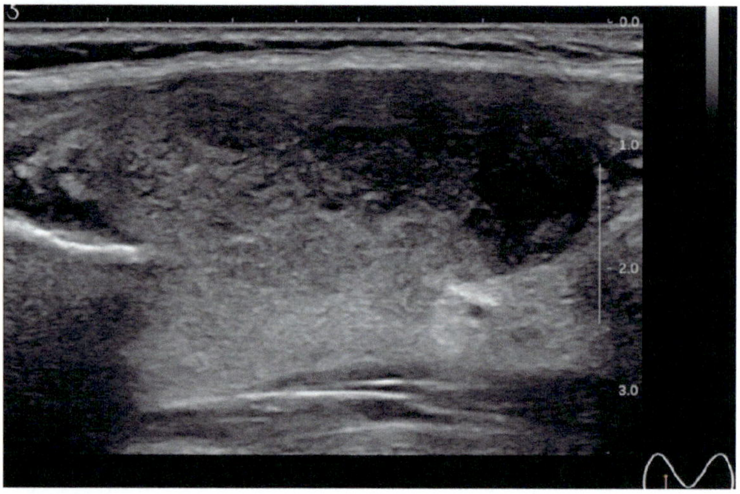

Fig. 4.100 On ultrasonogram, the right thyroid gland was diffusely enlarged and showed hypoechogenic irregular bordered lesion

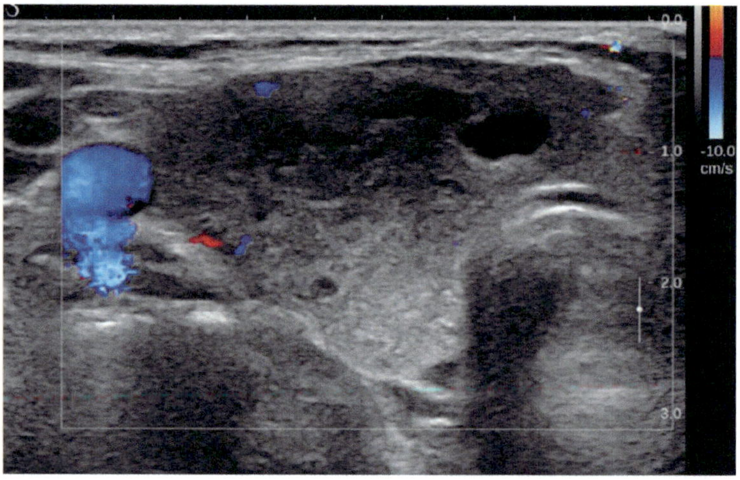

Fig. 4.101 Little internal vascularity was observed on color Doppler

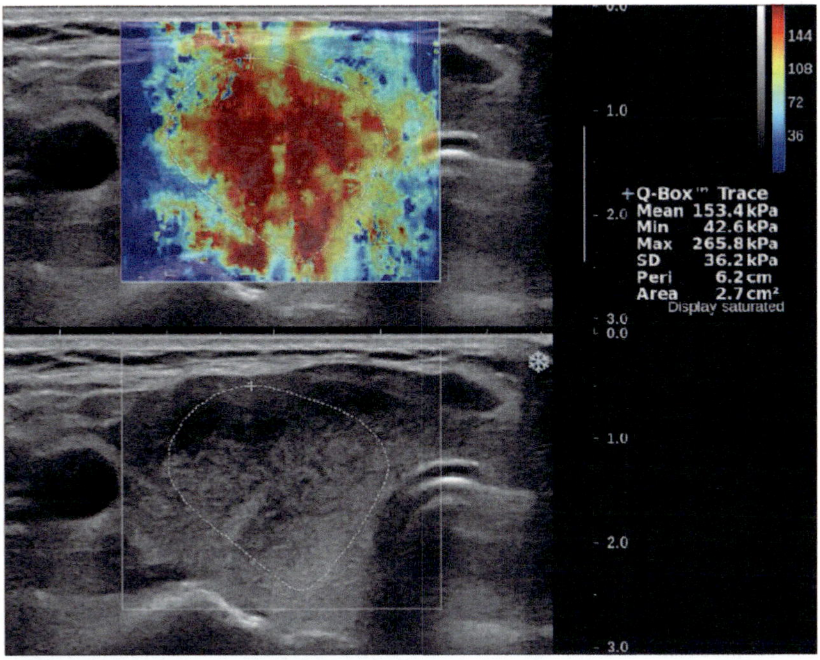

Fig. 4.102 Shear wave elastogram showed markedly increased elasticity and E_{Max} was 265.8 kPa

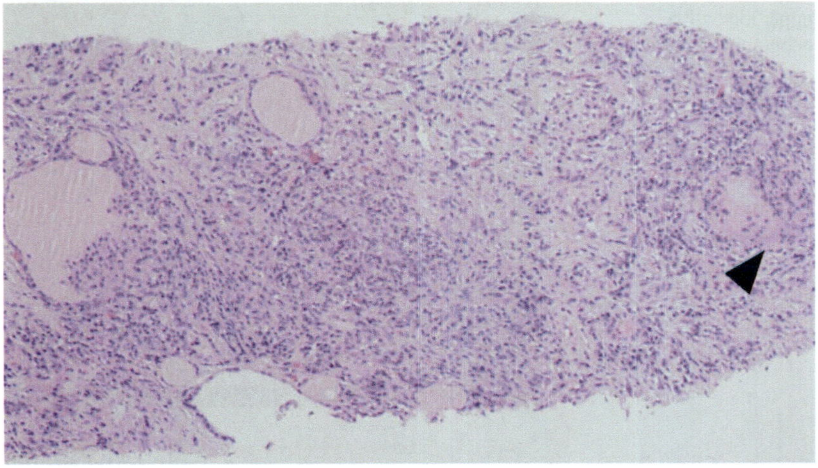

Fig. 4.103 CNB result was subacute granulomatous thyroiditis showing diffuse infiltration of inflammatory cells and giant cells (arrow)

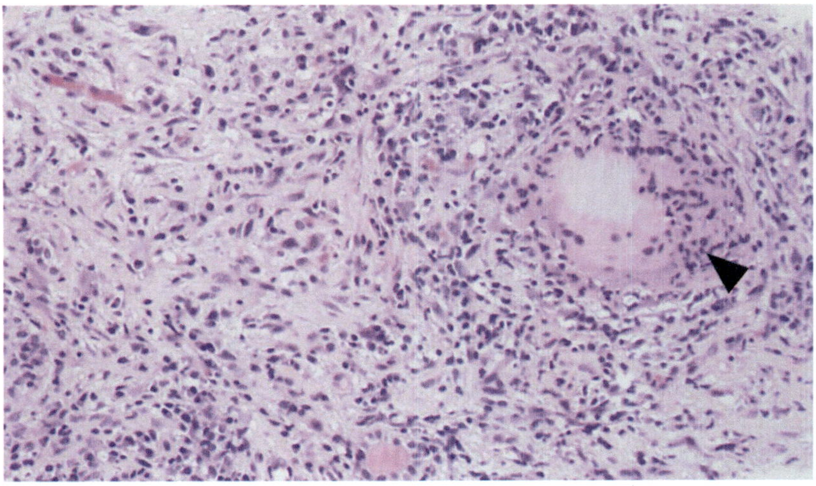

Fig. 4.104 CNB result was subacute granulomatous thyroiditis showing diffuse infiltration of inflammatory cells and giant cells (arrow)

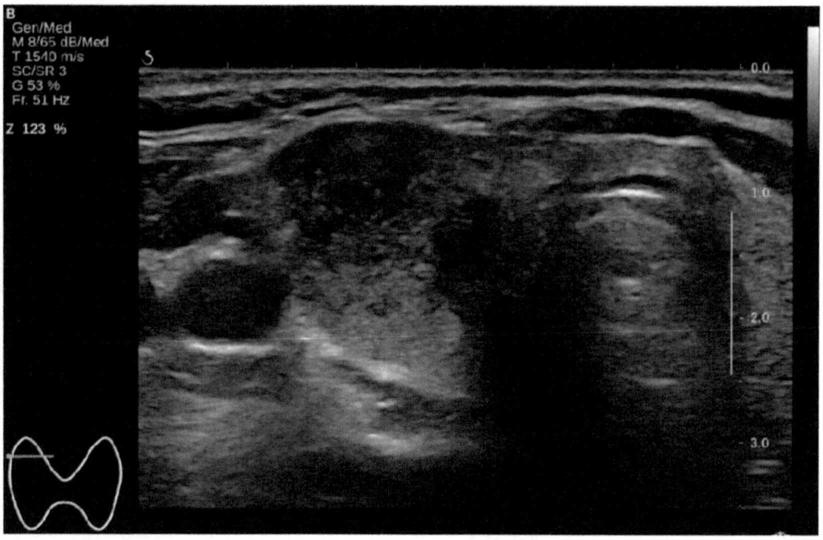

Fig. 4.105 Ultrasonogram showed focal hypoechoic parenchyma in the right upper lobe with geographic pattern

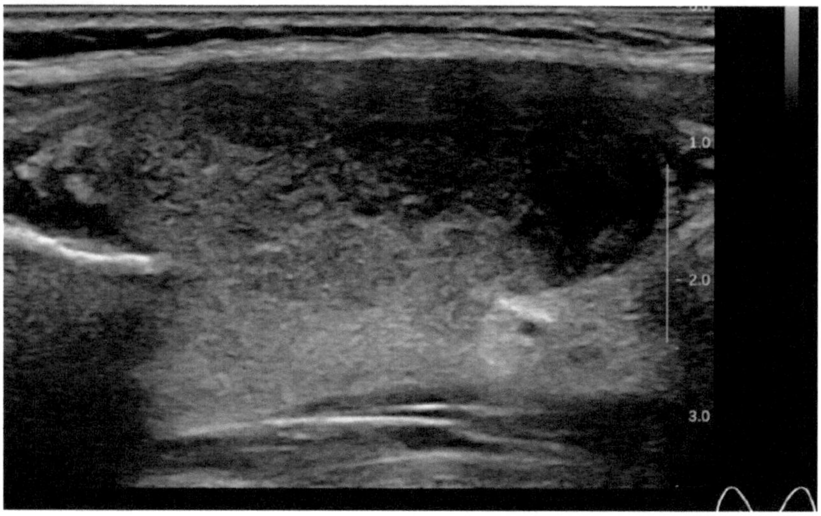

Fig. 4.106 Ultrasonogram showed focal hypoechoic parenchyma in the right upper lobe with geographic pattern

4.3.2 Case 2

A 52-year-old woman was referred for the evaluation of tender neck mass. She had a history of upper respiratory infection (two weeks earlier). Ultrasonogram showed focal hypoechoic parenchyma in the right upper lobe showing a geographic pattern with little blood flow on color Doppler (Figs. 4.105, 4.106, and 4.107). Shear wave elastogram showed markedly increased elasticity with E_{Max} 300 kPa (Fig. 4.108). The CNB result was subacute granulomatous thyroiditis with diffused infiltration of inflammatory cells and fibrotic change showing giant cells (arrows, Figs. 4.109 and 4.110).

4.3.3 Case 3

A 33-year-woman was referred for the evaluation of painful neck mass. She had fever and sore throat one week earlier, and on physical examination, tenderness was present on both lobes. On ultrasonogram, hypoechoic lesion with geo-

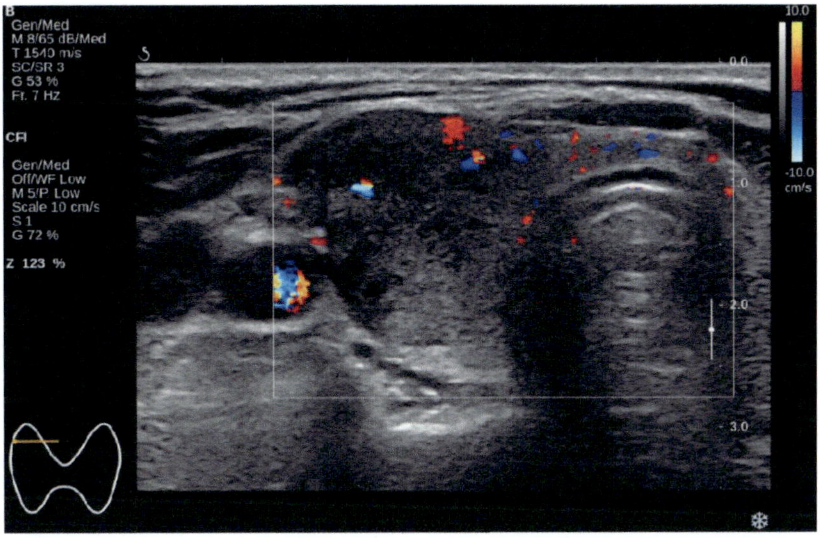

Fig. 4.107 Little internal vascularity was observed on color Doppler

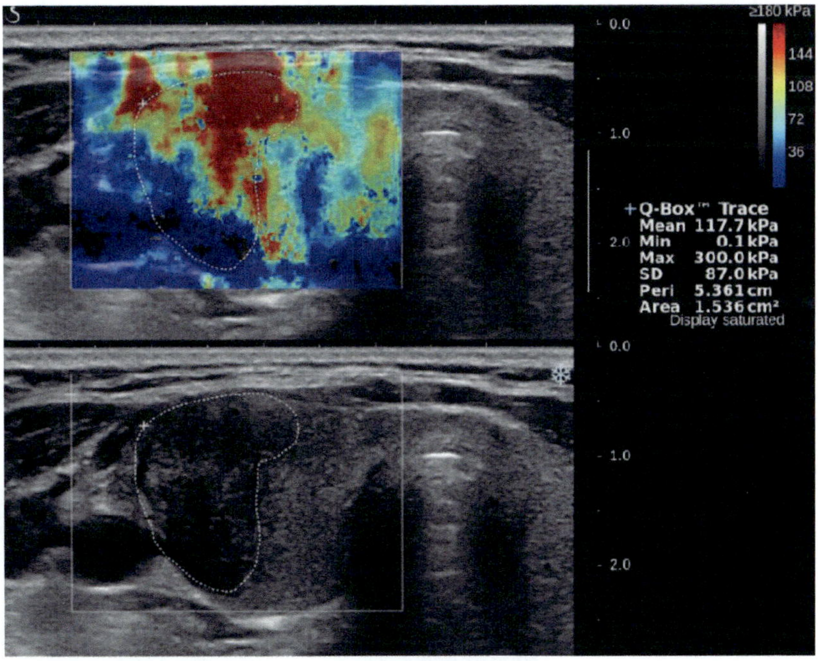

Fig. 4.108 Shear wave elastogram showed markedly increased elasticity with E_{Max} 300 kPa

graphic pattern was observed (Figs. 4.111, 4.112, and 4.113) in both lobes with little blood flow on color Doppler (Fig. 4.114). Shear wave elastogram showed markedly increased elasticity with E_{Max} 165.8 kPa (Fig. 4.115). The CNB result was subacute granulomatous thyroiditis showing diffuse infiltration of epithelioid cells and giant cells (arrow, Figs. 4.116, and 4.117) with diffuse fibrosis causing diffuse increased elasticity on SWE (Fig. 4.115).

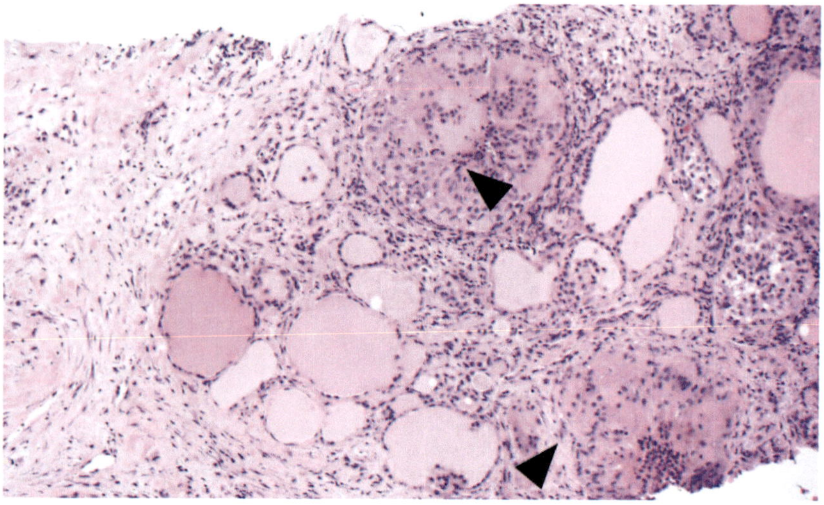

Fig. 4.109 CNB result was subacute granulomatous thyroiditis with diffuse infiltration of inflammatory cells and fibrotic change showing giant cells (arrows)

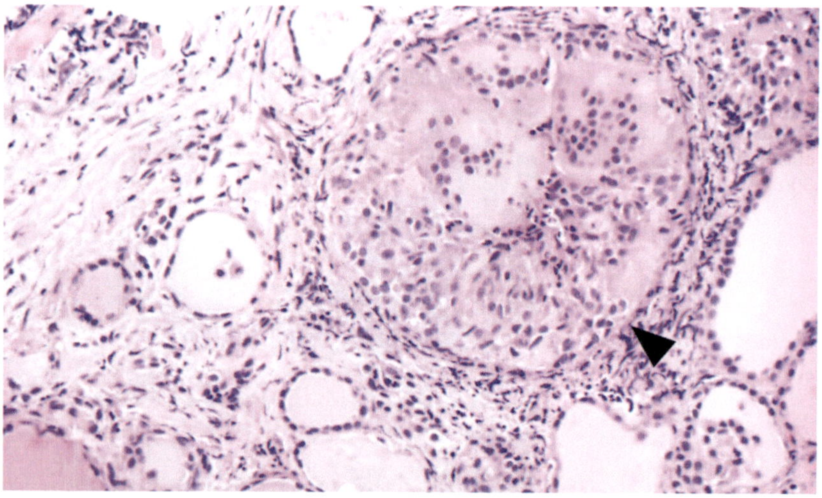

Fig. 4.110 CNB result was subacute granulomatous thyroiditis with diffuse infiltration of inflammatory cells and fibrotic change showing giant cells (arrow)

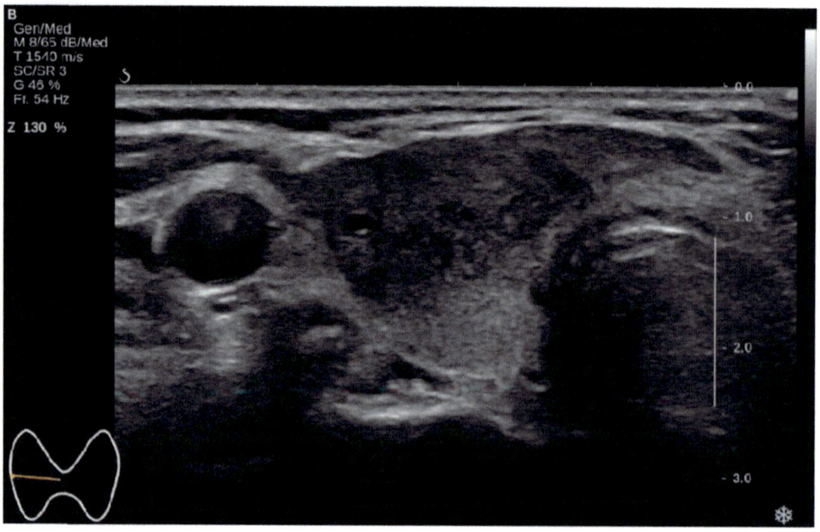

Fig. 4.111 On ultrasonogram, hypoechoic lesioin with geographic pattern was observed in the right lobe

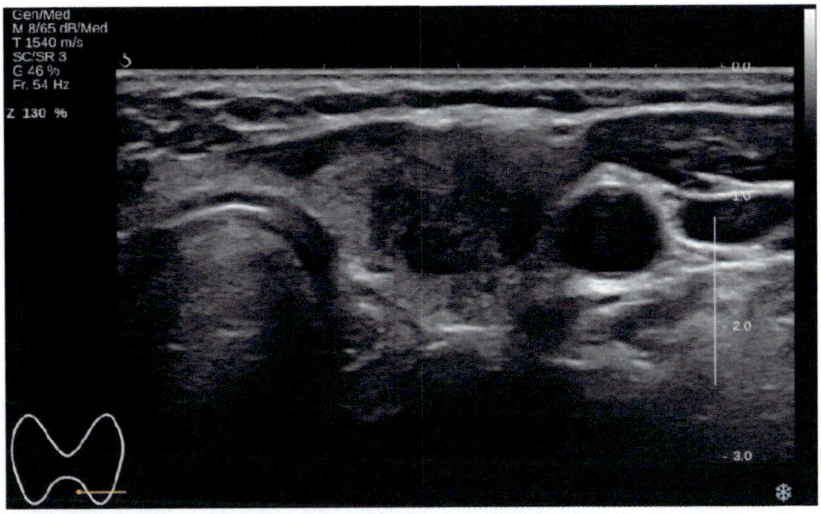

Fig. 4.112 On ultrasonogram, hypoechoic lesioin with geographic pattern was observed in the left lobe

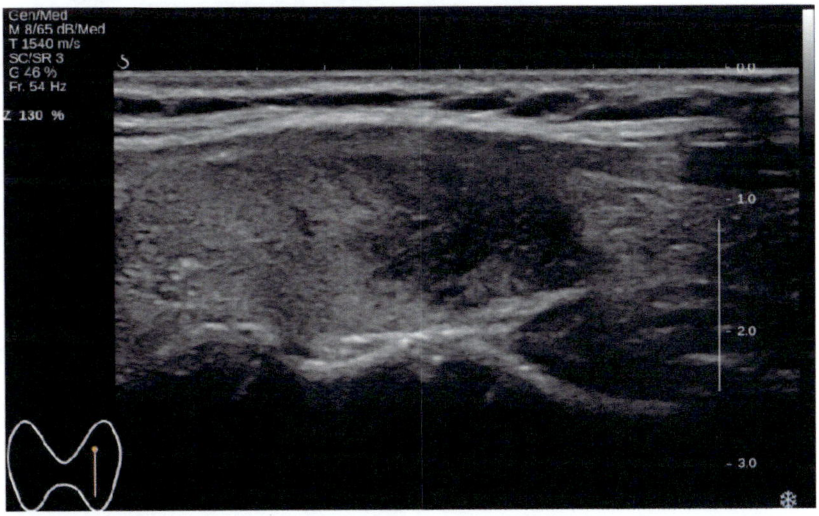

Fig. 4.113 On ultrasonogram, hypoechoic lesioin with geographic pattern was observed in the left lobe

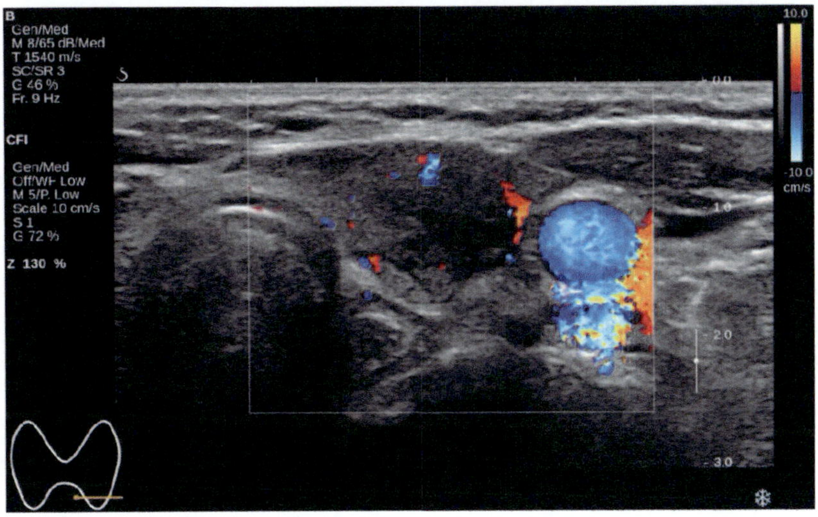

Fig. 4.114 Little internal vascularity was observed on color Doppler

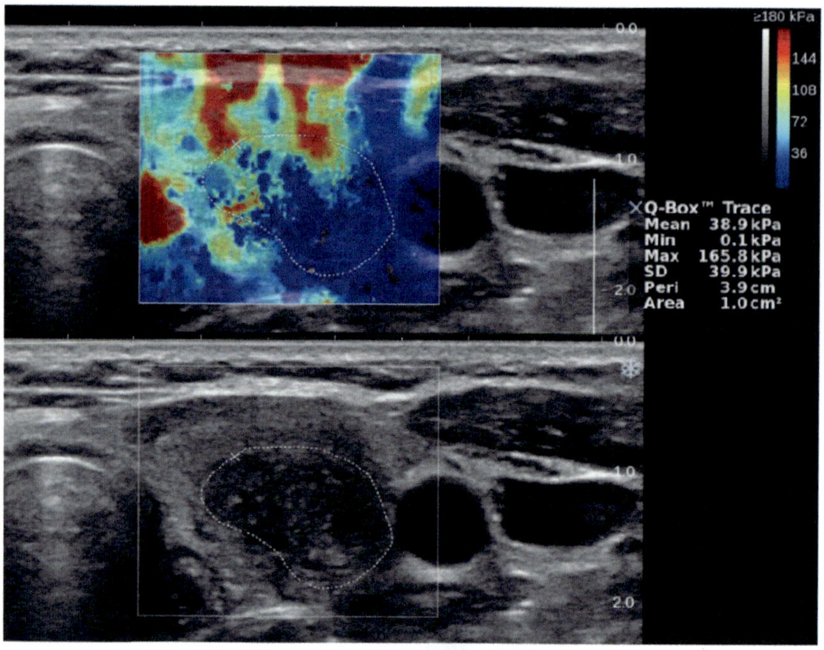

Fig. 4.115 Shear wave elastogram showed markedly increased elasticity with E_{Max} 165.8 kPa

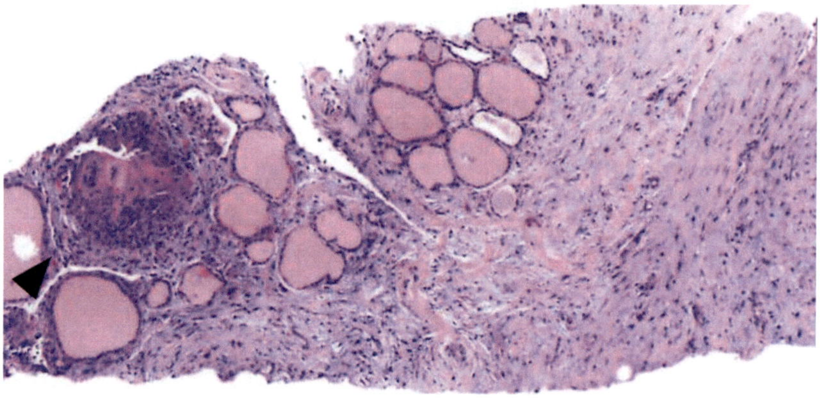

Fig. 4.116 CNB result was subacute granulomatous thyroiditis showing diffuse infiltration of epithelioid cells and giant cells (arrow)

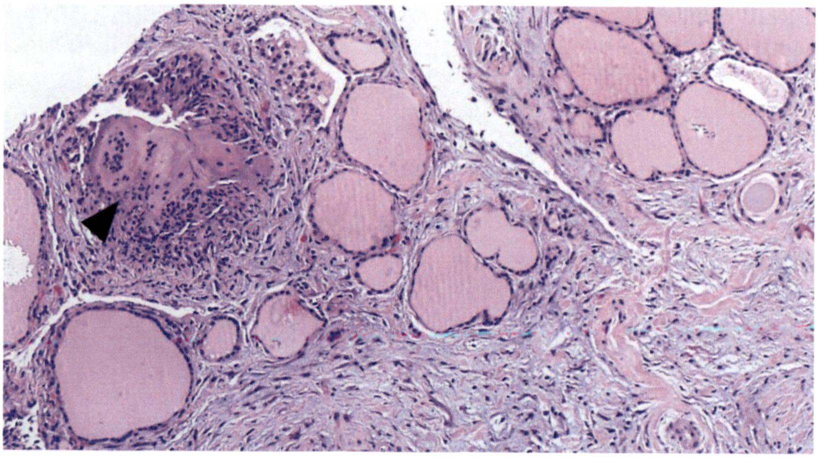

Fig. 4.117 CNB result was subacute granulomatous thyroiditis showing diffuse infiltration of epithelioid cells and giant cells (arrow)

4.3.4 Case 4

A 33-year-woman was referred for the evaluation of painful neck mass. She had fever two weeks earlier. On physical examination, both thyroid glands showed severe tenderness. On ultrasonogram, hypoechoic lesion with geographic pattern was observed (Figs. 4.118 and 4.119) with little blood flow on color Doppler (Fig. 4.120). Shear wave elastogram showed markedly increased elasticity with E_{Max} 173.5 kPa (Figs. 4.121 and 4.122). The CNB result was subacute granulomatous thyroiditis with diffuse infiltration of inflammatory cells and fibrosis showing giant cells (arrow, Fig. 4.123).

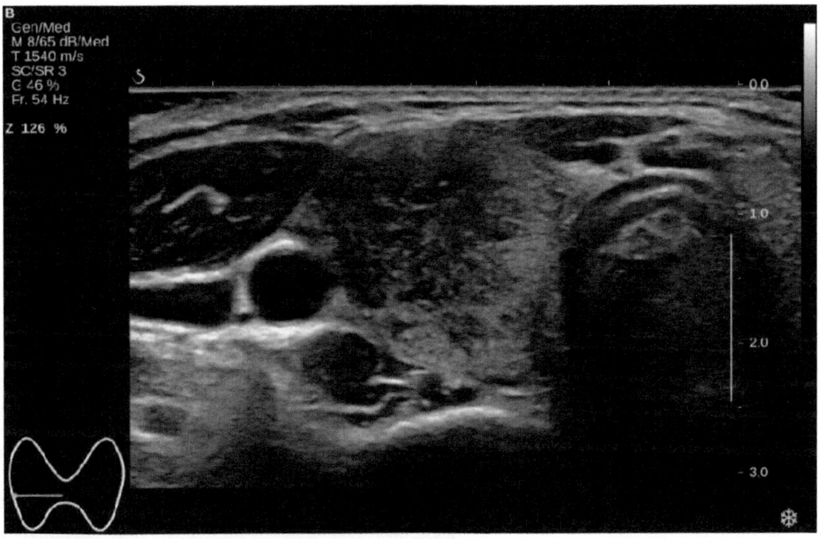

Fig. 4.118 On ultrasonogram, hypoechoic lesion with geographic pattern was observed

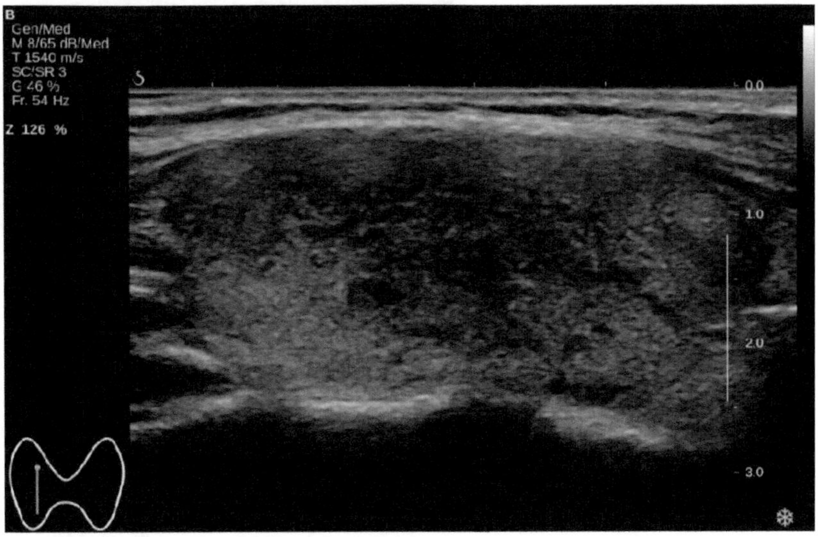

Fig. 4.119 On ultrasonogram, hypoechoic lesion with geographic pattern was observed

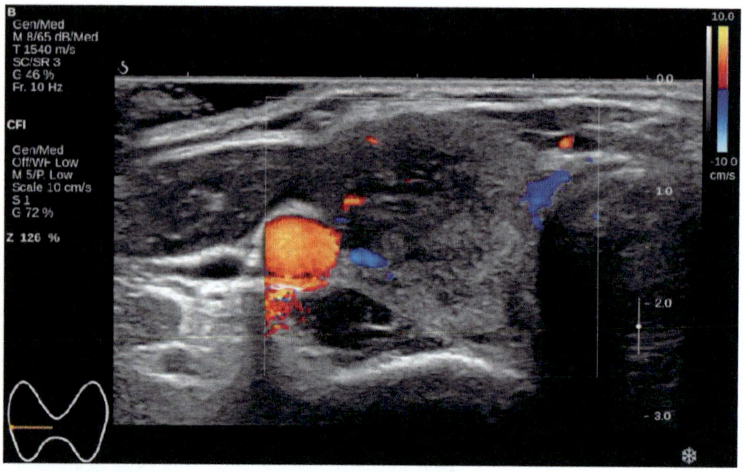

Fig. 4.120 Little internal vascularity was observed on color Doppler

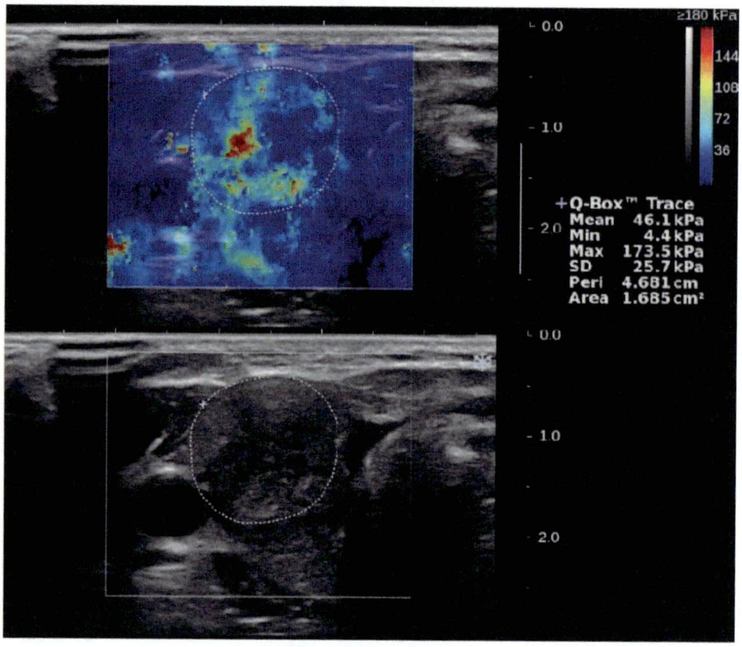

Fig. 4.121 Shear wave elastogram showed markedly increased elasticity with E_{Max} 173.5 kPa

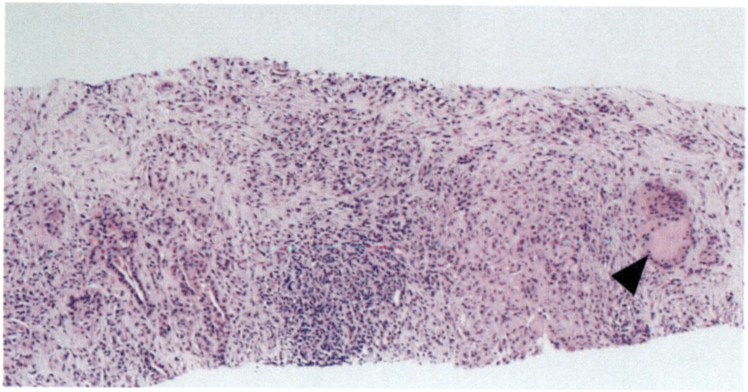

Fig. 4.122 CNB result was subacute granulomatous thyroiditis with diffuse infiltration of inflammatory cells and fibrosis showing giant cells (arrow)

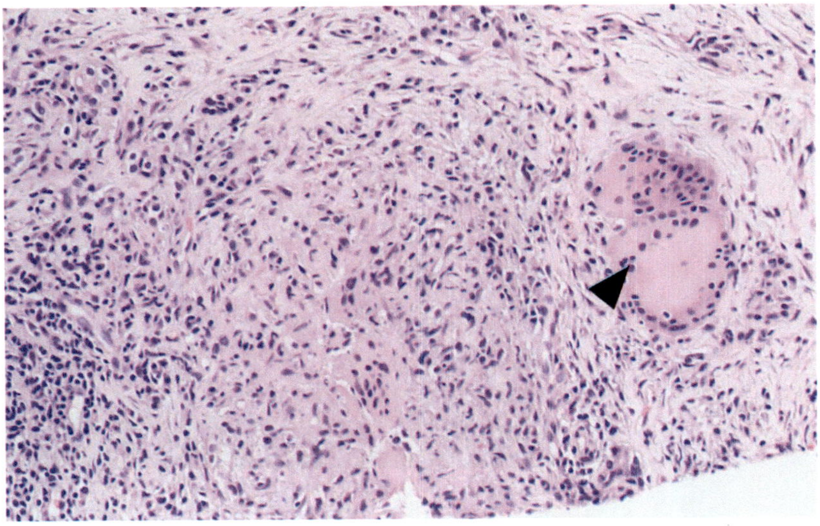

Fig. 4.123 CNB result was subacute granulomatous thyroiditis with diffuse infiltration of inflammatory cells and fibrosis showing giant cells (arrow)

4.4 Follicular Adenoma

Follicular adenoma is usually presented as a solitary round nodule. Histopathologically, follicular adenoma is a well encapsulated neoplastic nodule surrounded by the compressed adjacent thyroid parenchyma. Usually the capsule is thin or moderately thick. Neoplastic cells often form uniform follicles with little variation in cell morphology, and the architectural and cytologic features are usually different from those of the surrounding thyroid parenchyma. Follicular adenoma may show microfollicular, normofollicular, macrofollicular or trabecular patterns and mitotic figures are rare. Occasionally the neoplastic cells show eosinophilic granular cytoplasm (oxyphilic cells or Hürthle cells). The stromal component of follicular adenoma is typically scant (1) and usually devoid of degenerative changes (2), but sometimes stromal fibrosis, edema, hyalinization, hemorrhage and calcification may be seen (1). Careful evaluation of the capsular invasion and vascular invasion is needed to exclude follicular carcinoma. On B-mode ultrasound follicular adenoma is presented as hypoechic or isoechoic round nodule and accompanied sometimes with halo. SWE of follicular adenoma showed usually low elasticity. Samir et al. reported follicular adenoma showed lower elasticity than malignant follicular lesion and suggested cut-off value of Emean as 22.3 kPa [14]. Our study also showed follicular adenoma showed lower elasticity than NH.and cut off value of Emean was 23.5 kPa(51).

4.4.1 Case 1

A 56 year old man was found to have the left 2 cm thyroid nodule on routine check. FNA showed benign follicular nodule (BFN) and CNB result was nodular hyperplasia. During USG follow up after 3 years later, USG showed 3.12 cm round solid nodule in the left lobe with rich vascularity around the capsule on color Doppler (Figs. 4.124, 4.125, and 4.126). Shear wave elastography showed low EI (E_{Max} 35.8 kPa) in the whole region of the nodule and color coded entirely as deep blue (Fig. 4.127), suggesting follicular neoplasm. CNB was performed again and CNB(second) showed micro and macrofollicular patterned follicular proliferative lesion surrounded by the thin capsule (arrow, Fig. 4.128) favoring follicular neoplasm (Figs. 4.128 and 4.129). He underwent total thyroidectomy and surgical histopathology was follicular adenoma completely encapsulated by the thin capsule (Fig. 4.130) from the surrounding normal tissue

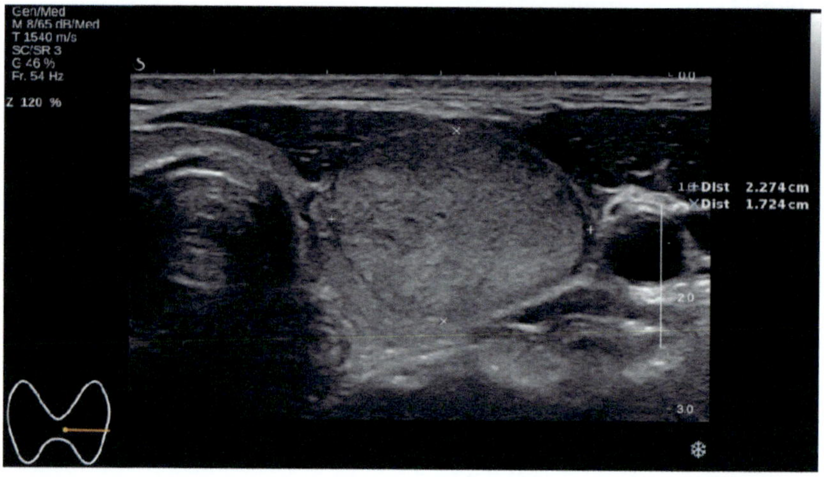

Fig. 4.124 During USG follow up after 3 years later, USG showed 3.12 cm round solid nodule with halo in the left lobe

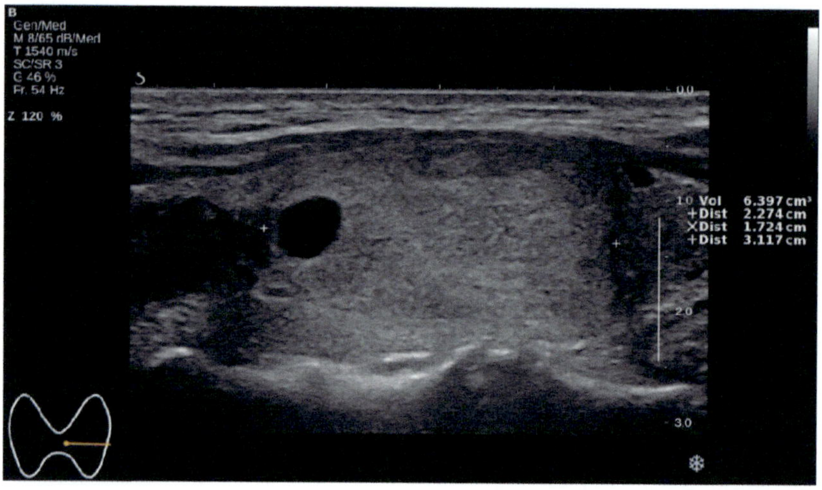

Fig. 4.125 USG showed 3.12 cm round solid nodule in the left lobe

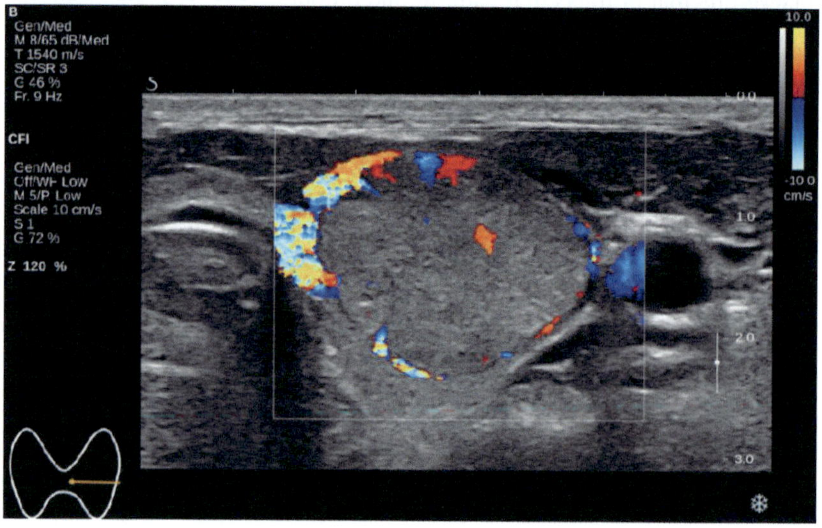

Fig. 4.126 Rich vascularity around the capsule was observed on color Doppler

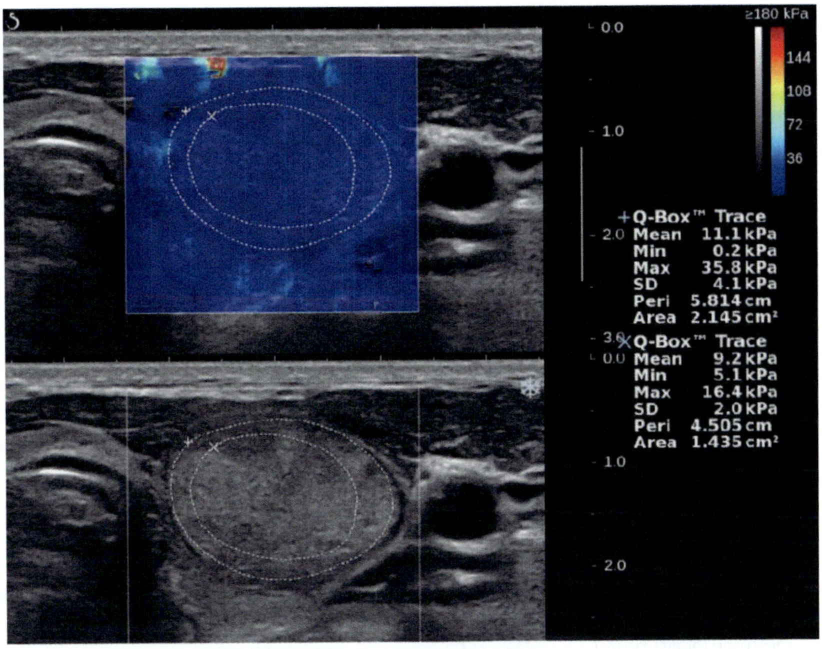

Fig. 4.127 Shear wave elastography showed low EI (E_{Max} 35.8 kPa) in the whole region of the nodule and color coded entirely as deep blue

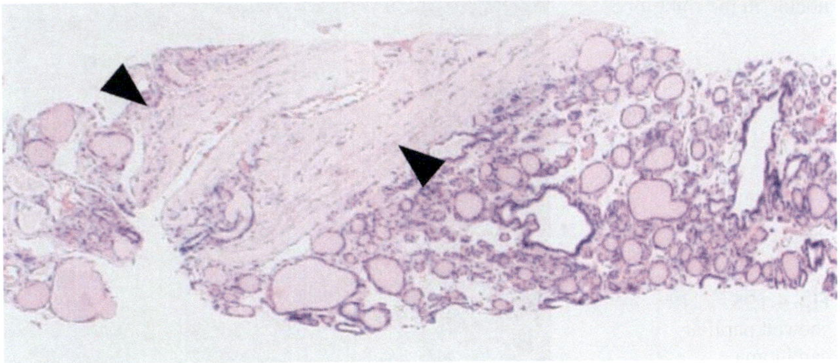

Fig. 4.128 CNB (second) showed micro and macrofollicular patterned follicular proliferative lesion separated from the nomal thyroid tissue by the thin capsule (arrow) favoring follicular neoplasm

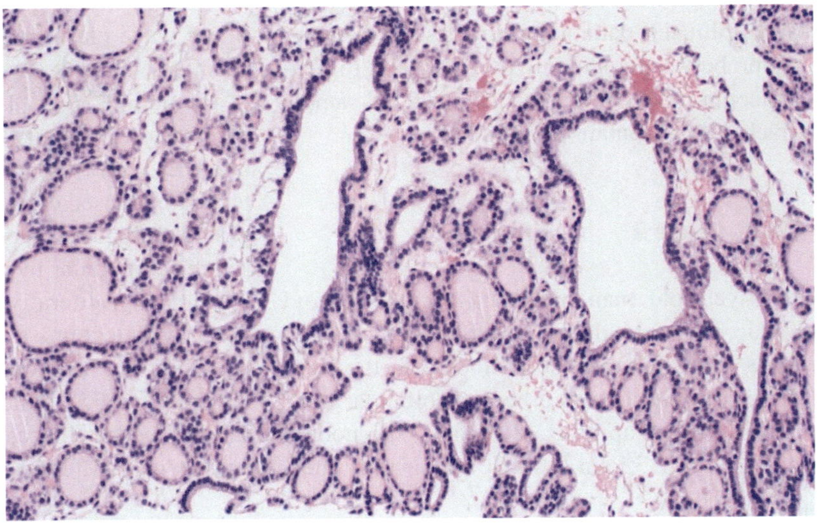

Fig. 4.129 CNB (second) showed micro and macrofollicular patterned follicular proliferative lesion

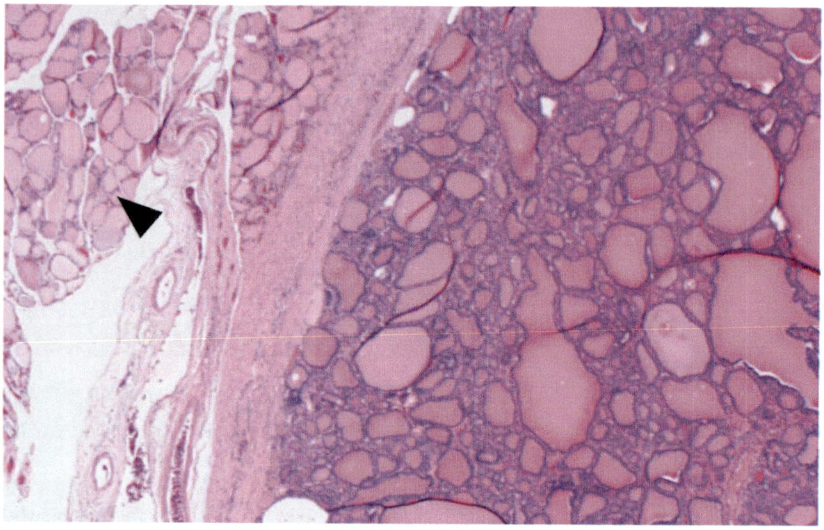

Fig. 4.130 Surgical histopathology was follicular adenoma completely encapsulated by the thin capsule which separate the tumor from the surrounding normal tissue (arrow). It was composed of mainly macrofollicular patterned follicules, so differenciation between nodular hyperplasia and follicular neoplasm was difficult in the first CNB sample which did not contain the capsule

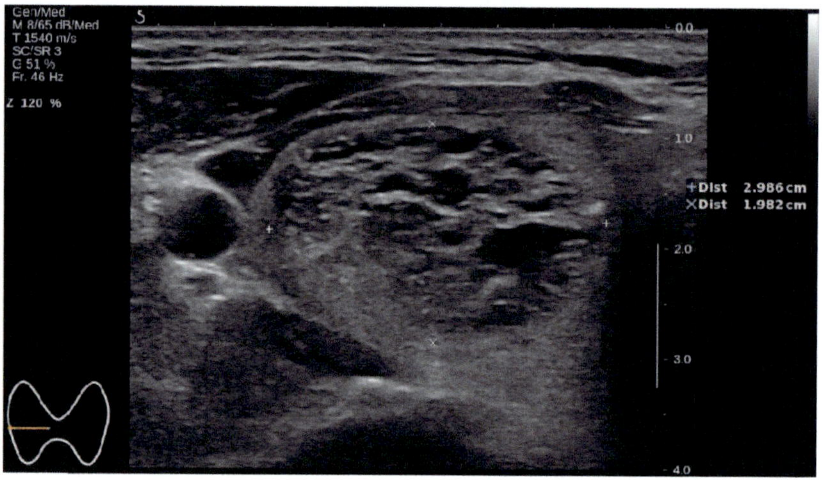

Fig. 4.131 Ultrasonogram showed 3.35 cm (10.4 cc) round partially cystic solid nodule in the right lobe

(arrow, Fig. 4.130) It was composed of mainly macrofollicular patterned follicules, so differenciation between nodular hyperplasia and follicular neoplasm was difficult in the first CNB sample which did not contain the capsule.

4.4.2 Case 2

A 59-year-old man presented a right thyroid nodule. Ultrasonogram showed a 2.7 cm (6.1 cc) round partially cystic solid nodule in the right lobe and FNA showed a benign follicular nodule. On follow-up after 18 months, the nodule increased to 3.35 cm (10.4 cc) with little internal vascularity (Figs. 4.131, 4.132, and 4.133). Shear wave elastography showed that areas of elevated elasticity are mainly around the margin of the nodule (E_{Max}, 116 kPa) and central parts reveled low elasticity with color coded as deep blue (E_{Max}: 28.4 kPa) showing a marginal pattern of increased elasticity (Fig. 4.134) and suggested follicular neoplasm. The CNB result suggested nodular hyperplasia, showing macrofollicular proliferative lesion. He underwent total thyroidectomy and surgical histopathology was follicular adenoma of macrofollicular pattern (Fig. 4.135), which was completely encapsulated by the thin capsule (arrow, Fig. 4.135) and showed different architecture from the sur-

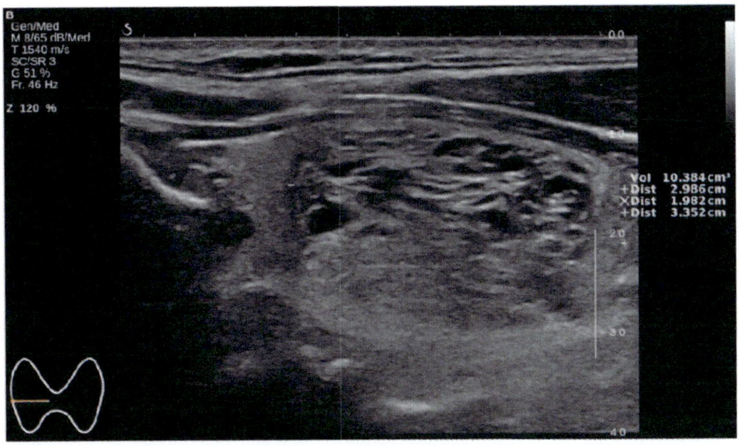

Fig. 4.132 Ultrasonogram showed 3.35 cm (10.4 cc) round partially cystic solid nodule in the right lobe

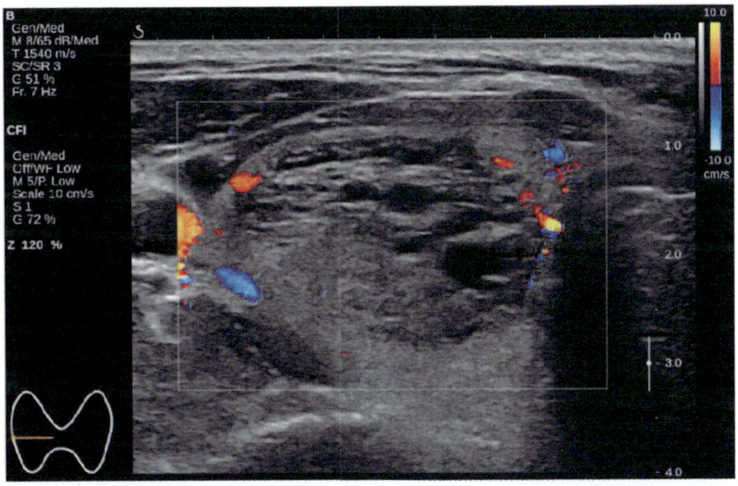

Fig. 4.133 Color Doppler showed little internal vascularity within the nodule

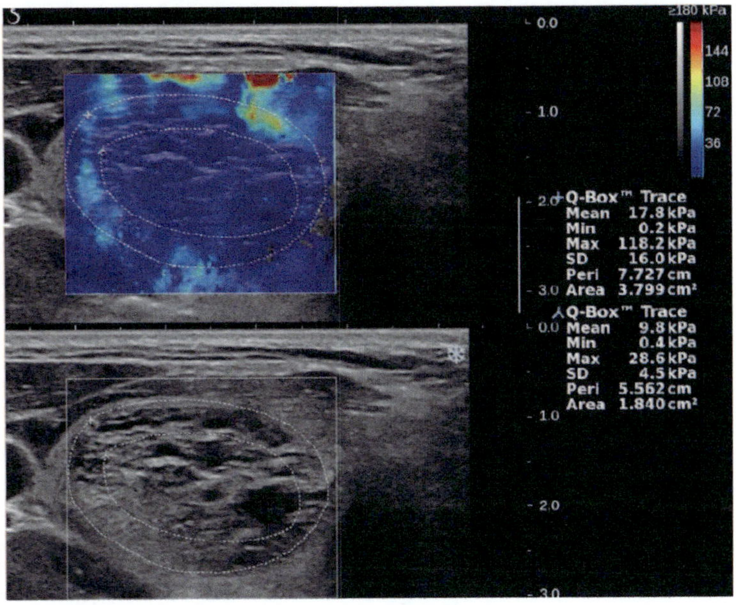

Fig. 4.134 Shear wave elastography showed areas of elevated elasticity are mainly around the margin of the nodule (E_{Max}, 118 kPa) and central parts reveled low elasticity with color coded as deep blue (E_{Max}: 28.6 kPa) showing marginal pattern of the increased elasticity and suggested follicular neoplasm

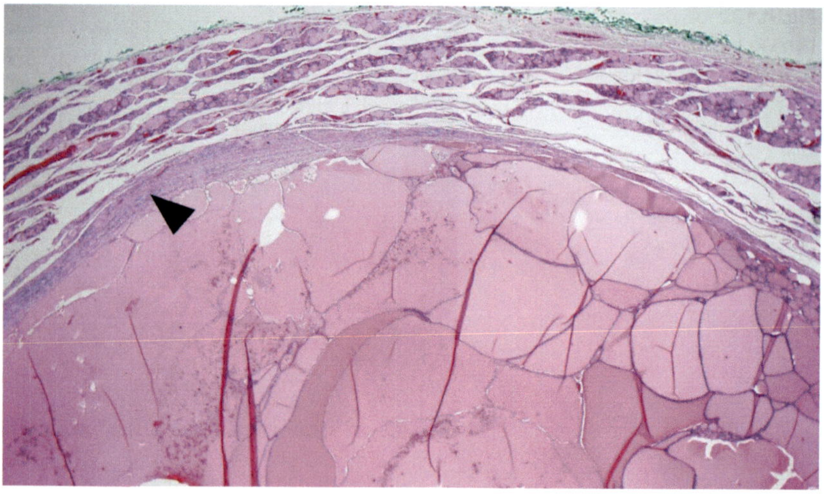

Fig. 4.135 Surgical histopathology was follicular adenoma of macrofollicular pattern which was completely encapsulated by the thin capsule (arrow) and showed different architecture from the surrounding normal tissue

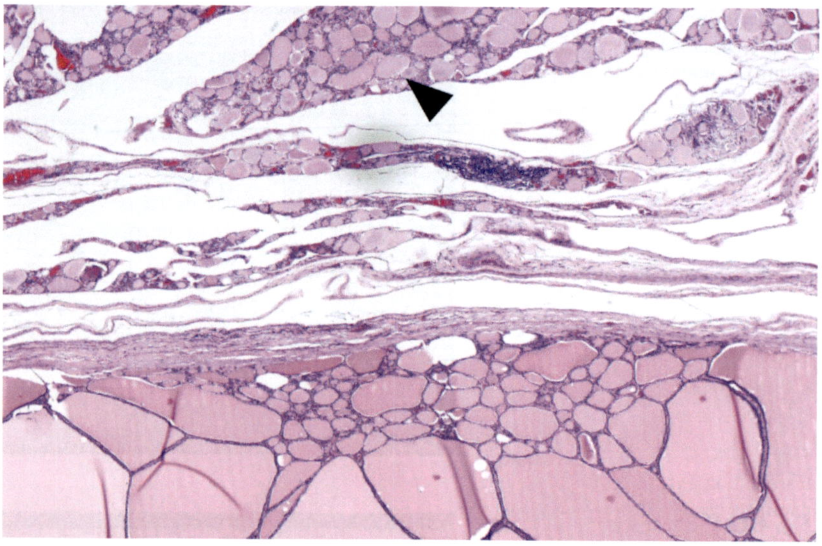

Fig. 4.136 Surgical histopathology was follicular adenoma of macrofollicular pattern which was completely encapsulated by the thin capsule and showed different architecture from the surrounding normal tissue (arrow)

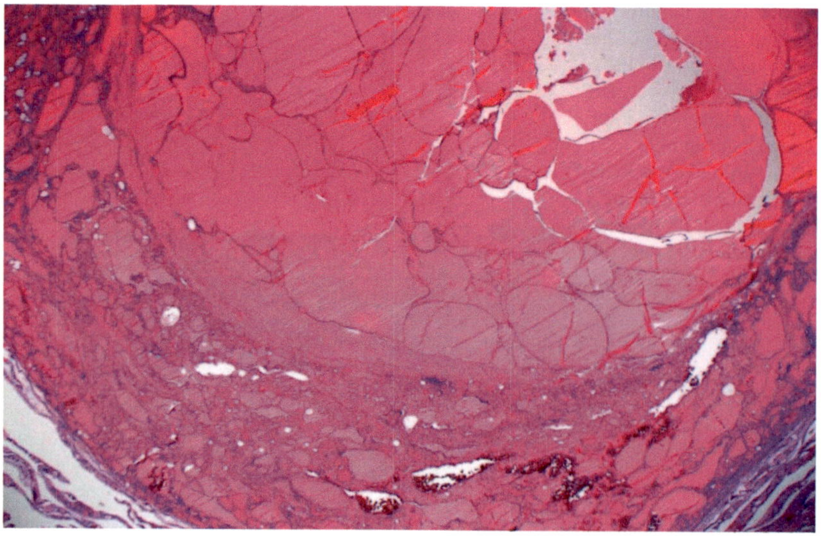

Fig. 4.137 Surgical histopathology was follicular adenoma of macrofollicular pattern which was completely encapsulated by the thin capsule

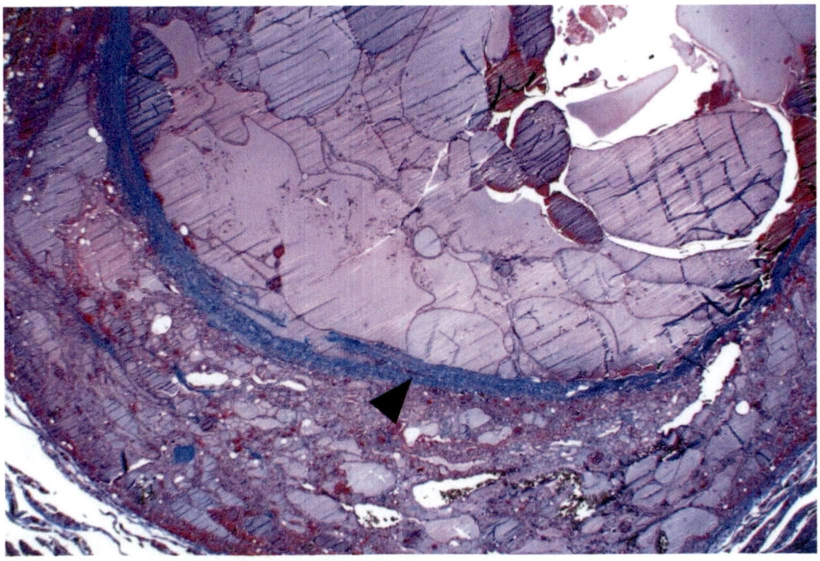

Fig. 4.138 Masson Trichrome stain showed fibrous areas were present only around the capsule (arrow) which match the shear wave elastogram (Fig. 4.134)

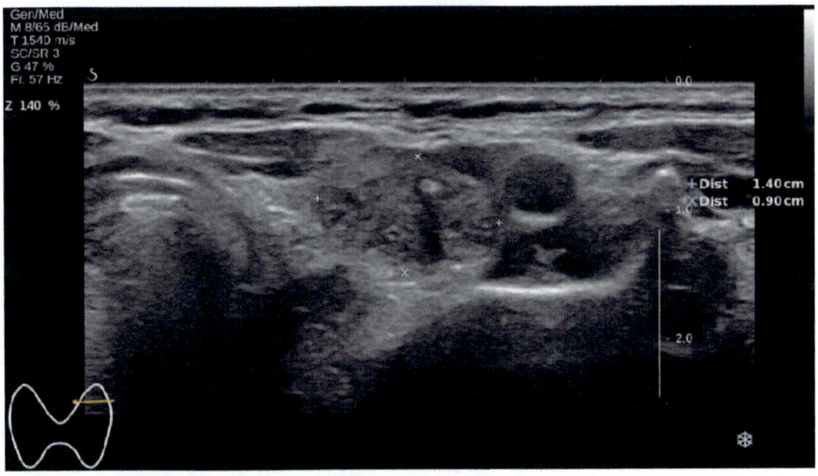

Fig. 4.139 B-mode USG showed isoechoic solidnodule in the left upper lobe

rounding normal tissue (arrow, Figs. 4.136 and 4.137). Masson Trichrome stain showed fibrous areas were present only around the capsule (arrow, Fig. 4.138), which match the shear wave elastogram (Fig. 4.134).

4.4.3 Case 3

A 48-year-old woman was found to have a left upper 1.0 cm thyroid nodule, and FNA showed follicular lesion. During follow-up after three years, the nodule increased to 1.54 cm in size. B-mode USG showed an isoechoic solid nodule in the left upper lobe with moderate internal vascularity on color Doppler (Figs. 4.139, 4.140, and 4.141). On shear wave elastogram, the nodule showed low elasticity, color coded with deep blue, and E_{Max} was 32 kPa (Fig. 4.142). CNB suggested follicular neoplasm with a thick capsule (arrow, Fig. 4.143). She underwent total thyroidectomy and surgical histopathology revealed follicular adenoma encapsulated with a fibrous capsule (arrow, Figs. 4.144 and 4.145) similar to CNB,

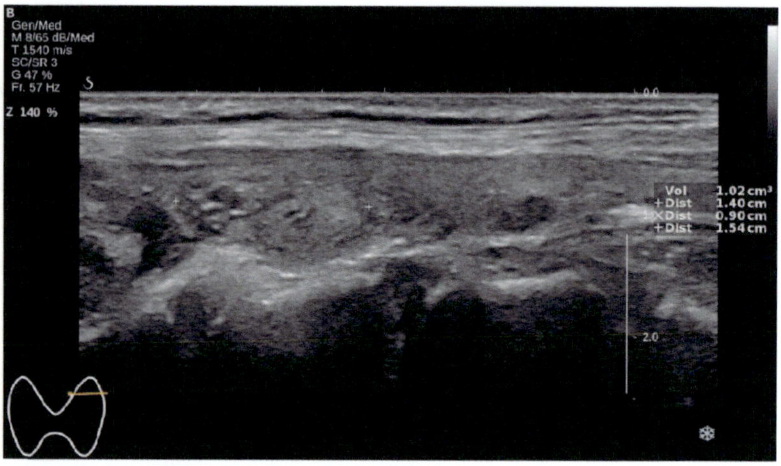

Fig. 4.140 B-mode USG showed isoechoic solidnodule in the left upper lobe

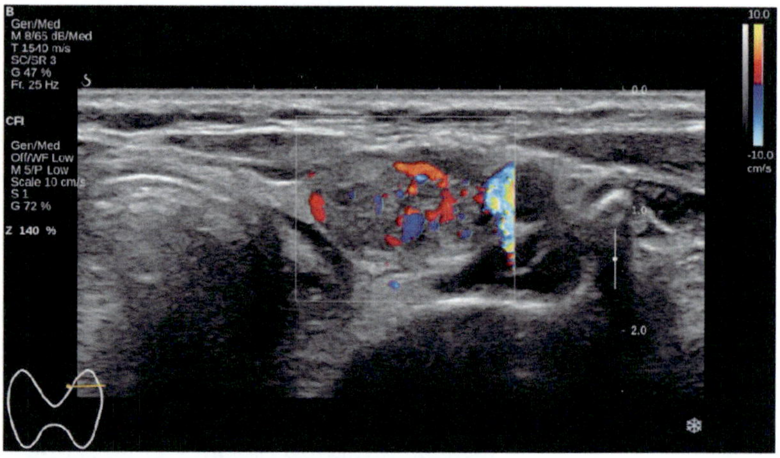

Fig. 4.141 Color Doppler showed moderately increased internal vascularity within the nodule

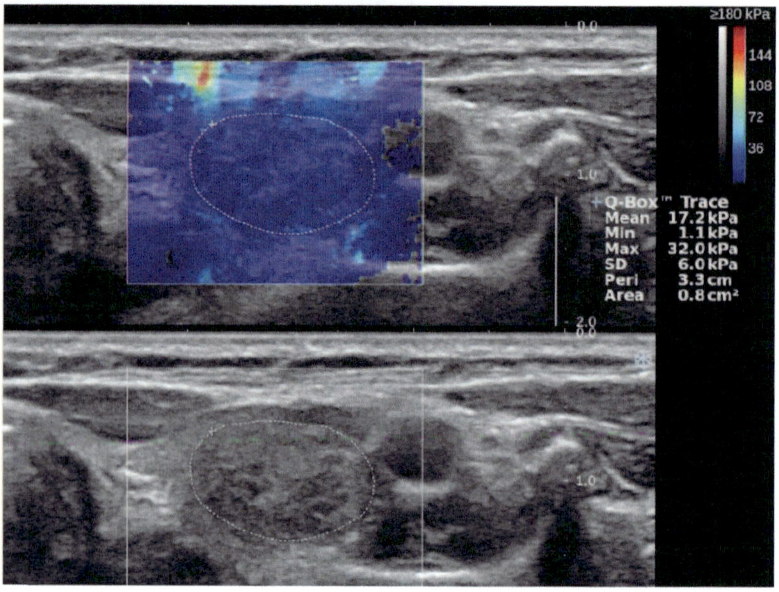

Fig. 4.142 On shear wave elastogram, the nodule showed low elasticity, color coded with deep blue and E_{Max} was 32 kPa

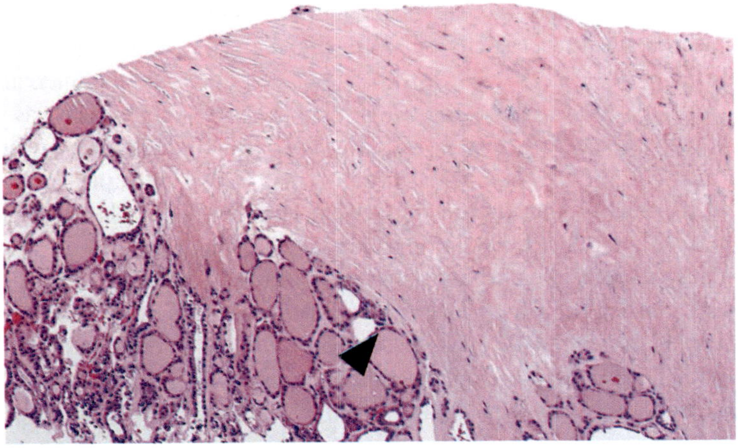

Fig. 4.143 CNB suggested follicular neoplasm with thick capsule (arrow)

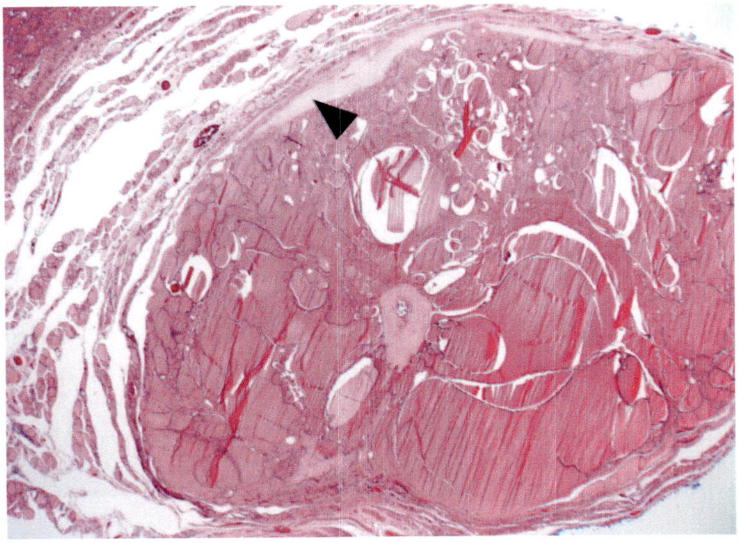

Fig. 4.144 Surgical histopathology revealed follicular adenoma encapsulated with fibrous capsule (arrow) similar to CNB, and showed scanty amount of interstitial tissue within the tumor, matching the low elasticity on SWE (Fig. 4.142)

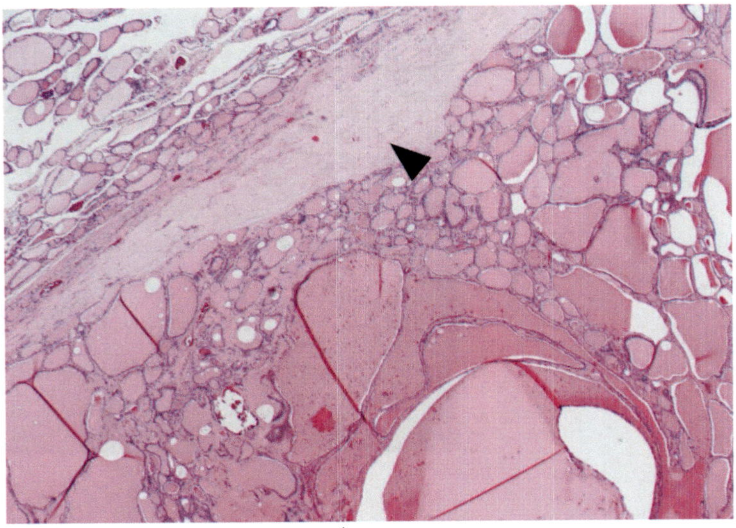

Fig. 4.145 Surgical histopathology revealed follicular adenoma encapsulated with fibrous capsule (arrow) similar to CNB, and showed scanty amount of interstitial tissue within the tumor

and showed scanty amount of interstitial tissue, matching the low elasticity on SWE (Fig. 4.142).

4.4.4 Case 4

49 year old woman was found to have a 2 cm thyroid nodule in the left lobe on routine check. On ultrasonogram, a 2.1 cm round predominantly solid isoechoic nodule with rim calcification (Figs. 4.146 and 4.147) was observed in the left lower lobe and color Doppler scan showed little internal vascularity (Fig. 4.148). Shear wave elastogram showed that the elevated EI area is mainly around the margin of the nodule (marginal pattern) and the internal parts of the nodule show low EI, color coded as deep blue (EI lower than 36 kPa) (Figs. 4.149 and 4.150). CNB suggested nodular hyperplasia showing macrofollicular patterned follicles without capsule. She underwent total thyroidectomy and surgical histopathology showed mainly macrofollicular patterned follicular adenoma, surrounded by thick calcified capsule (Figs. 4.151, 4.152, 4.153, 4.154, and 4.155), causing increased EI around the margin of the nodule on shear wave elastogram (Figs. 4.149 and

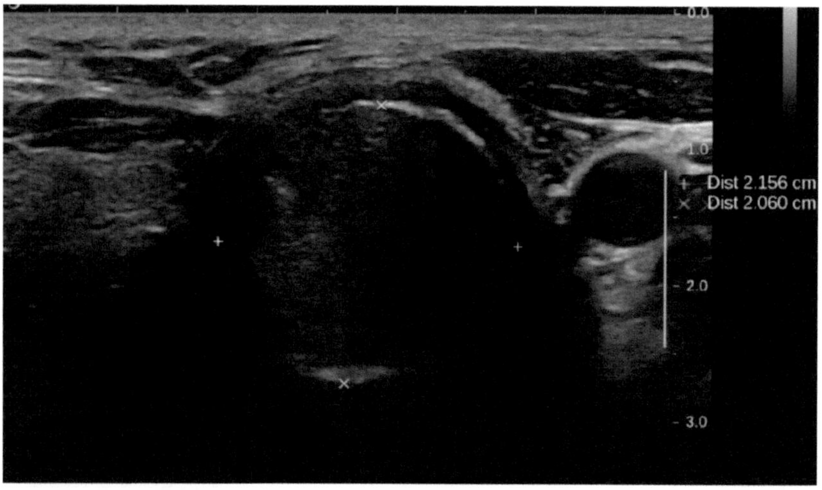

Fig. 4.146 On ultrasonogram, 2.1 cm round predominantly solid isoechoic nodule with rim calcification was observed in the left lower lobe

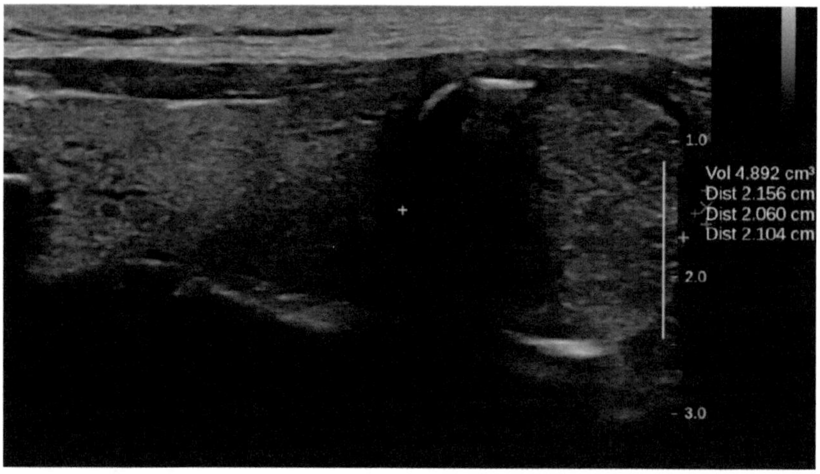

Fig. 4.147 On ultrasonogram, 2.1 cm round predominantly solid isoechoic nodule with rim calcification was observed in the left lower lobe

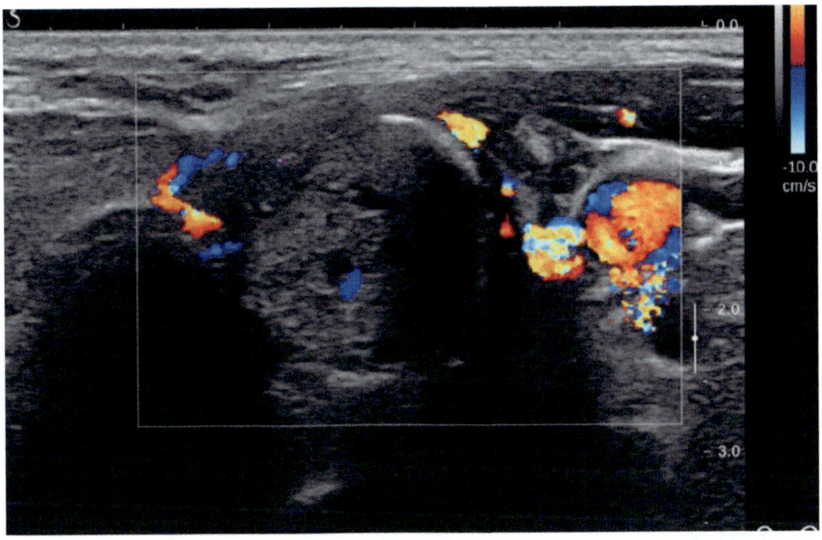

Fig. 4.148 Color Doppler showed little internal vascularity within the nodule

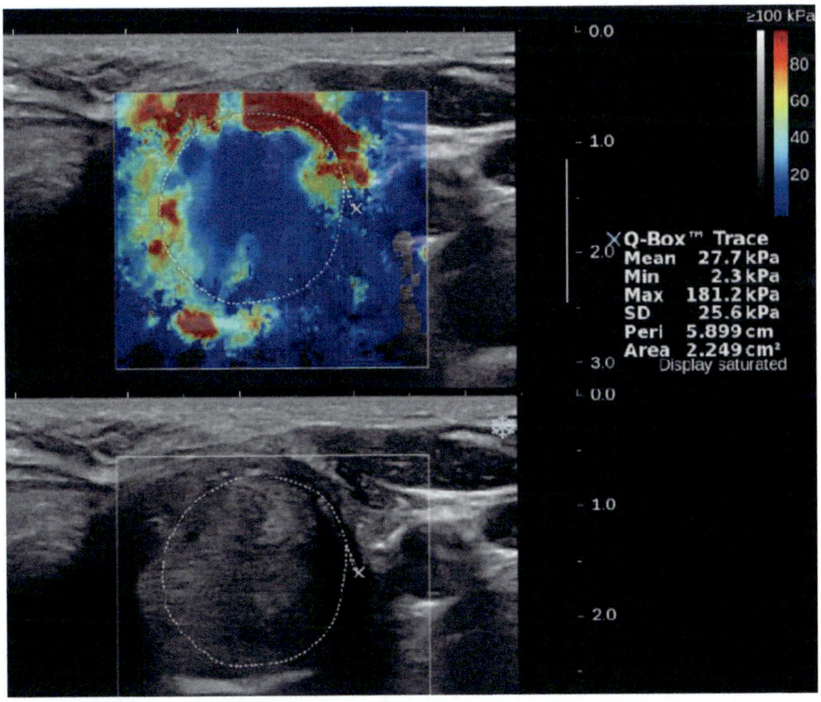

Fig. 4.149 Shear wave elastogram showed elevated EI area is mainly around the margin of the nodule (marginal pattern) and internal parts of the nodule show low EI, color coded as deep blue (EI lower than 36 KPa)

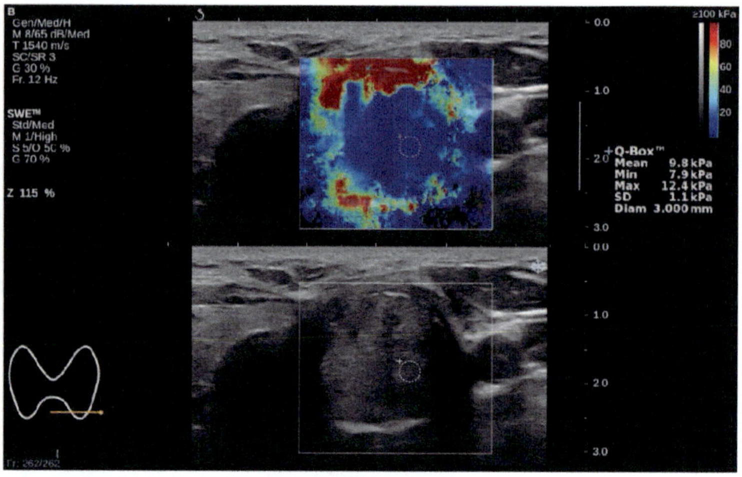

Fig. 4.150 Shear wave elastogram showed elevated EI area is mainly around the margin of the nodule (marginal pattern) and internal parts of the nodule show low EI, color coded as deep blue (EI lower than 36 KPa)

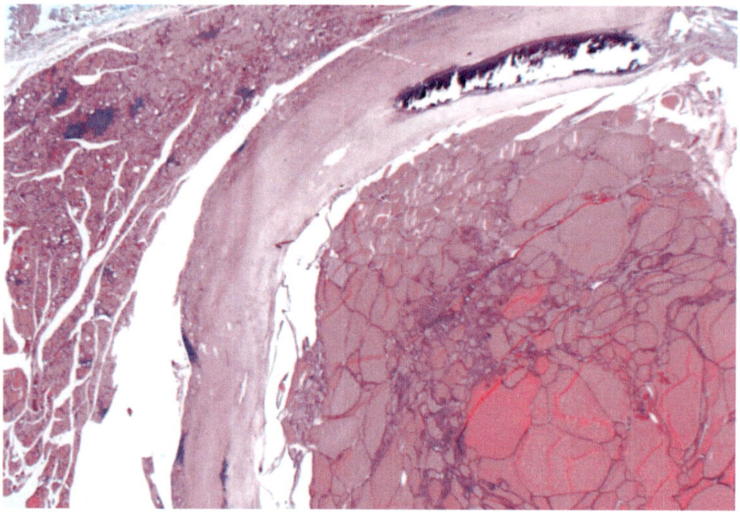

Fig. 4.151 Surgical histopathology showed mainly macrofollicular patterned follicular adenoma, surrounded by thick calcified capsule causing increased EI around the margin of the nodule on shear wave elastogram (Figs. 4.149 and 4.150)

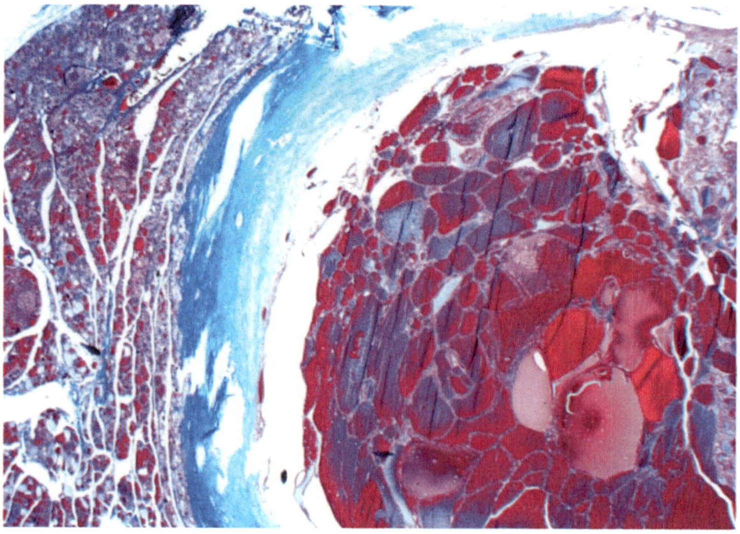

Fig. 4.152 Masson Trichrome stain also showed little fibrosis in internal parts of the tumor matching the low elasticity in the central parts of the nodule on SWE

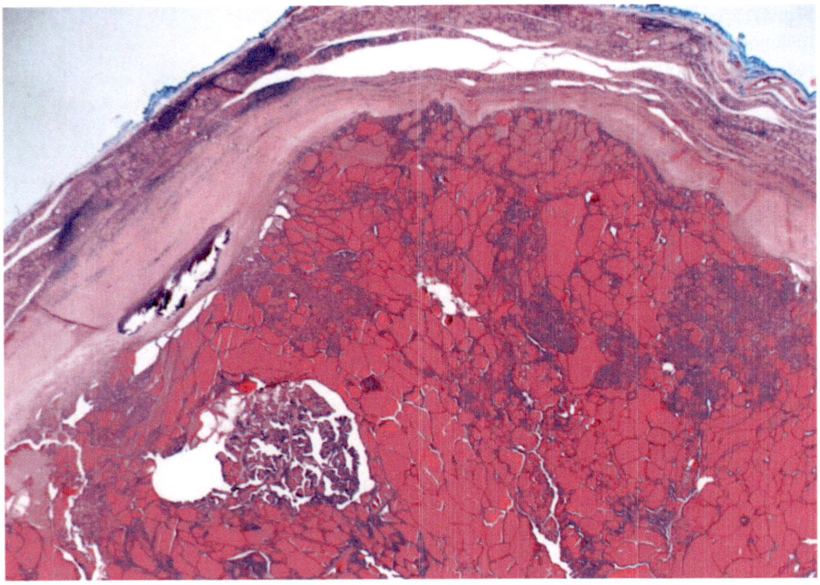

Fig. 4.153 H & E stain showed little fibrosis in internal parts of the tumor

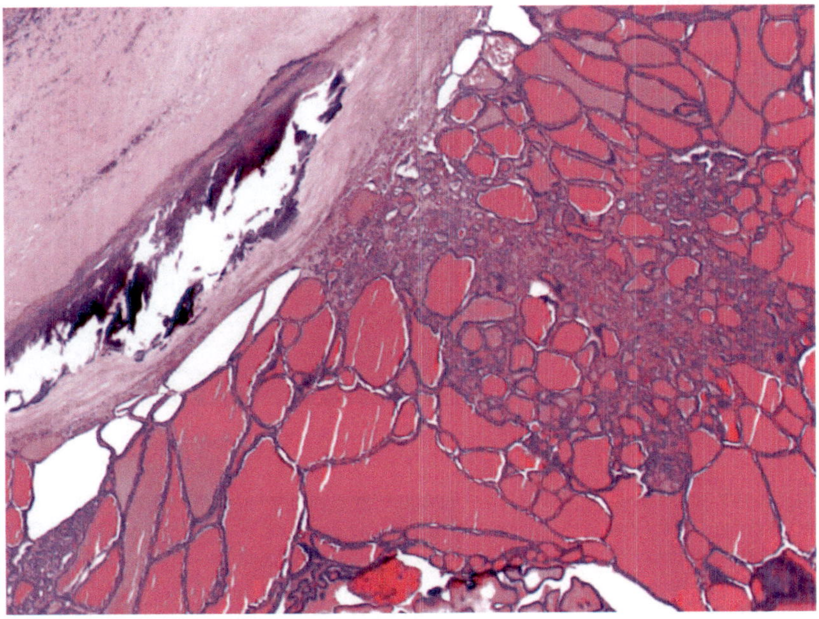

Fig. 4.154 Surgical histopathology showed mainly macrofollicular patterned follicular adenoma, surrounded by thick calcified capsule

4.150). H & E and Masson Trichrome stain also showed little fibrosis in internal parts of the tumor (Figs. 4.151 and 4.152), matching the low elasticity in the central parts of the nodule on SWE.

4.4.5 Case 5

A 52-year-old woman was found to have a thyroid nodule in the left lobe on routine check. On ultrasonogram, a 1.4 cm round solid hypoechoic nodule with rim calcification in the upper margin of the nodule (Figs. 4.156 and 4.157) was observed and color Doppler scan showed moder-

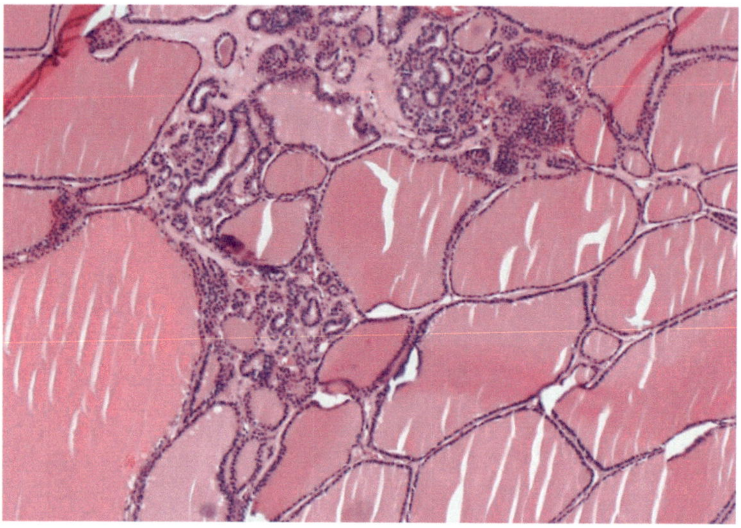

Fig. 4.155 Surgical histopathology showed mainly macrofollicular patterned follicular adenoma

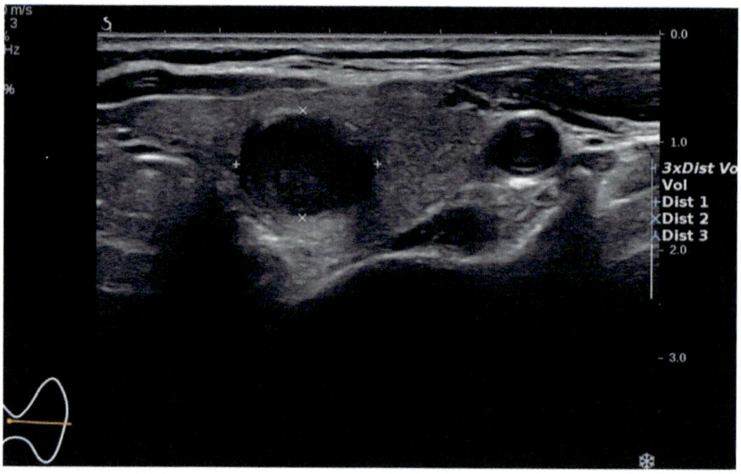

Fig. 4.156 On ultrasonogram, 1.4 cm round solid hypoechoic nodule with rim calcification in the upper margin of the nodule was observed

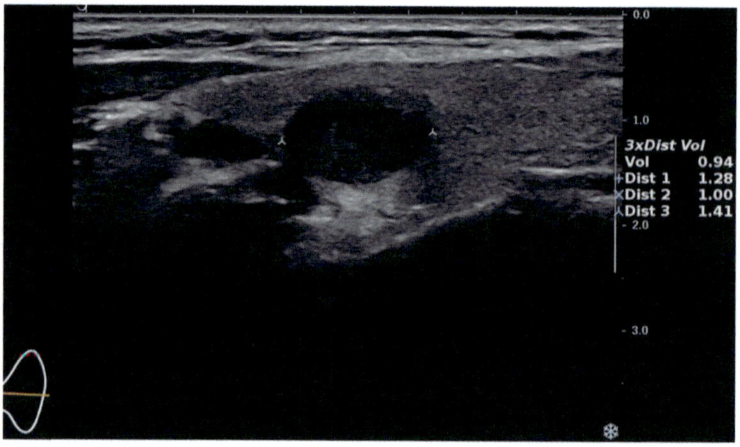

Fig. 4.157 On ultrasonogram, 1.4 cm round solid hypoechoic nodule with rim calcification in the upper margin of the nodule was observed

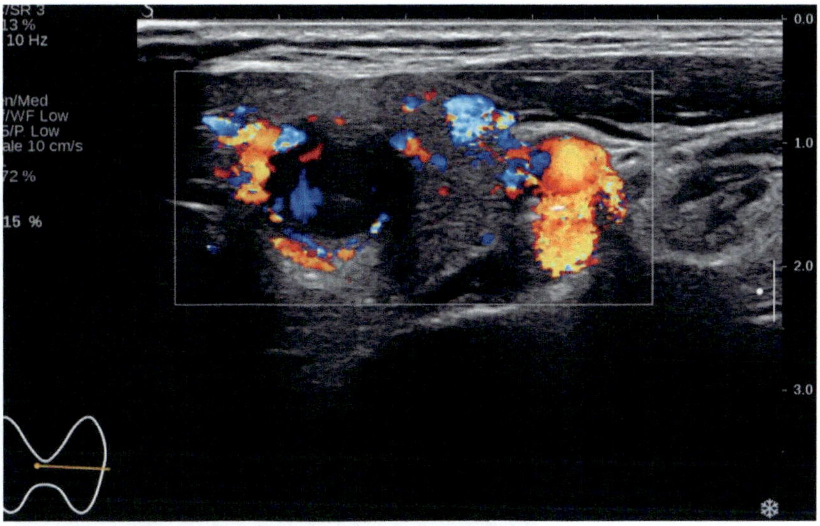

Fig. 4.158 Color Doppler showed moderately increased internal blood flow within the nodule

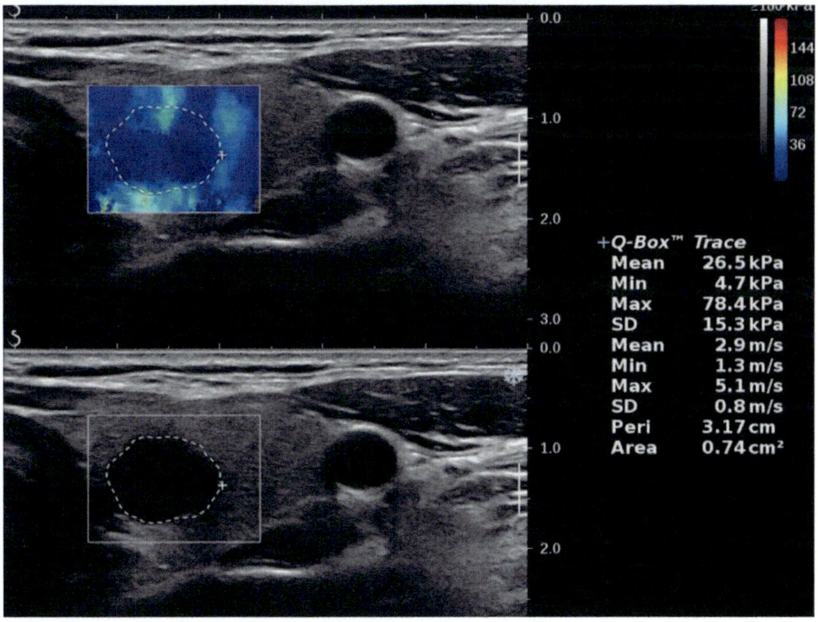

Fig. 4.159 Shear wave elastogram showed elevated EI area is only around the upper margin of the nodule (E_{Max} 78.2 kPa, marginal pattern) and internal parts of the nodule show low EI, color coded as deep blue (E_{Max} 25.2 kPa)

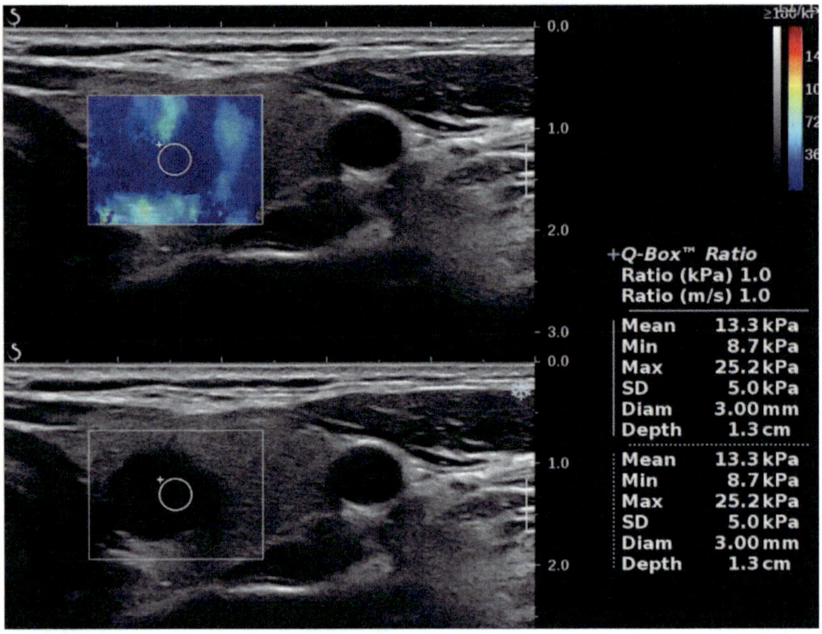

Fig. 4.160 Shear wave elastogram showed elevated EI area is only around the upper margin of the nodule (E_{Max} 78.2 kPa, marginal pattern) and internal parts of the nodule show low EI, color coded as deep blue (E_{Max} 25.2 kPa)

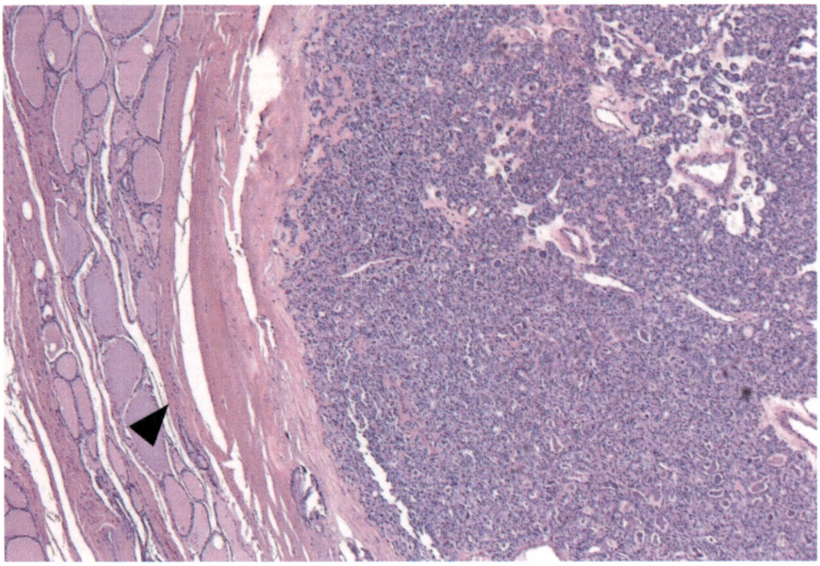

Fig. 4.161 Surgical histopathology showed follicular adenoma which was surrounded by intact capsule (arrow)

ate internal vascularity (Fig. 4.158). Shear wave elastogram showed the elevated EI area is only around the upper margin of the nodule (E_{Max} 78.2 kPa, marginal pattern) and the internal parts of the nodule show low EI, color coded as deep blue (E_{Max} 25.2 kPa, Figs. 4.159 and 4.160). FNA and CNB suggested follicular neoplasm showing microfollicles. She underwent total thyroidectomy and surgical histopathology showed follicular adenoma, which was surrounded by an intact capsule (arrow, Fig. 4.161) with the calcified upper margin. And the tumor was composed of microfollicular patterned follicular structure (Fig. 4.162) with little fibrosis, which matched the low elasticity inside the nodule except the upper margin of the nodule on shear wave elastogram (Figs. 4.159 and 4.160).

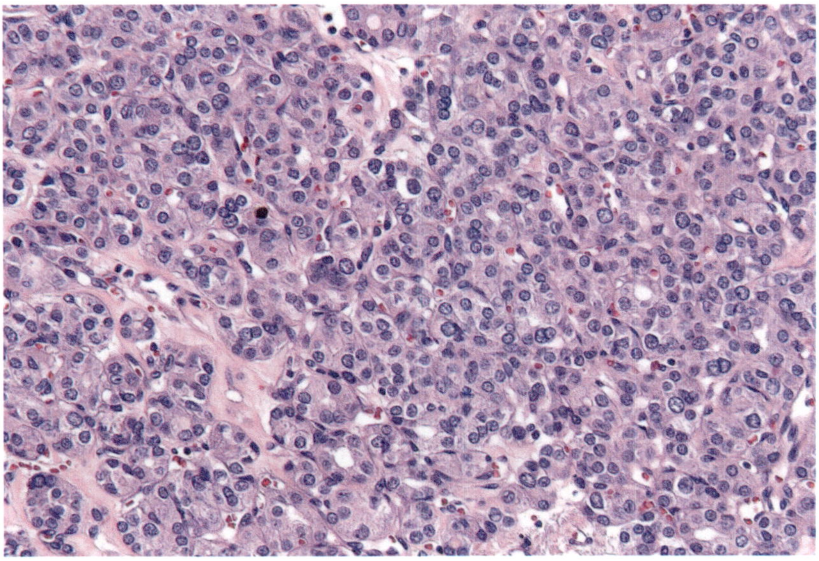

Fig. 4.162 Surgical histopathology showed follicular adenoma with the calcified upper margin and composed of microfollicular patterned follicular structure with little fibrosis which matched the low elasticity inside the nodule

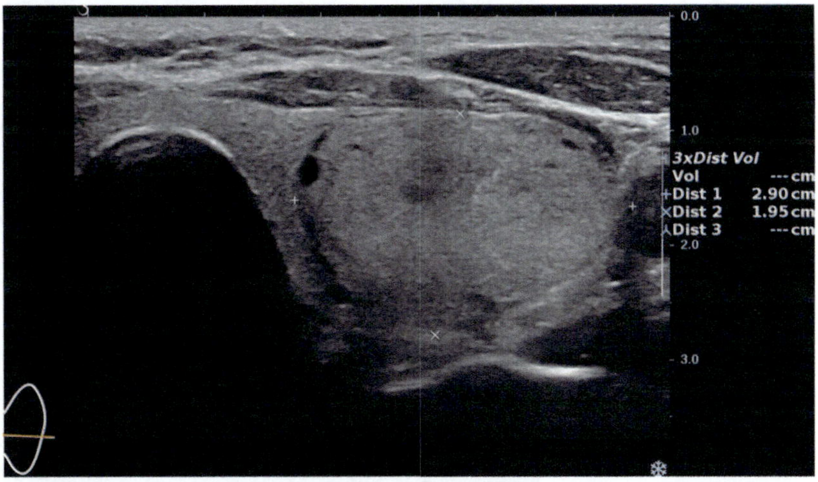

Fig. 4.163 On USG, 4.71 cm round isoechoic nodule with halo was observed in the left middle lobe

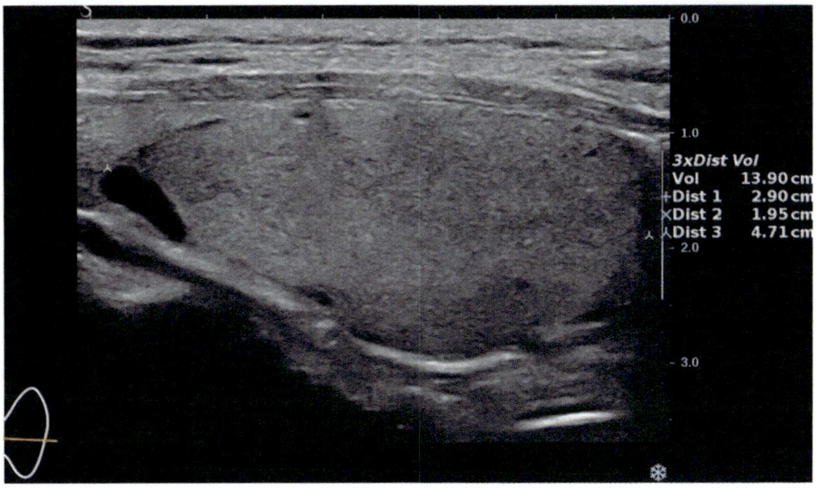

Fig. 4.164 On USG, 4.71 cm round isoechoic nodule with halo was observed in the left middle lobe

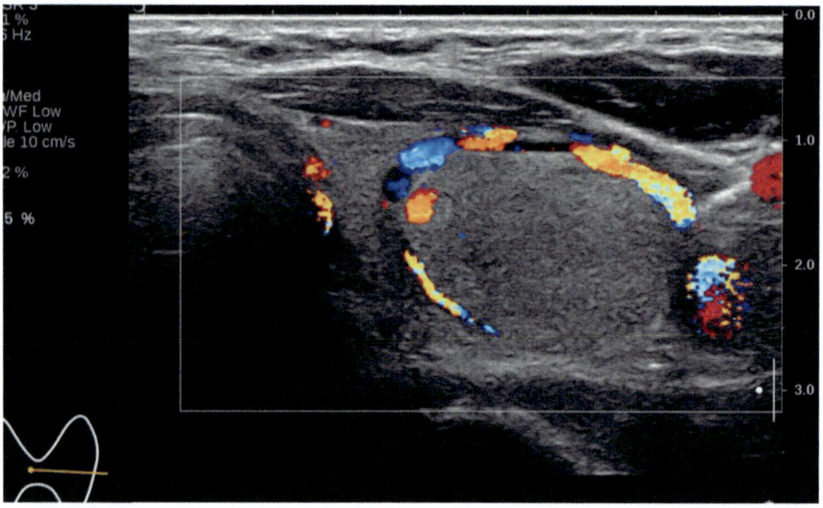

Fig. 4.165 Rich vascularity was observed around the margin of the nodule on color Doppler

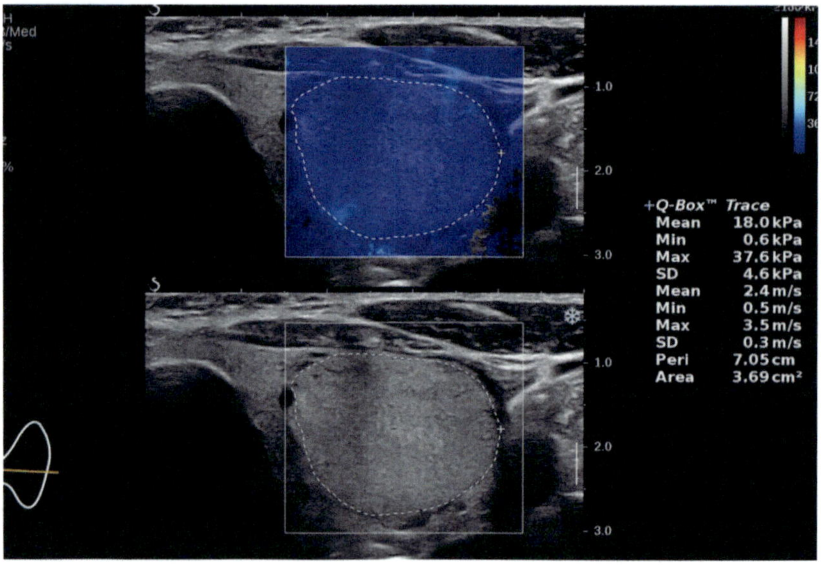

Fig. 4.166 On SWE, whole nodule showed low ela6ticity and color coded with deep blue E_{Max} 37.6 kPa

4.4.6 Case 6

A 60-year-old man was found to have a thyroid nodule on routine check and was referred for evaluation. On USG, a 4.71 cm round isoechoic nodule with halo was observed in the left middle lobe with little internal vascularity (Figs. 4.163, 4.164, and 4.165). On SWE, the whole nodule showed low elasticity and was color coded with deep blue (E_{Max} 37.6 kPa, Fig. 4.166). FNA showed a benign follicular nodule (Fig. 4.167) and CNB showed macro and microfollicular follicular proliferation surrounded by the capsule and suggested follicular neoplasm (Figs. 4.168 and 4.169). He underwent total thyroidectomy without complication and surgical histopathology revealed follicular adenoma surrounded by the intact capsule (arrow, Fig. 4.170), with scanty amount of interstitial tissue, resulting in low elasticity on shear wave elastogram (Fig. 4.166).

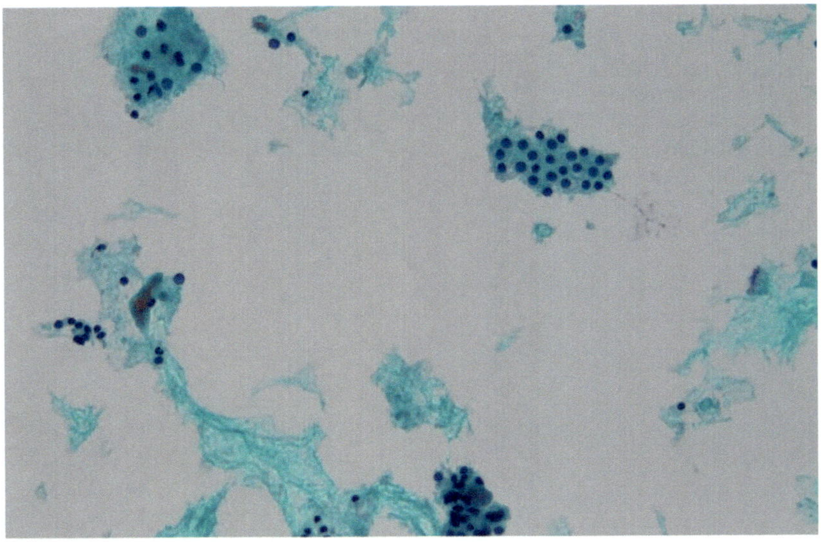

Fig. 4.167 FNA showed benign follicular nodule

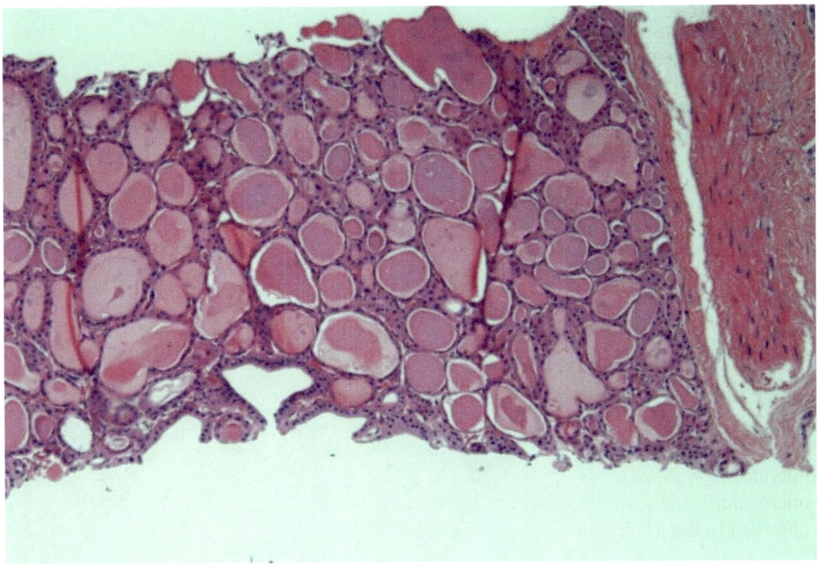

Fig. 4.168 CNB showed macro and microfollicular follicular proliferation surrounded by the capsule and suggested follicular neoplasm

4.5 Papillary Carcinoma

Papillary carcinoma (PTC) is the most common form of thyroid cancer, accounting for 80–90% of all thyroid cancers. PTC is usually invasive, shows papillae and has characteristic nuclear features. The papillae have a central fibrovascular stalk covered by neoplastic epithelial cells. The nuclei of PTC cells show elongated irregularly shaped nuclei and contain finely dispersed chromatin and optically clear or empty appearance designated as ground glass or Orphan Annie eye nuclei. Invagination of the cytoplasm to the nucleus gives the appearance of intranuclear cytoplasmic pseudo inclusions. Longitudinal nuclear groove may be seen resulting from a nucleus folded on to itself [3]. Psammoma bodies are often present usually within the core of papillae. An abundant fibrous stroma is a common feature of PTC and is particularly evident at the advancing edge [1]. Metastasis to cervical lymph nodes occurs in up to 30–50% of the patients with PTC [1].

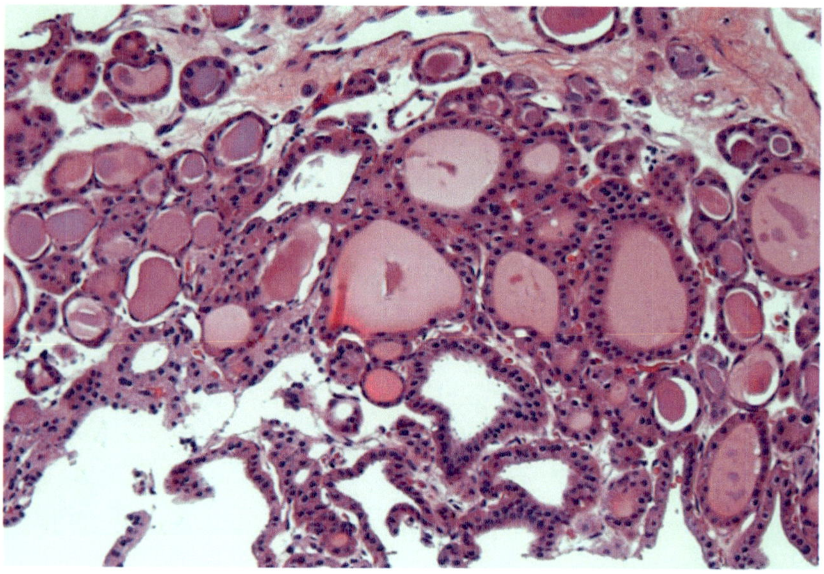

Fig. 4.169 CNB showed macro and microfollicular follicular proliferation surrounded by the capsule and suggested follicular neoplasm

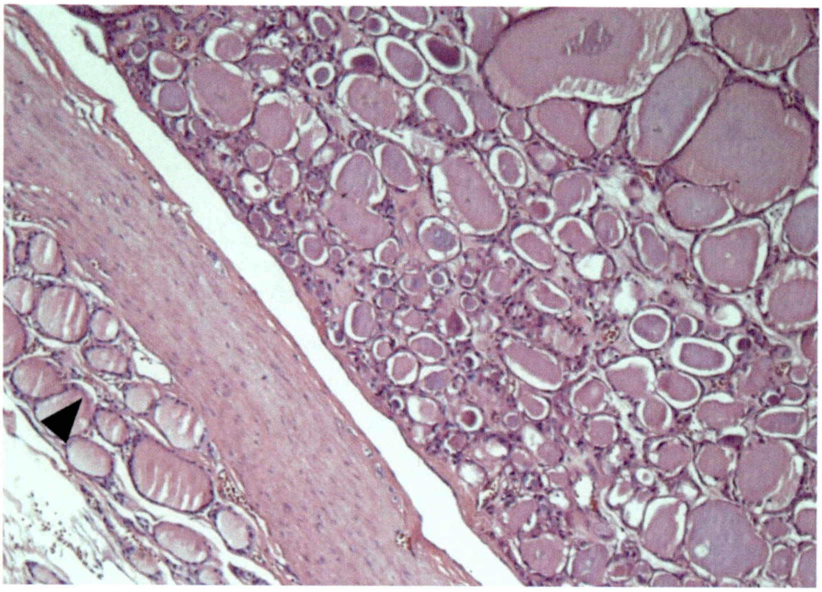

Fig. 4.170 Surgical histopathology revealed follicular adenoma separated by the intact capsule from the surrounding normal tissue (arrow). Follicular adenoma showed scanty amount of interstitial tissue resulting low elasticity on shear wave elastogram (Fig. 4.166)

A diffuse sclerosing variant of PTC shows diffuse involvement of the thyroid gland, with dense sclerosis and changes of chronic lymphocytic thyroiditis. The diffuse sclerosing variant is associated with a higher incidence of extrathyroidal extension, cervical lymph node metastasis and distant metastasis [1].

Follicular variant PTC (FVPTC) has the nuclear characteristics of PTC and shows an almost exclusively follicular architecture. FV PTC is infiltrative or is encapsulated with invasion, and the latter has generally more favorable prognosis.

On B-mode ultrasound, PTC shows several characteristic features including microcalcification, hypoechogenicity, irregular margins and taller-than-wide shape. The SWE of PTC showed usually increased elasticity. Many research reported diverse cut-off values of 34–90 kPa [15],

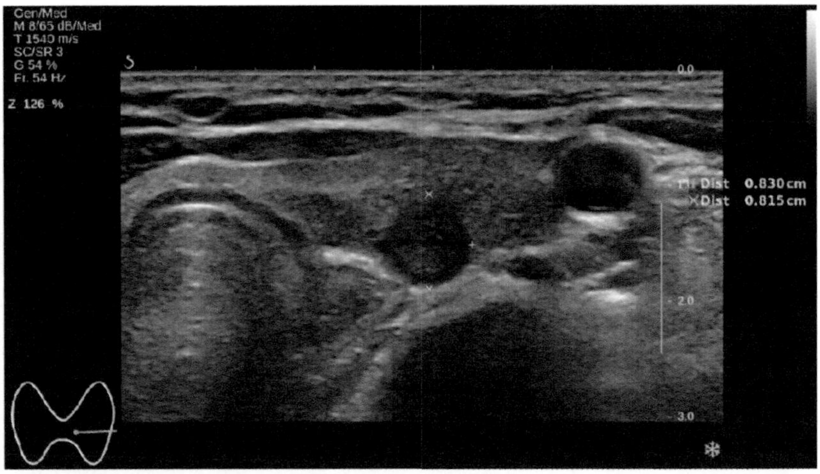

Fig. 4.171 On ultrasonogram, a 0.8 cm hypoechoic suspicious malignant nodule with irregular border was found in the left middle lobe

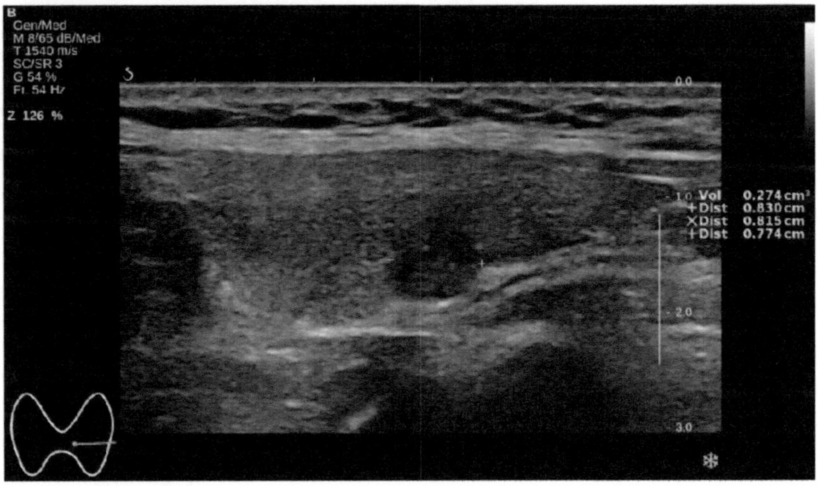

Fig. 4.172 On ultrasonogram, a 0.8 cm hypoechoic suspicious malignant nodule with irregular border was found in the left middle lobe

detecting malignancy, probably due to variable degrees of fibrosis of the malignant thyroid tumors, especially of PTC.

4.5.1 Case 1

A 51-year-old woman was found to have a thyroid nodule on routine check and was referred for evaluation. On ultrasonogram, a 0.8 cm hypoechoic suspicious malignant nodule with irregular border was found in the left middle lobe (Figs. 4.171 and 4.172), and shear wave elastogram showed increased E1 (E_{Max}; 112.3 kPa) in the upper portion of the nodule (Fig. 4.173). The FNA and CNB results were papillary carcinoma (Figs. 4.174 and 4.175). Total thyroidectomy was performed and surgical histopathology was papillary carcinoma (Figs. 4.176, 4.177, 4.178, and 4.179) with increased fibrotic areas in the upper portion of the nodule on Masson Tricrom stain (arrow, Fig. 4.177), consistent with the shear wave elastography.

4.5.2 Case 2

44 year-old man was referred for an enlarging thyroid nodule during the past 5 years (6 mm > 18 mm). B mode ultrasonoram revealed 1.63cm hypoechoic suspicious malignant nodule with lobulated margin in the left middle lobe with

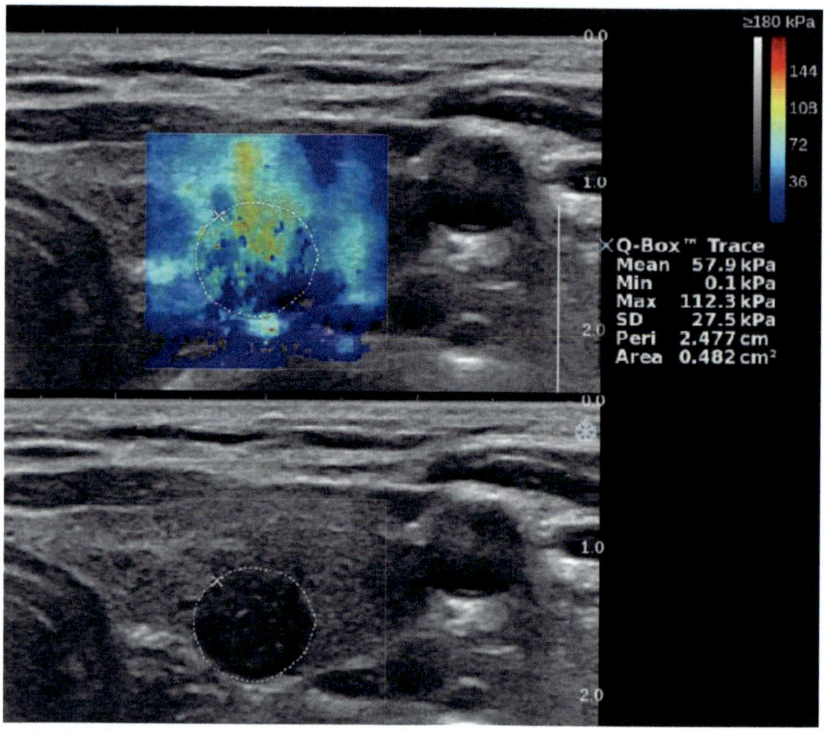

Fig. 4.173 Shear wave elastogram showed increased E1 (E_{Max}; 112.3 kPa) in the upper portion of the nodule

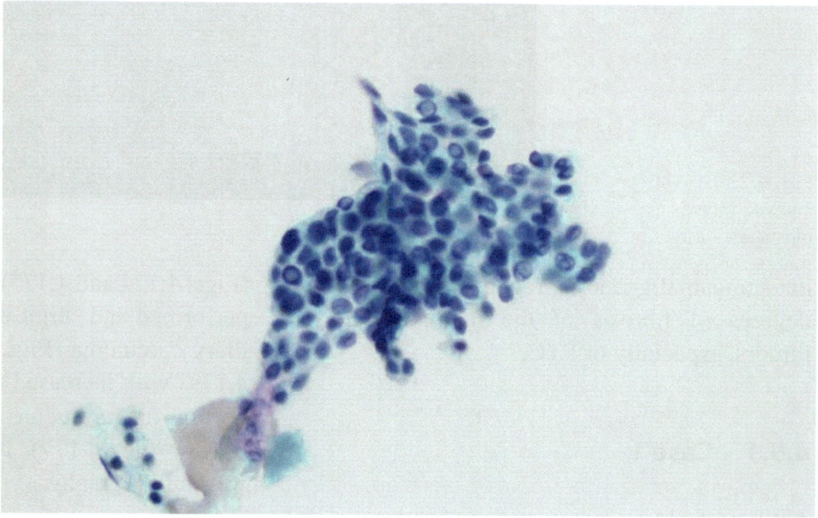

Fig. 4.174 FNA result was papillary carcinoma

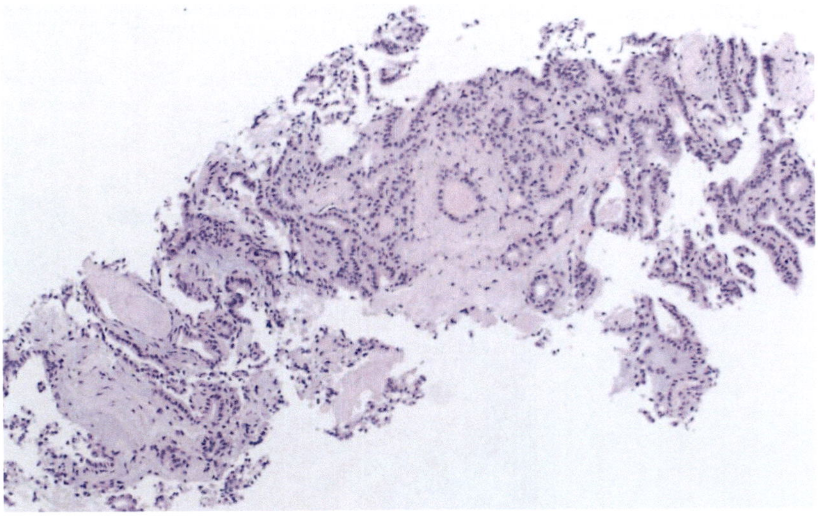

Fig. 4.175 CNB result was papillary carcinoma

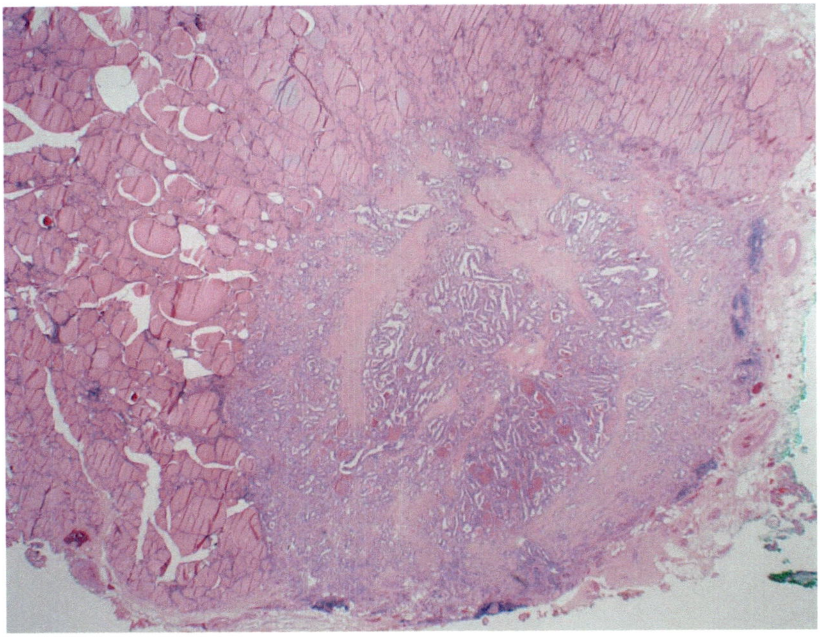

Fig. 4.176 Surgical histopathology was papillary carcinoma with increased fibrotic areas in the upper portion of the nodule

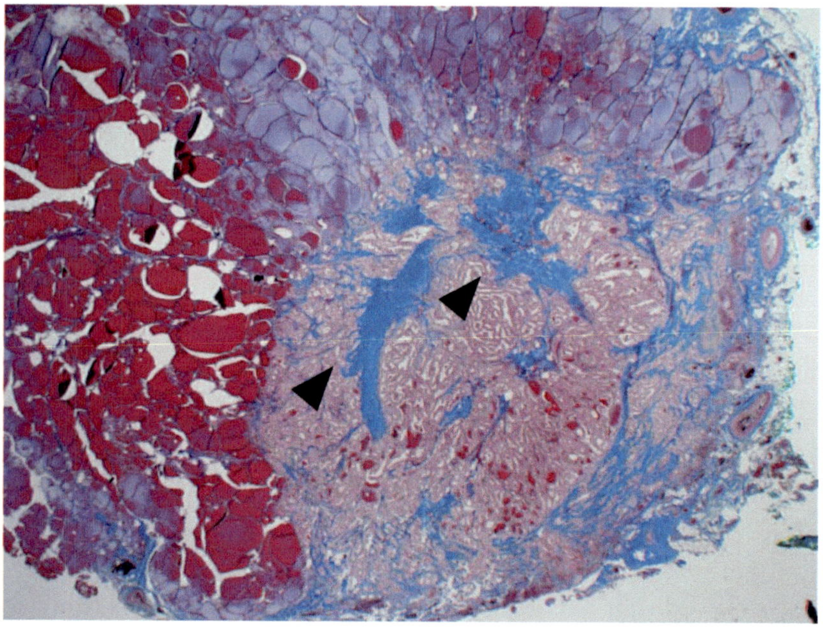

Fig. 4.177 Surgical histopathology was papillary carcinoma with increased fibrotic areas in the upper portion of the nodule on Masson Tricrom stain (arrow) consistent with the shear wave elastography

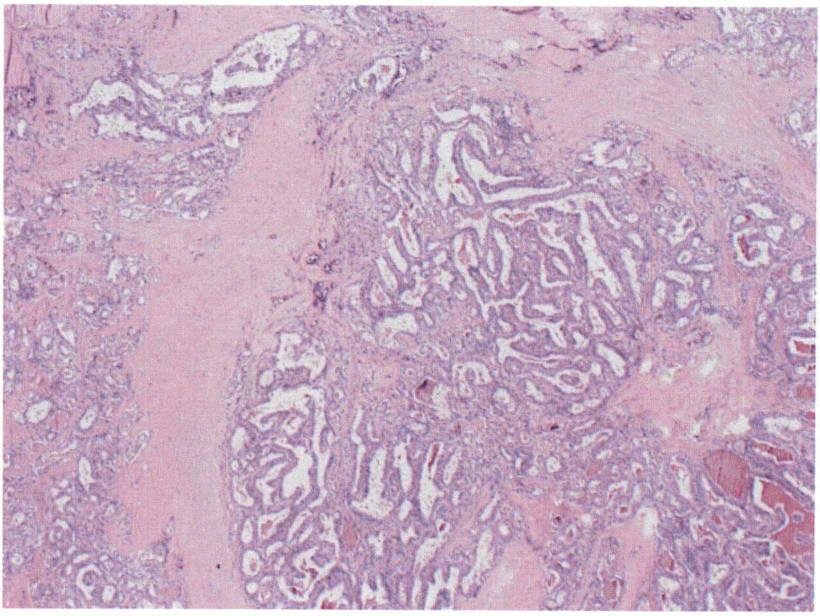

Fig. 4.178 Surgical histopathology showing increased fibrotic areas

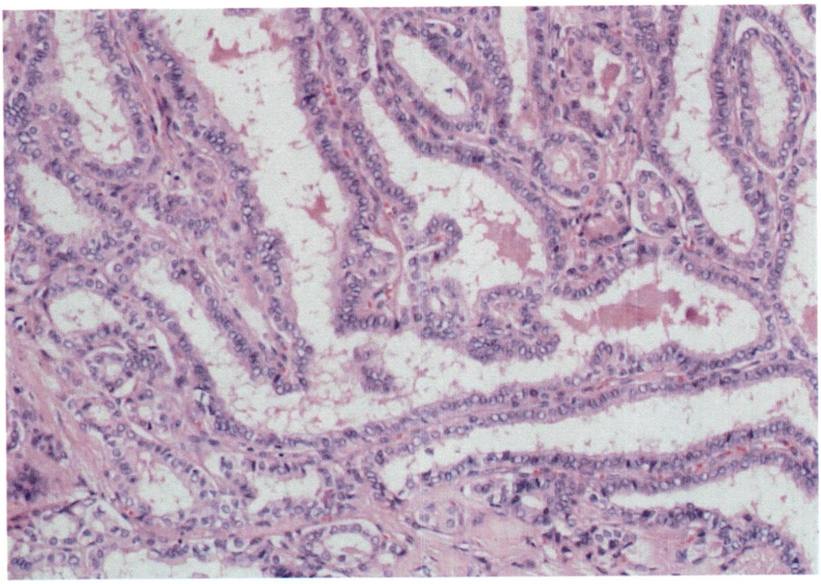

Fig. 4.179 Surgical histopathology showing papillae in papillary carcinoma

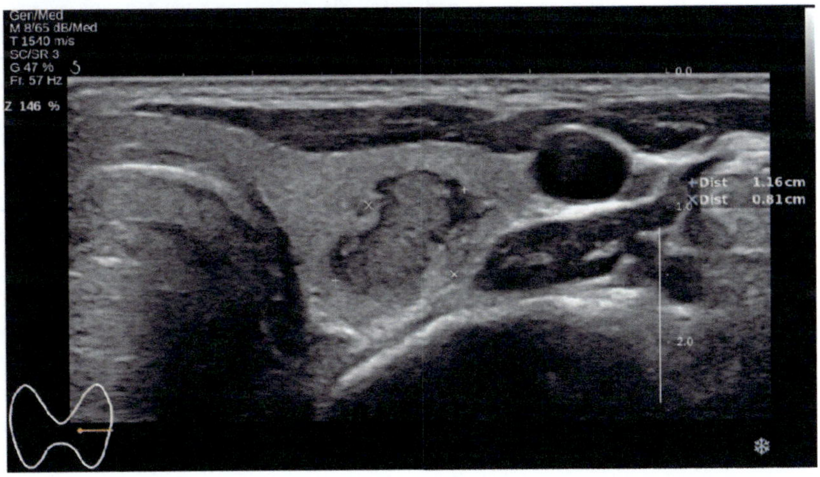

Fig. 4.180 B mode ultrasonoram revealed 1.63 cm hypoechoic suspicious malignant nodule with lobulated margin in the left middle lobe

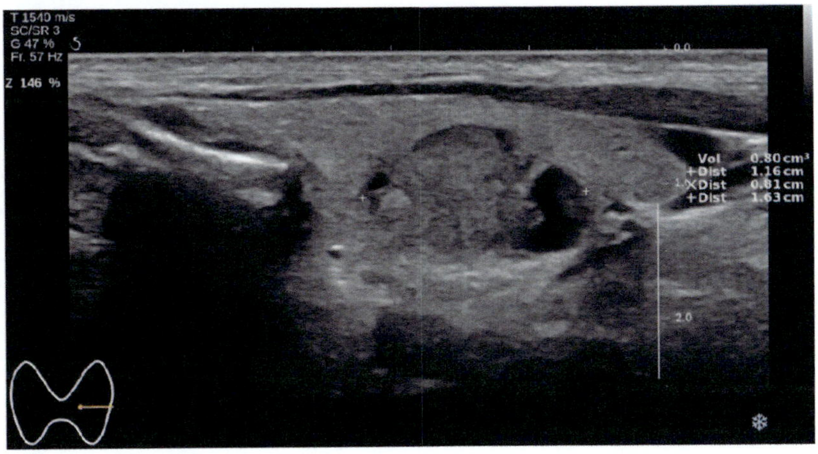

Fig. 4.181 B mode ultrasonoram revealed 1.63cm hypoechoic suspicious malignant nodule with lobulated margin in the left middle lobe

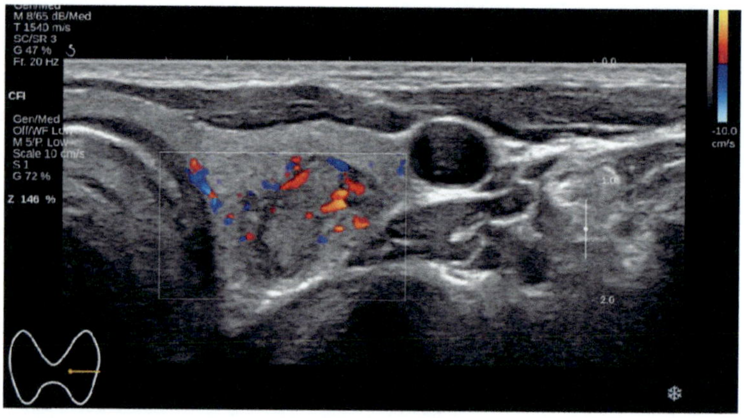

Fig. 4.182 Color Doppler showed moderately increased internal vascularity within the nodule

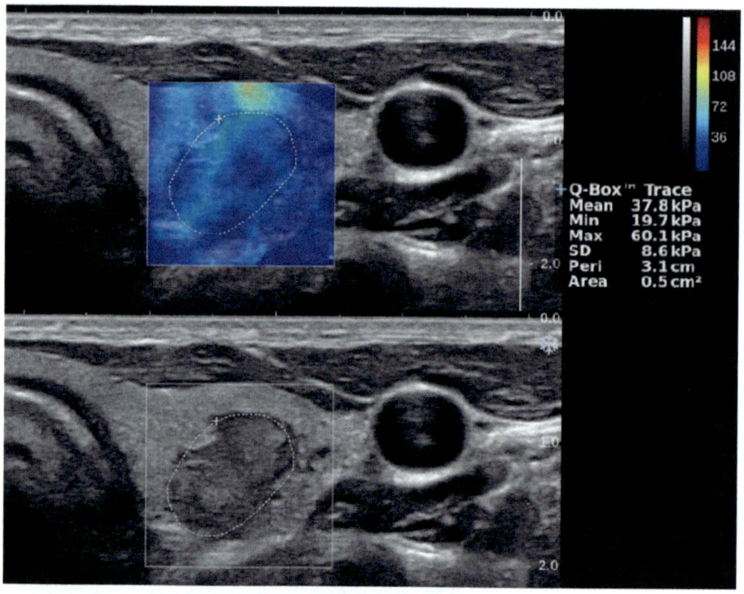

Fig. 4.183 On shear wave elastogram distribution of high EI area (E_{Max}, 60.1 kPa) was observed as the encircling pattern within the nodule

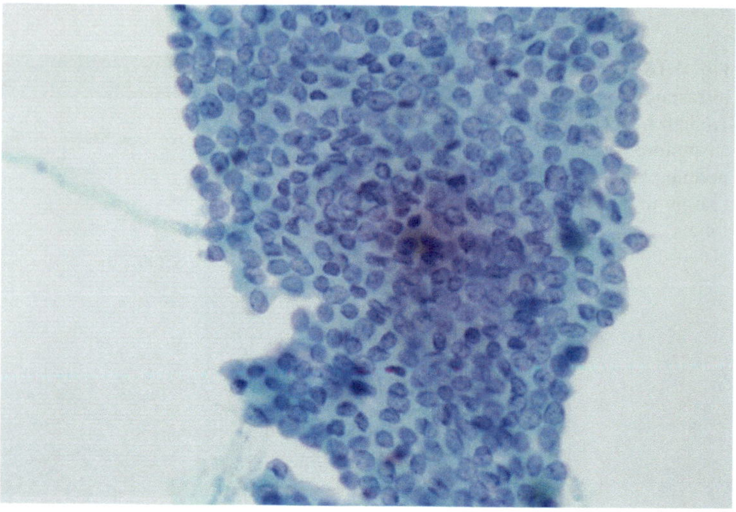

Fig. 4.184 FNA showed papillary carcinoma

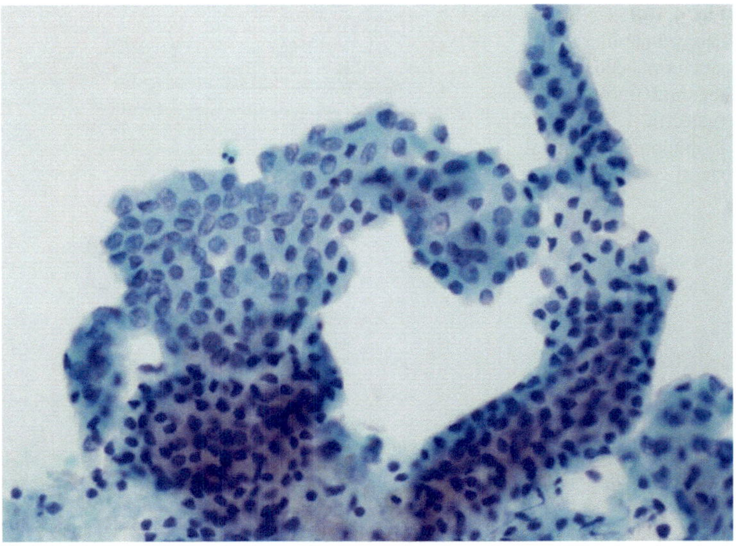

Fig. 4.185 FNA showed papillary carcinoma

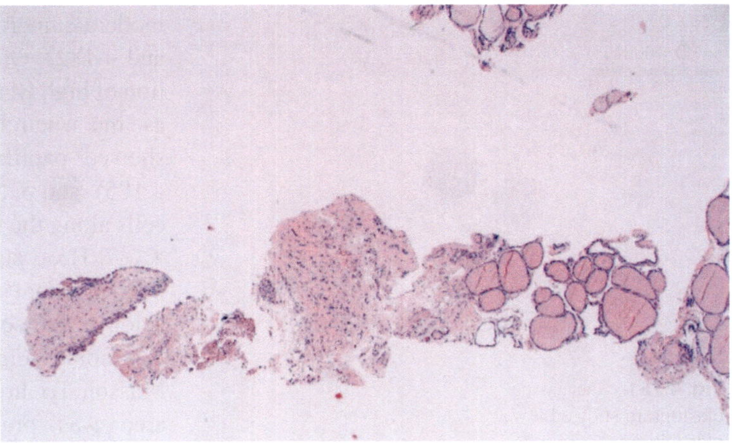

Fig. 4.186 CNB showed papillary carcinoma cells along the thick fibrous core

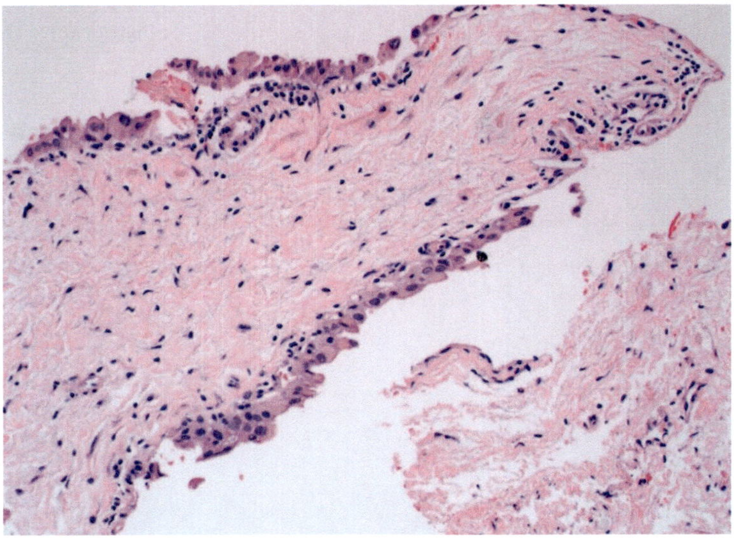

Fig. 4.187 CNB showed papillary carcinoma cells along the thick fibrous core

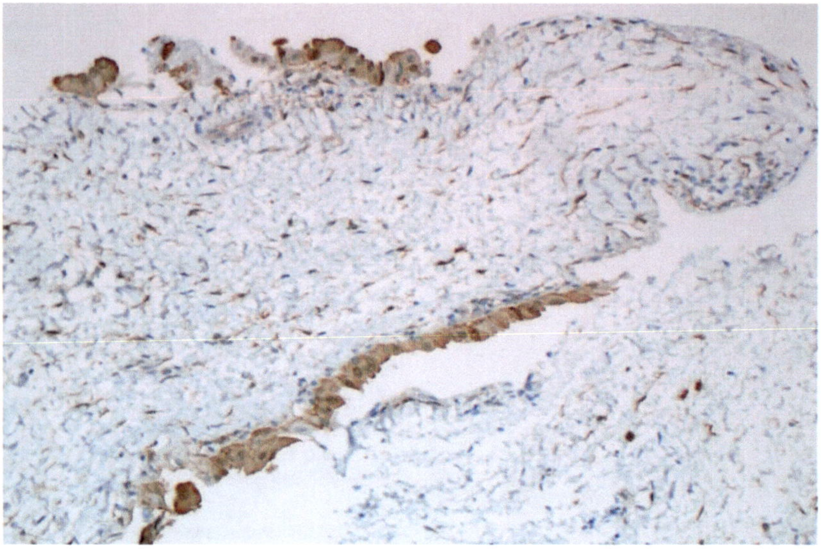

Fig. 4.188 CNB showed papillary carcinoma cells along the thick fibrous core (galectin immunohistochemical stain)

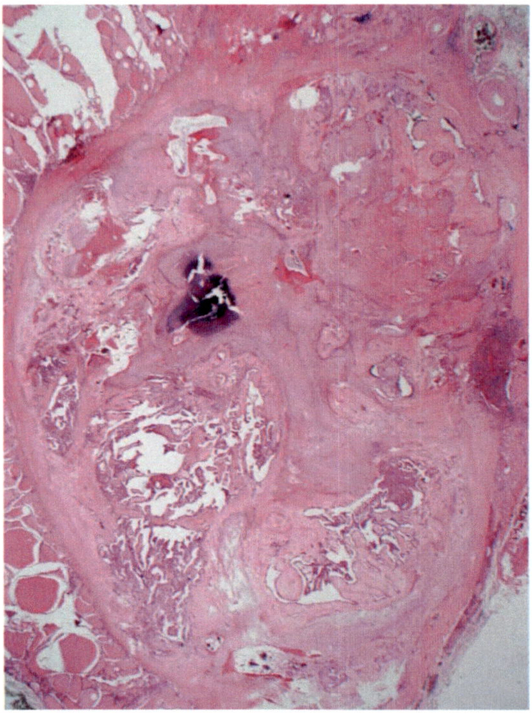

Fig. 4.189 Surgical histopathogy was papillary carcinoma

moderate internal vascularity (Figs. 4.180, 4.181, and 4.182). On shear wave elastogram distribution of high EI area (E_{Max}, 60.1 kPa) was observed as the encircling pattern (Fig. 4.183). FNA showed papillary carcinoma (Figs. 4.184 and 4.185) and CNB showed papillary carcinoma cells along the thick fibrous core (Figs. 4.186 and 4.187, H&E stain, Fig. 4.188, galectin immunohistochemical stain). He underwent total thyroidectomy, and surgical histopathogy was papillary carcinoma (Figs. 4.189, 4.190, and 4.191). On Masson Trichrome stain, distribution of fibrotic area was present in the encircling pattern (Fig. 4.190) within the nodule which was similar to the patterns of the high E1 area in shear wave elastography (Fig. 4.183).

4.5.3 Case 3

A 40-year-old man presented a 0.6 cm nodule with microcalcification. Ultrasonogram revealed a hypoechoic irregularly bordered nodule in the

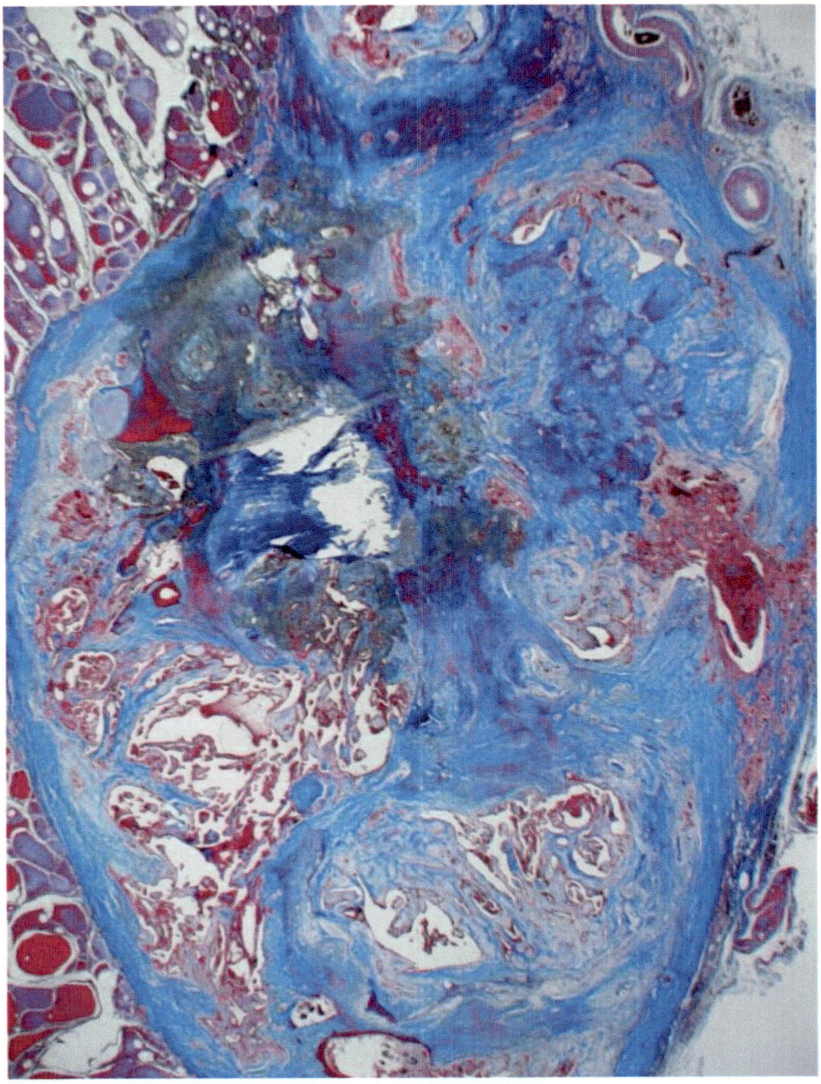

Fig. 4.190 Surgical histopathogy was papillary carcinoma. On Masson Trichrome stain, distribution of fibrotic area was present in the encircling pattern within the nodule which was similar to the patterns of the high El area on shear wave elastography (Fig. 4.183)

left middle lobe (Figs. 4.192 and 4.193). Shear wave elastogram showed increased EI area in the upper, lower and lateral margin of the nodule and E_{Max} was 79.1 kPa (Fig. 4.194). FNA suggested atypia, Bethesda category III, and CNB showed papillary carcinoma (Fig. 4.195). Thyroidectomy was performed and surgical histopathology was papillary carcinoma (Figs. 4.196, 4.197, 4.198, 4.199, and 4.200), showing a fibrotic area in the upper, lower and lateral borders of the tumor on the Masson Trichrome stain (Fig. 4.197), compatible with the high EI area on shear wave elastography (Fig. 4.194).

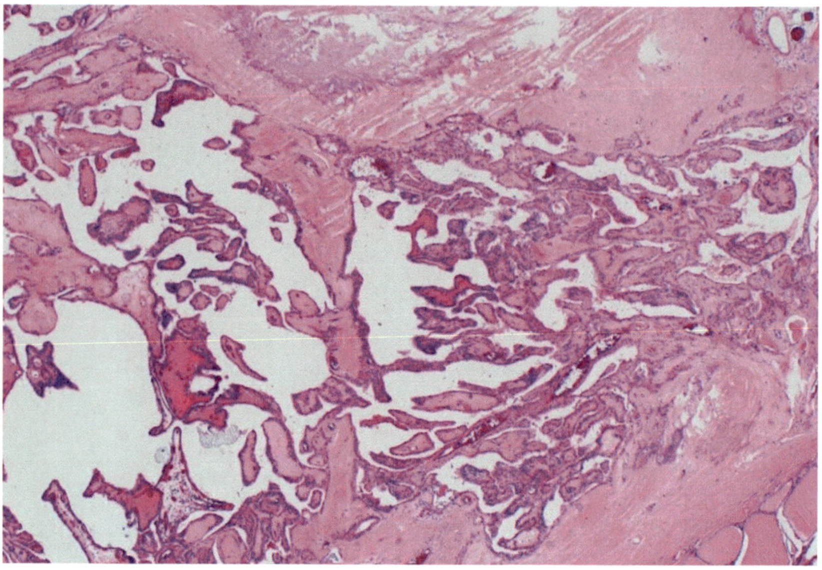

Fig. 4.191 Surgical histopathology showing papillae in papillary carcinoma

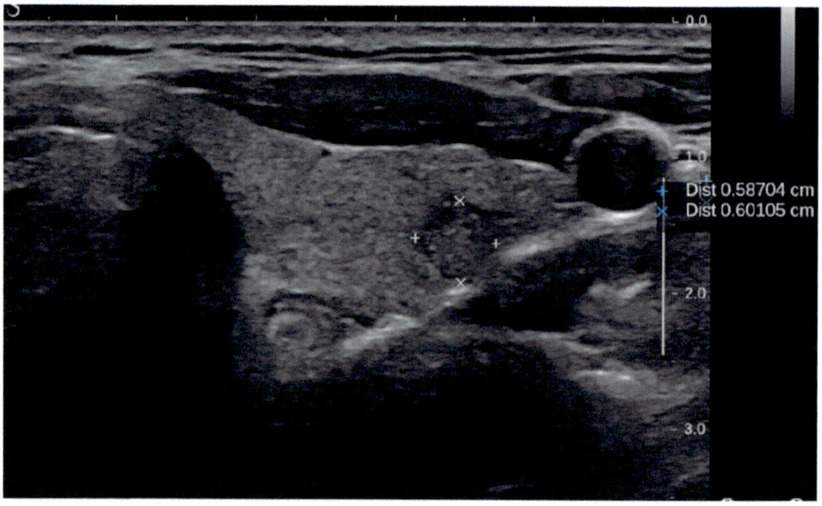

Fig. 4.192 Ultrasonogram revealed 0.6cm hypoechoic irregularly bordered nodule in the left middle lobe with microcalcification

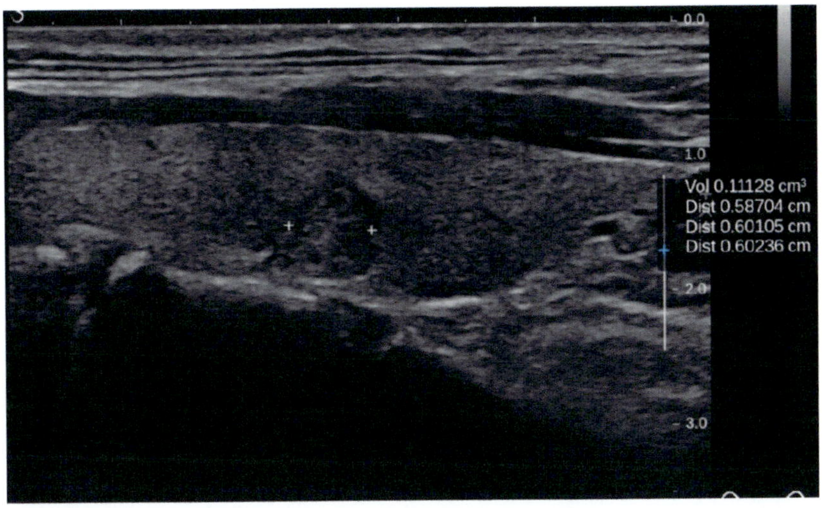

Fig. 4.193 Ultrasonogram revealed 0.6cm hypoechoic irregularly bordered nodule in the left middle lobe with microcalcification

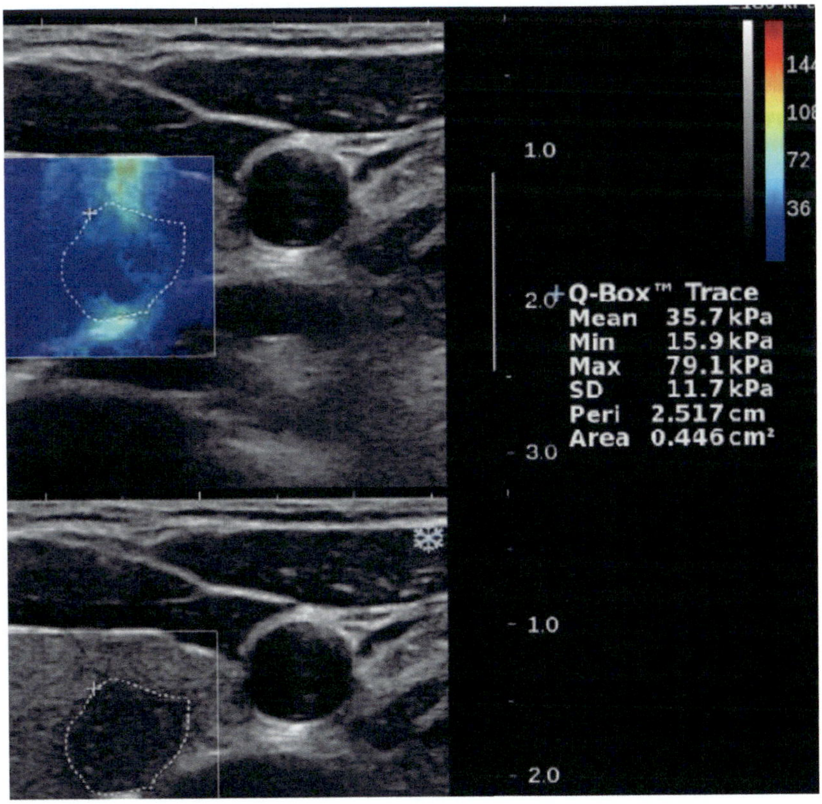

Fig. 4.194 Shear wave elastogram showed increased EI area in the upper. lower and lateral margin of the nodule and E_{Max} was 79.1 kPa

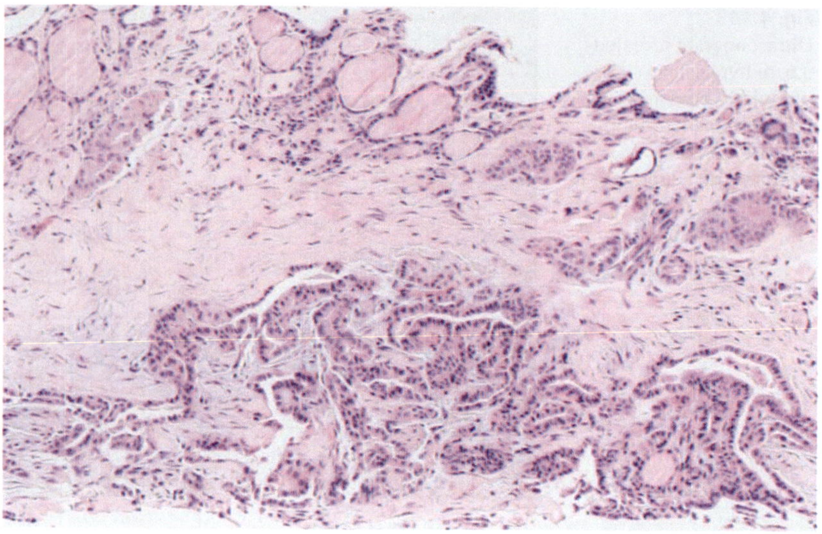

Fig. 4.195 CNB showed papillary carcinoma

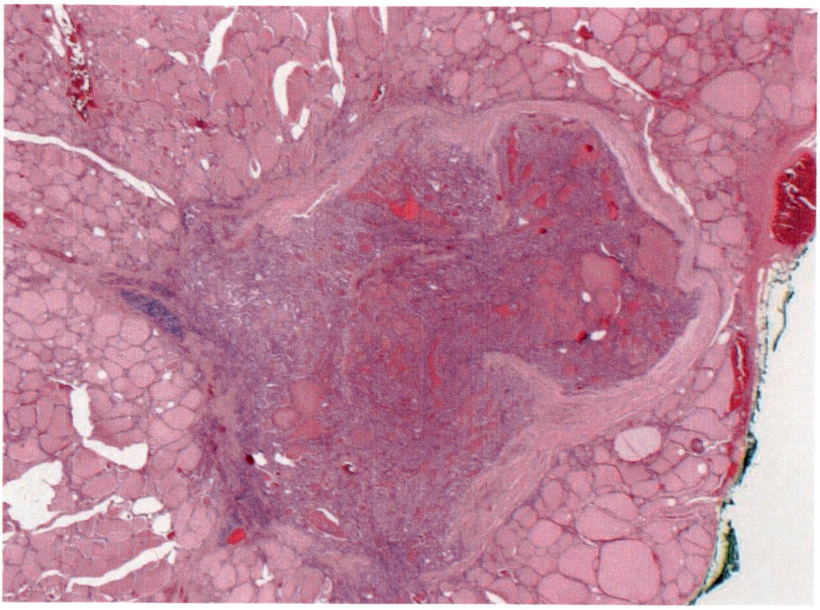

Fig. 4.196 Surgical histopathology was papillary carcinoma showing fibrotic area in the upper, lower and lateral borders of the tumor

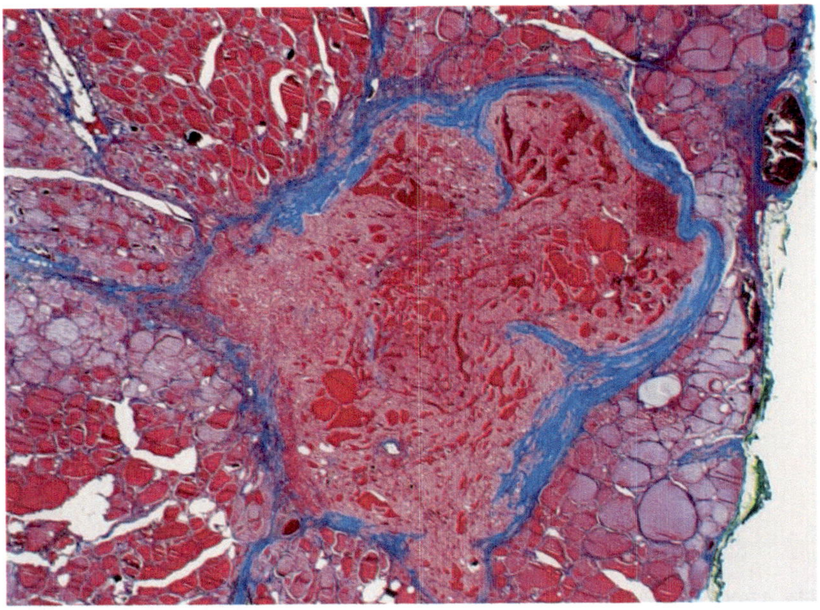

Fig. 4.197 Surgical histopathology was papillary carcinoma showing fibrotic area in the upper, lower and lateral borders of the tumor on Masson Trichrome stain compatible with the high EI area on shear wave elastography (Fig. 4.194)

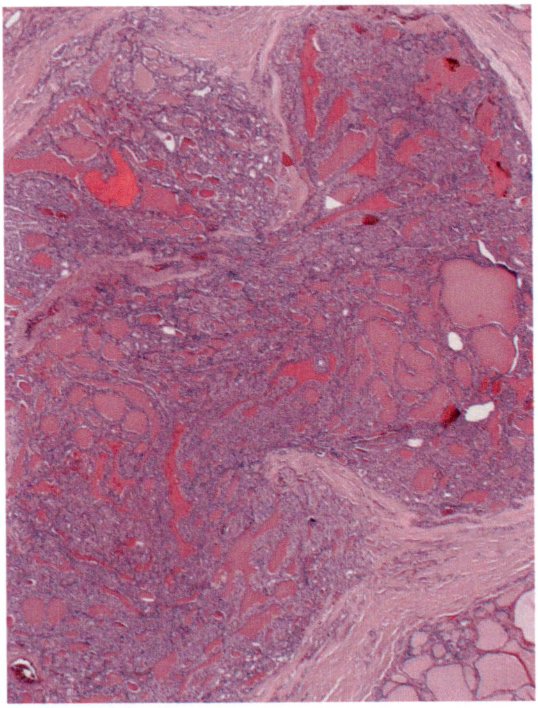

Fig. 4.198 Surgical histopathology was papillary carcinoma showing fibrotic area in the upper, lower and lateral borders of the tumor

4.5.4 Case 4

A 67-year-old woman presented for the evaluation of the thyroid nodule found incidentally. On ultrasonogram, a 3.1 cm hypoechoic suspicious malignant nodule was found in the right middle lobe (Figs. 4.201 and 4.202). Shear wave elastogram showed increased EI areas in the whole region of the nodule and E_{Max} was 109.3 kPa (Fig. 4.203). FNA and CNB showed papillary carcinoma with fibrosis (Figs. 4.204, 4.205, and 4.206). Total thyroidectomy was done and surgical histopathology was papillary carcinoma with extensive fibrosis and calcification (Figs. 4.207, 4.208, and 4.209), and on the Masson-Trichrome stain, diffuse fibrosis was observed in the whole area of the nodule (Fig. 4.210), compatible with the 2D shear wave elastography.

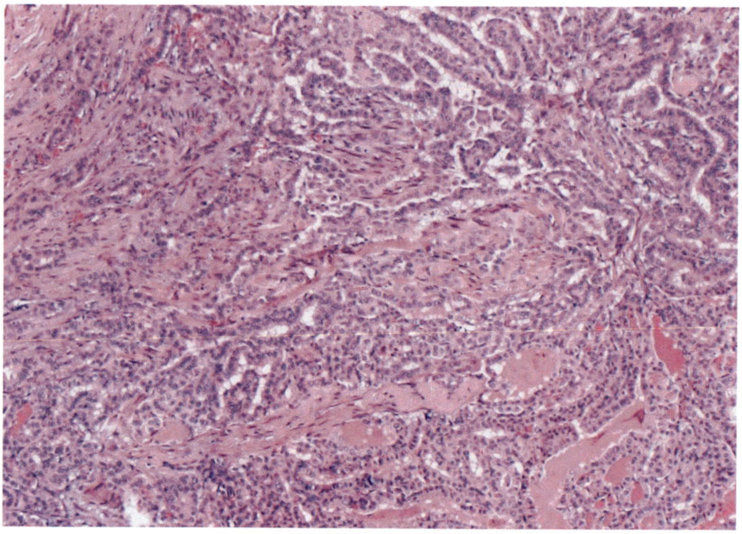

Fig. 4.199 Surgical histopathology showing papillae in papillary carcinoma

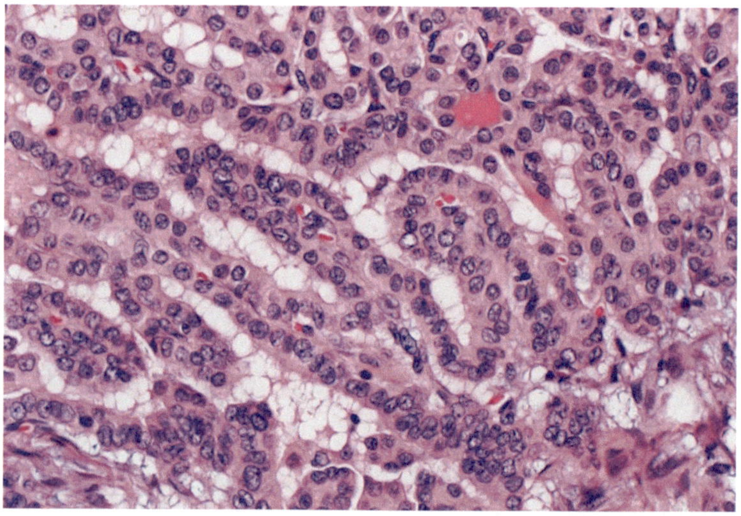

Fig. 4.200 Surgical histopathology showing papillae in papillary carcinoma.

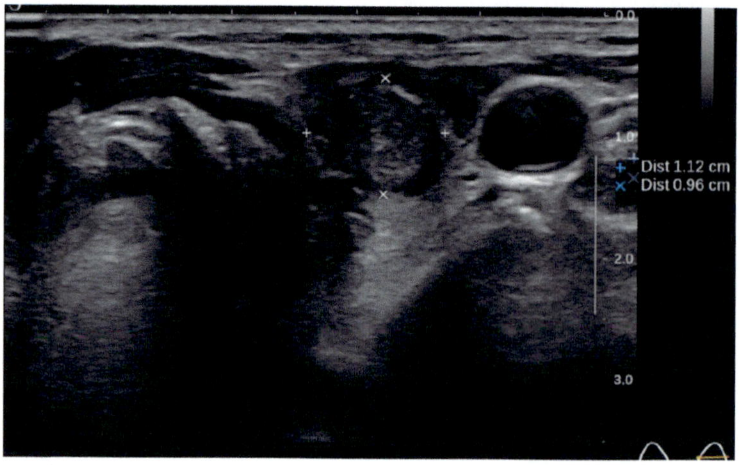

Fig. 4.201 On ultrasonogram, a 3.1 cm hypoechoic suspicious malignant nodule was found in the right middle lobe

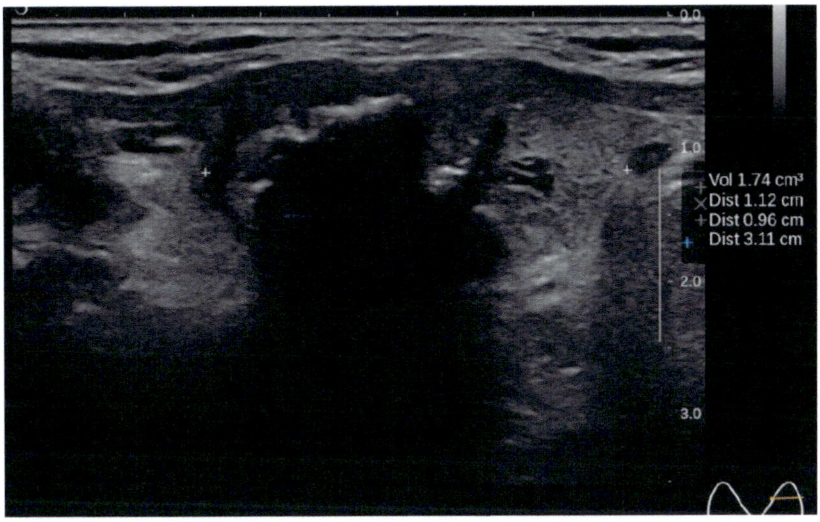

Fig. 4.202 On ultrasonogram, a 3.1 cm hypoechoic suspicious malignant nodule was found in the right middle lobe

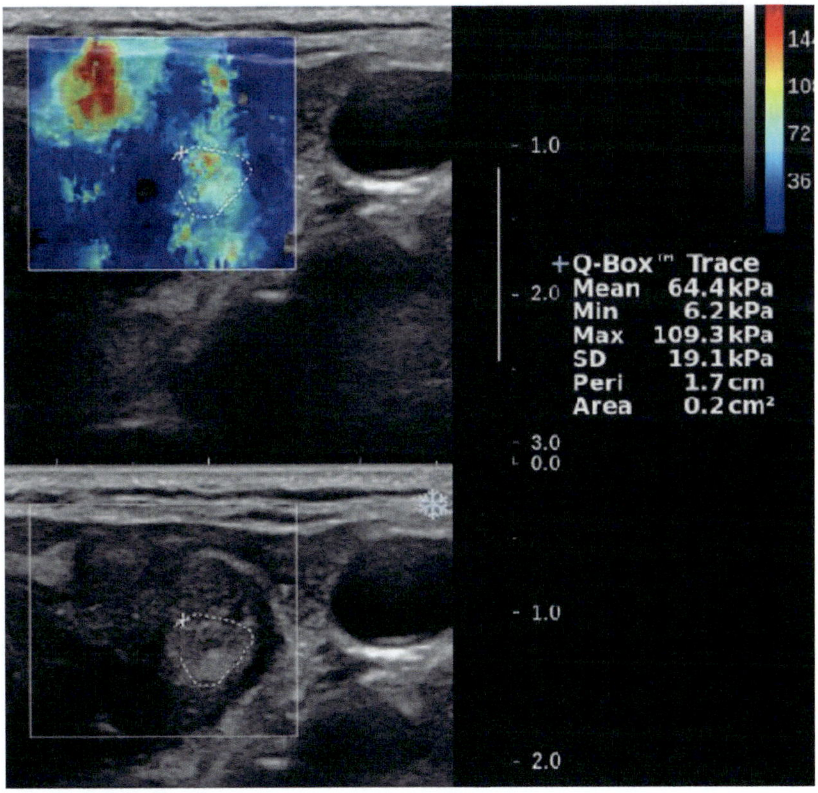

Fig. 4.203 Shear wave elastogram showed increased EI areas in the whole region of the nodule and E_{Max} was 109.3 kPa

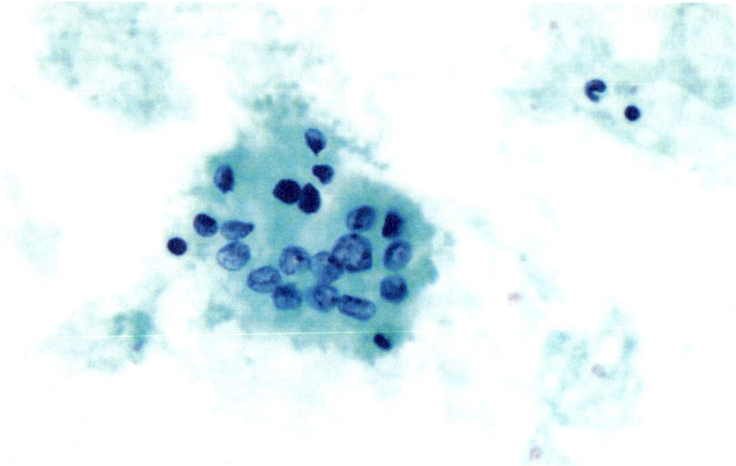

Fig. 4.204 FNA showed papillary carcinoma

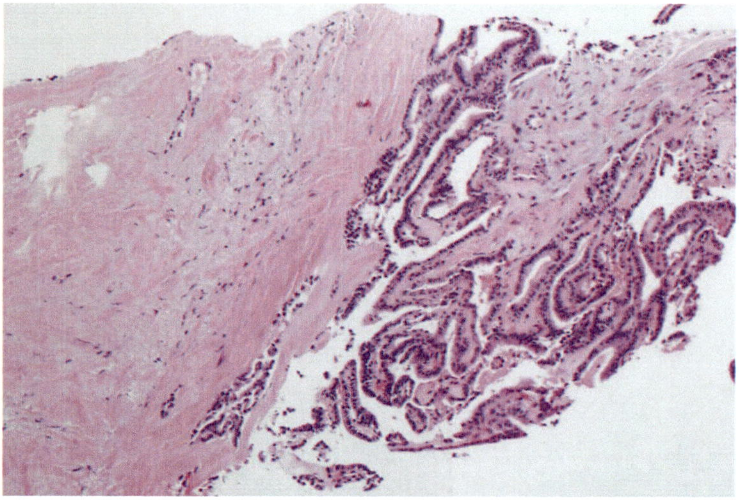

Fig. 4.205 CNB showed papillary carcinoma with fibrosis

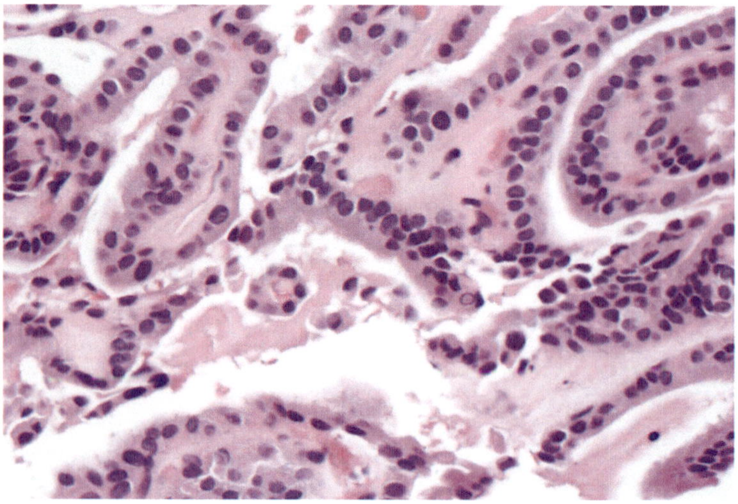

Fig. 4.206 CNB showed papillary carcinoma

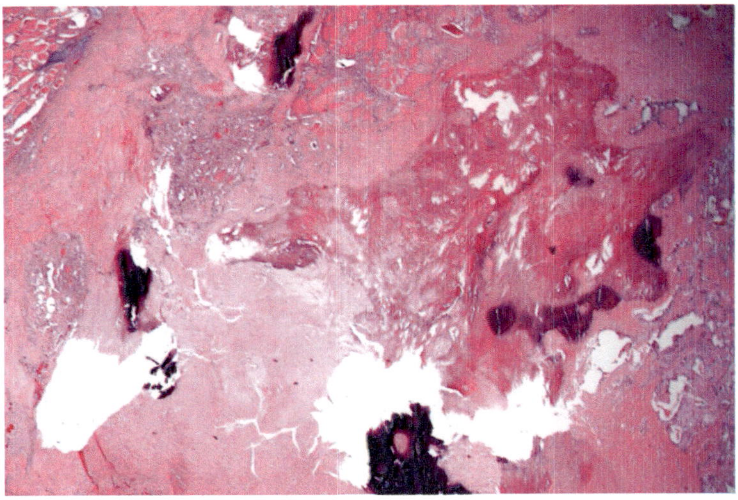

Fig. 4.207 Surgical histopathology was papillary carcinoma with extensive fibrosis and calcification

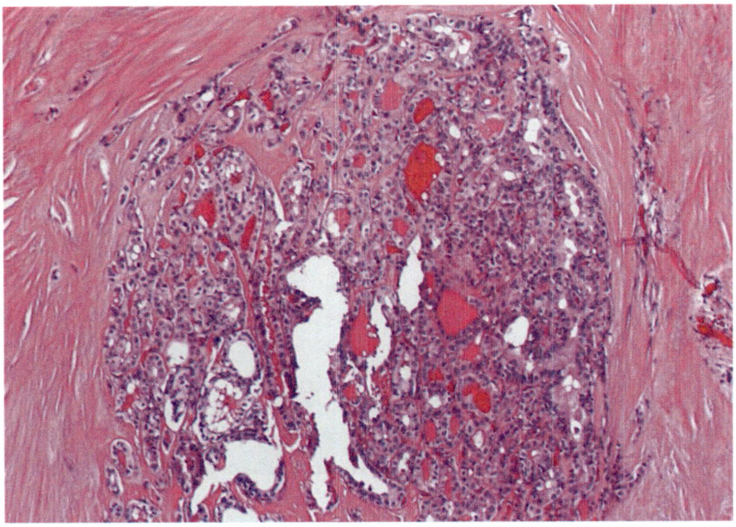

Fig. 4.208 Surgical histopathology was papillary carcinoma with extensive fibrosis

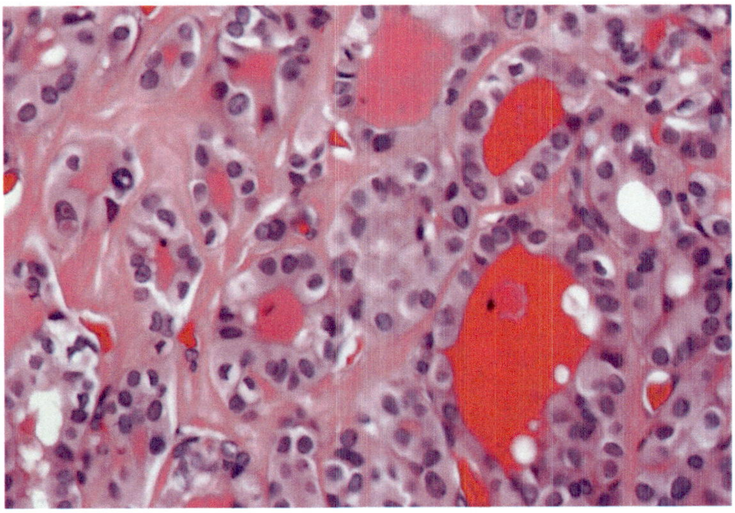

Fig. 4.209 Surgical histopathology showing papillary carcinoma

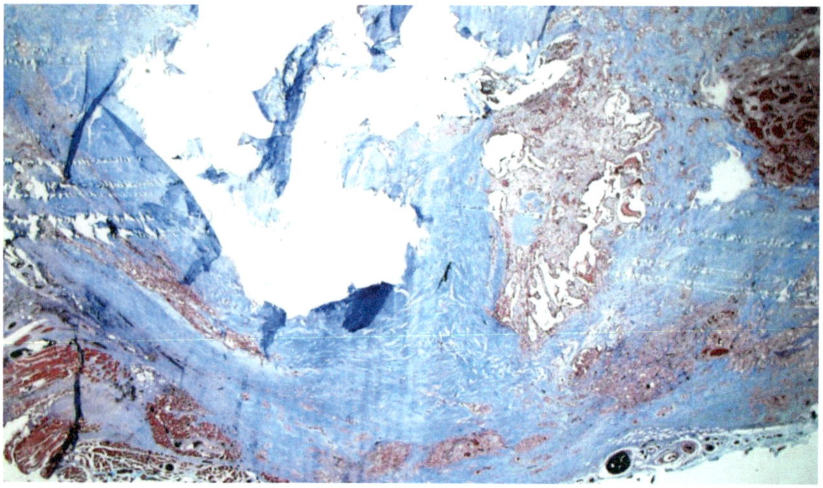

Fig. 4.210 Surgical histopathology was papillary carcinoma with extensive fibrosis and calcification and on Masson-Trichrome stain, diffuse fibrosis was observed in the whole area of the nodule compatible with the 2D shear wave elastography

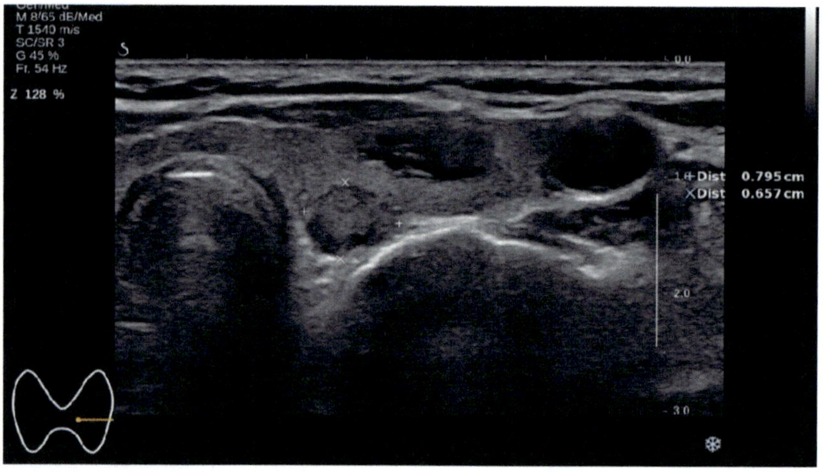

Fig. 4.211 On ultrasonogram 0.795cm hypochoic irregularly bordered nodule was found in the left middle lobe

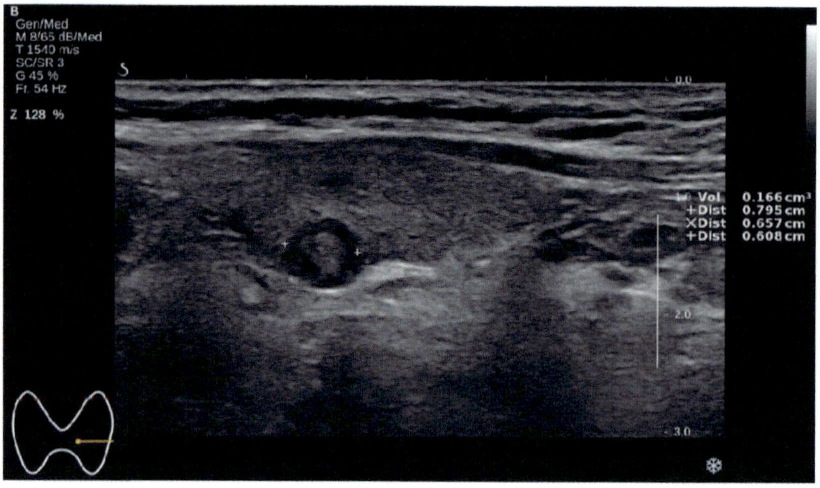

Fig. 4.212 On ultrasonogram 0.795cm hypochoic irregularly bordered nodule was found in the left middle lobe

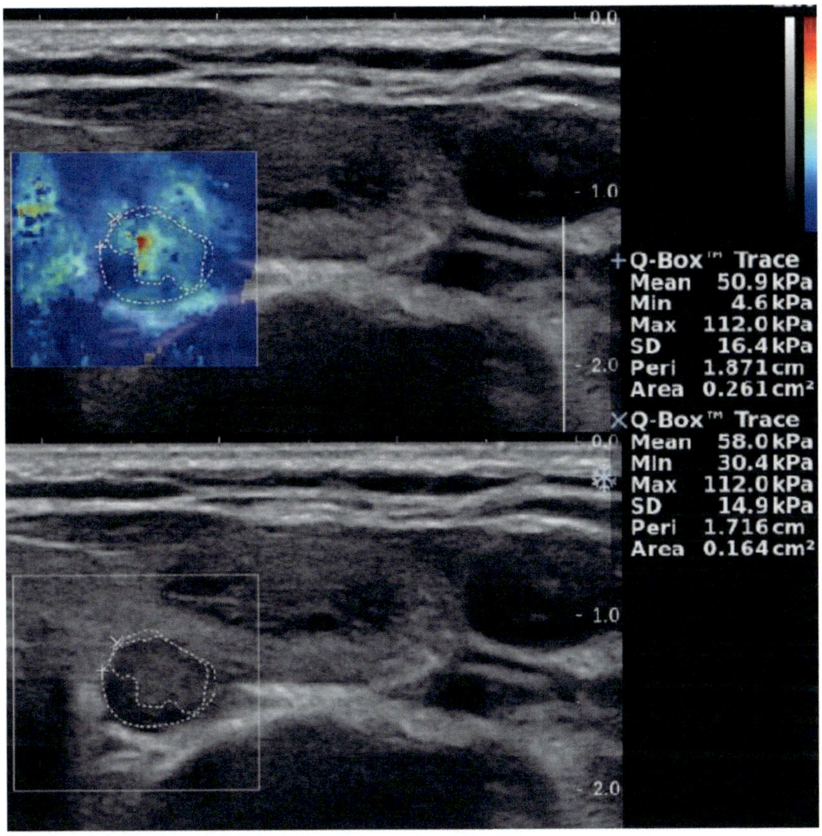

Fig. 4.213 Shear wave elastogram showed diffusely elevated elasticity with E_{Max} 112.0 kPa

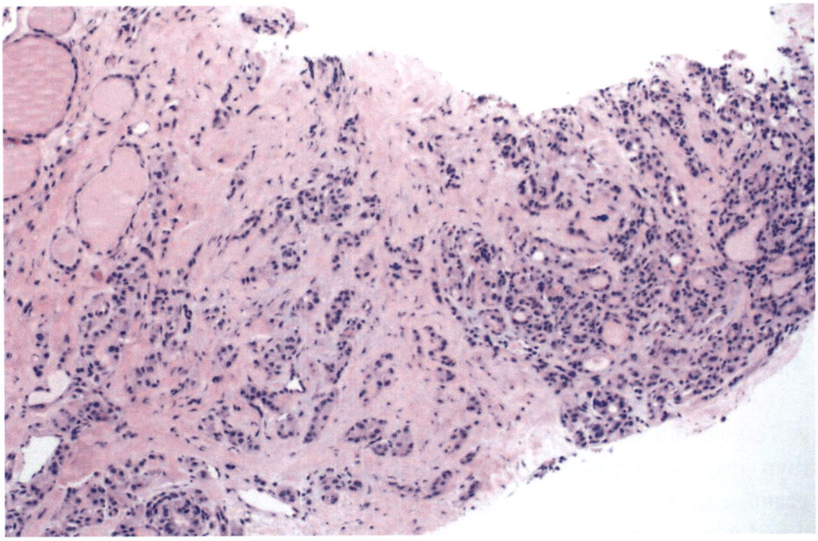

Fig. 4.214 CNB showed papillary carcinoma with fibrotic change

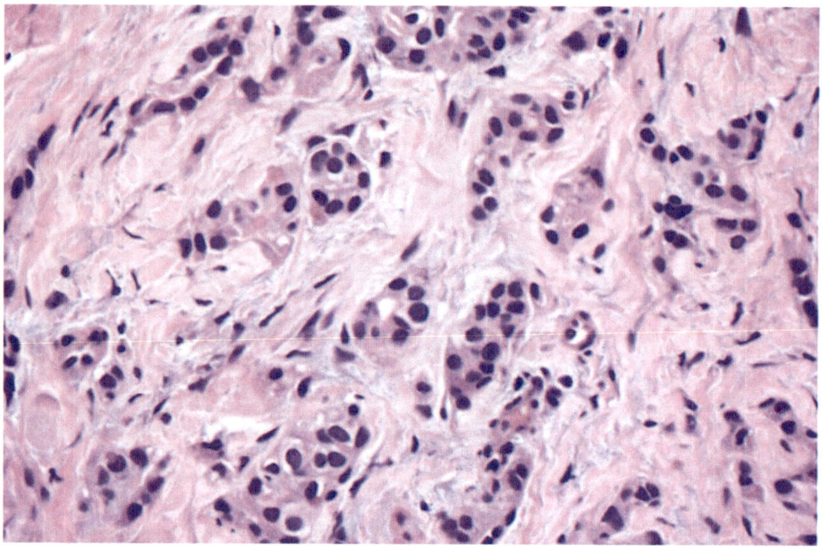

Fig. 4.215 CNB showed papillary carcinoma with fibrotic change

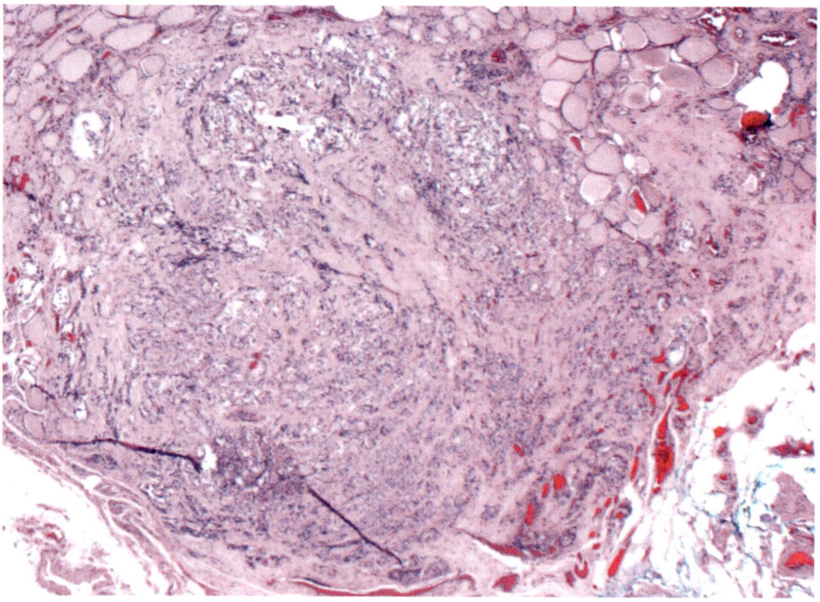

Fig. 4.216 Surgical histopathology revealed papillary carcinoma

4.5.5 Case 5

A 72-year-old woman was found to have a left thyroid nodule on routine check. On ultrasonogram, a 0.795 cm hypoechoic irregularly bordered nodule was found in the left middle lobe (Figs. 4.211 and 4.212). Shear wave elastogram showed diffusely elevated elasticity with E_{Max} 112.0 kPa (Fig. 4.213). CNB showed papillary carcinoma with fibrotic change (Figs. 4.214 and 4.215). She underwent thyroidectomy and histopathology revealed papillary carcinoma (Fig. 4.216) and the Masson Trichrome stain

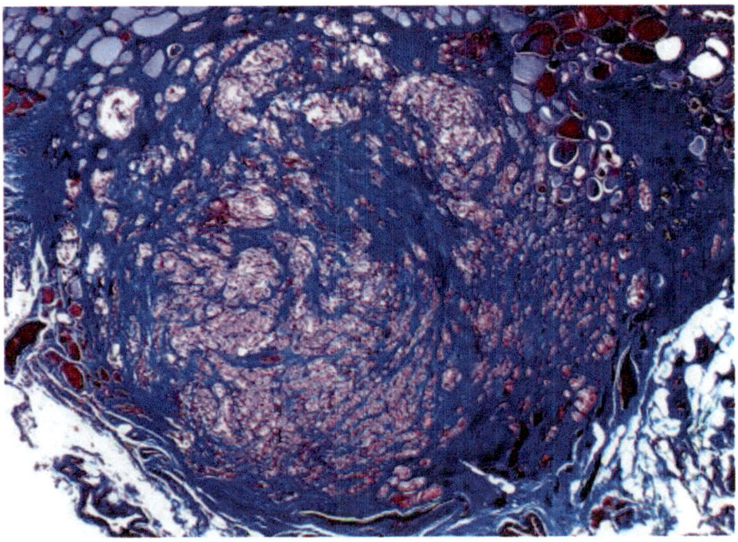

Fig. 4.217 Surgical histopathology revealed papillary carcinoma (Fig. 4.216) and Masson Trichrome stain showed extensive fibrosis except the partial portion in the lower part of the nodule which was compatible with low EI area on SWE (Fig. 4.213)

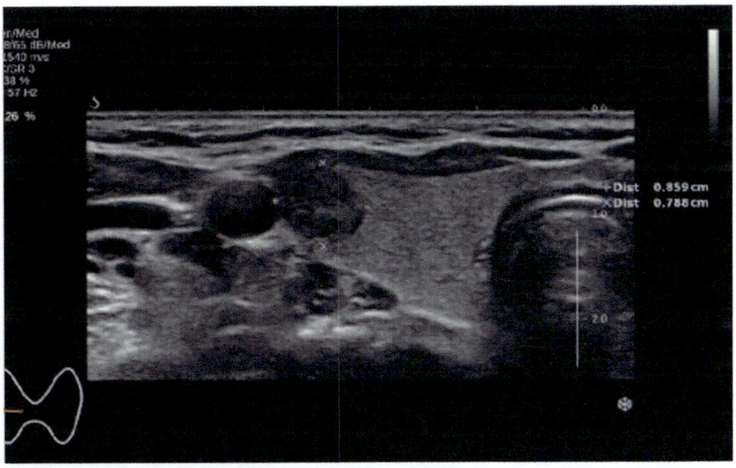

Fig. 4.218 On ultrasonogram 0.88 cm hypoechoic suspicious malignant nodule was found in the right middle lobe

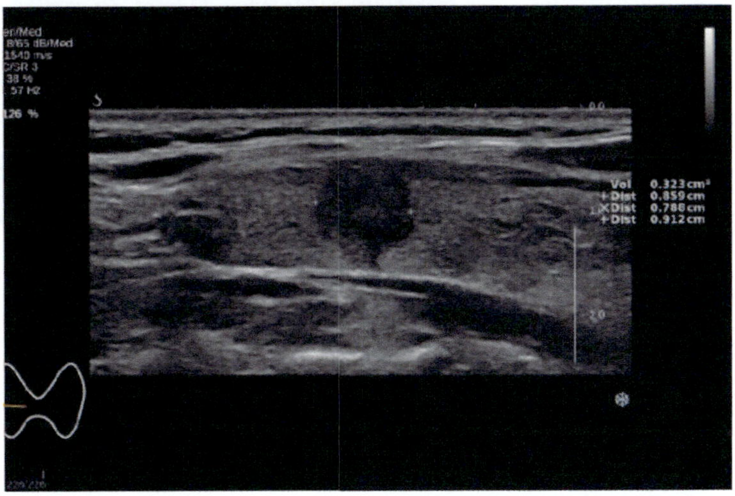

Fig. 4.219 On ultrasonogram 0.88 cm hypoechoic suspicious malignant nodule was found in the right middle lobe

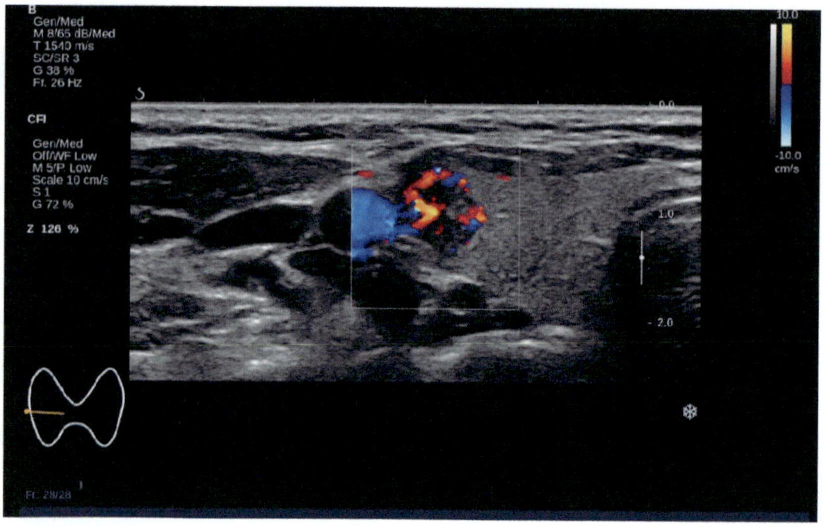

Fig. 4.220 Color Doppler showed increased internal vascularity

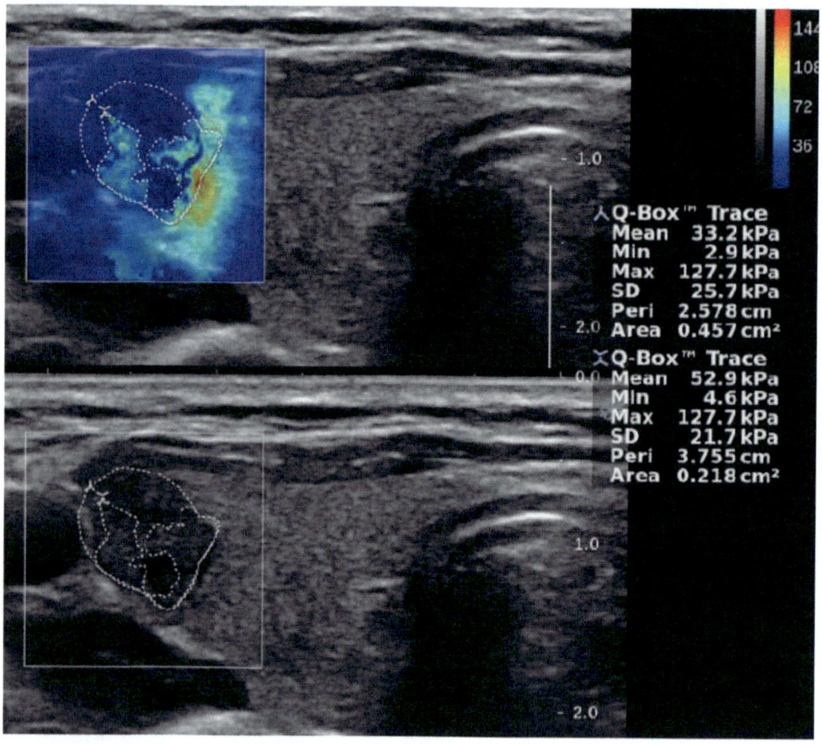

Fig. 4.221 Shear wave elastogram showed increased EI areas in the medial and lateral borders of the nodule (E_{Max} 127.7 kPa)

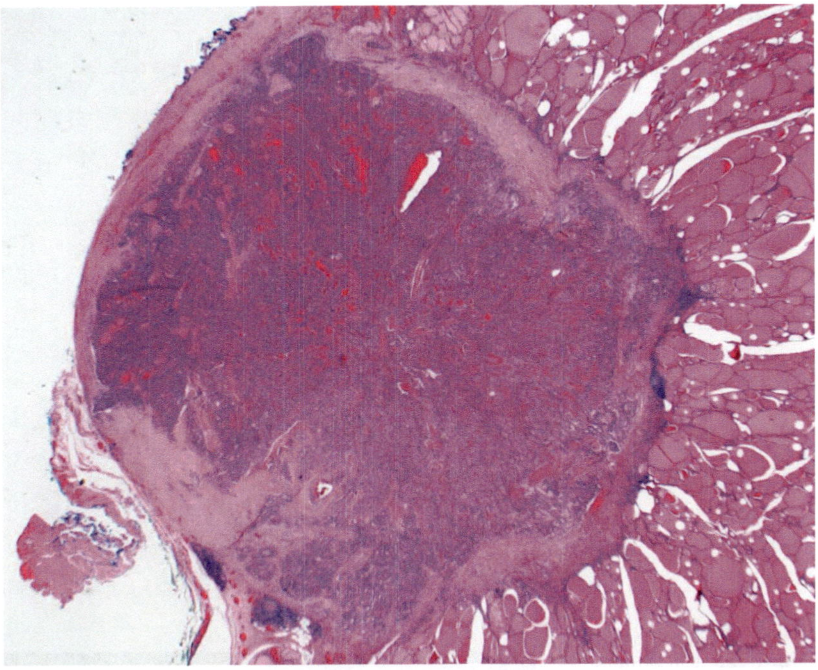

Fig. 4.222 Surgical histopathology was papillary carcinoma

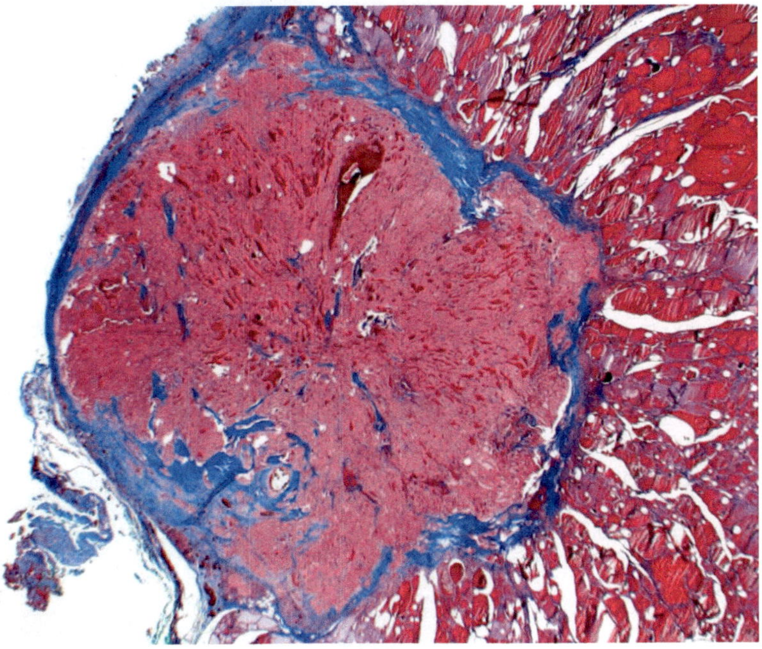

Fig. 4.223 Surgical histopathology was papillary carcinoma and on Masson Trichrome stain, areas of fibrosis were observed in the medial and lateral borders of the nodule (Fig. 4.224), compatible with the 2D shear wave elastography

showed extensive fibrosis (Fig. 4.217), except in the lower part of the nodule which was compatible with low EI area on SWE (Fig. 4.213).

4.5.6 Case 6

A 48-year-old man presented for the evaluation of the thyroid nodule found incidentally. On ultrasonogram, a 0.88 cm hypoechoic suspicious malignant nodule was found in the right middle lobe (Figs. 4.218, 4.219, and 4.220), and Color

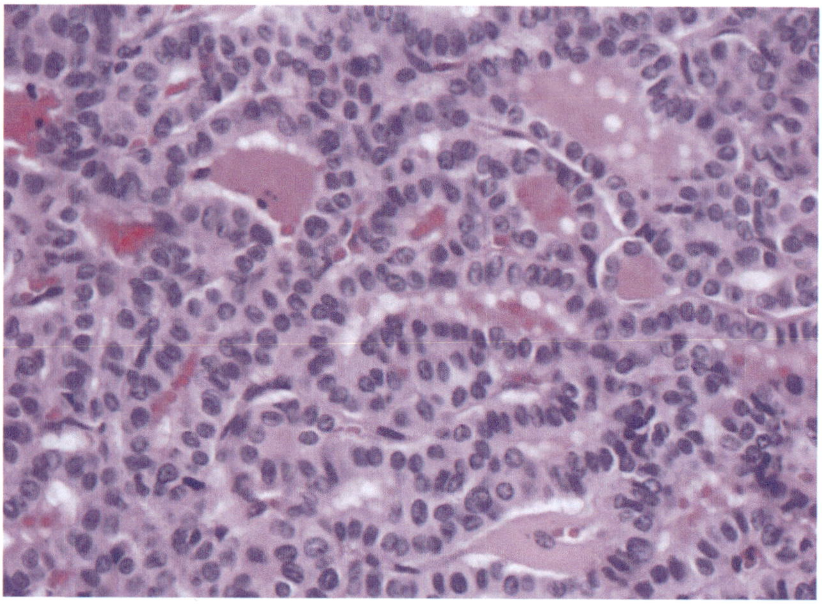

Fig. 4.224 Surgical histopathology showing papillary carcinoma

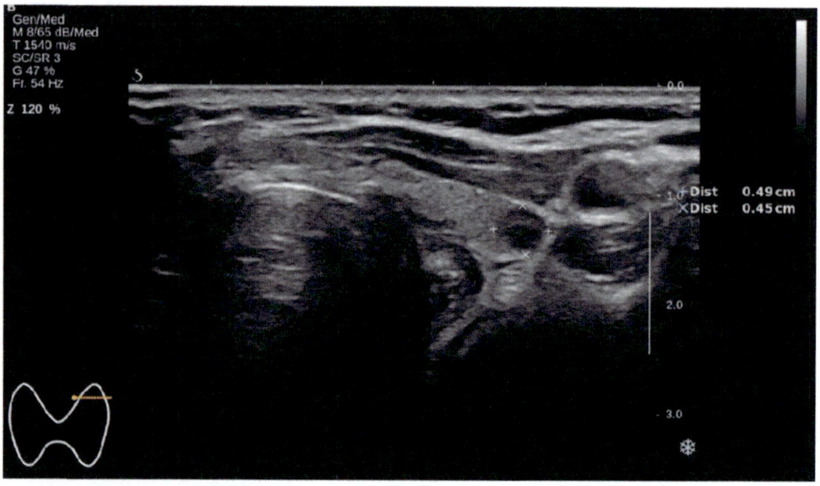

Fig. 4.225 On B mode USG, 0.49 cm hypoechoic nodule was found in the left upper lobe

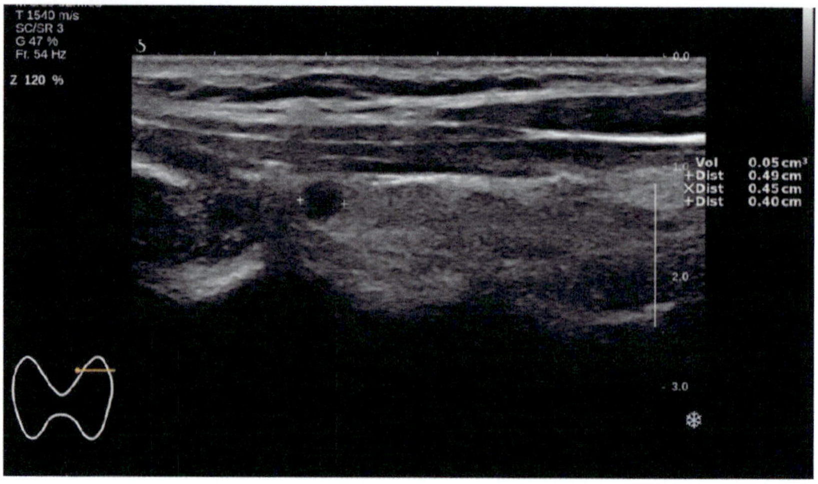

Fig. 4.226 On B mode USG, 0.49 cm hypoechoic nodule was found in the left upper lobe

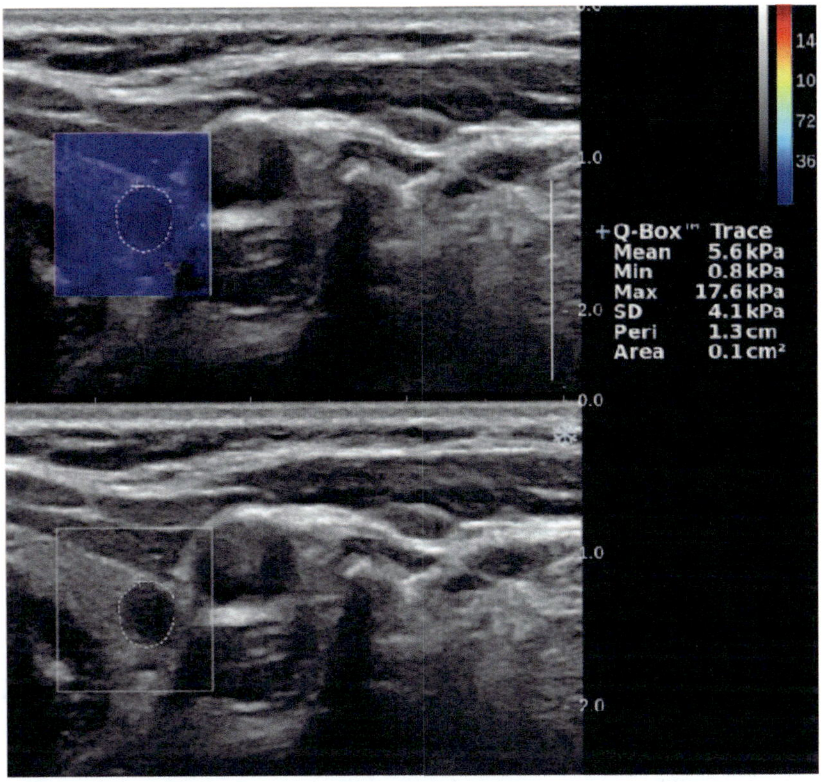

Fig. 4.227 SWE showed low elasticity with E_{Max} 17.6 kPa

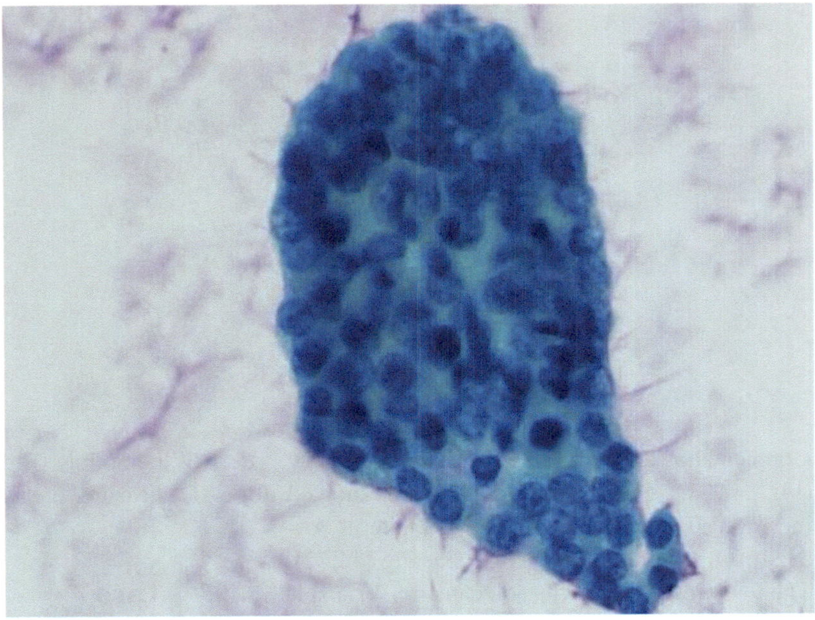

Fig. 4.227 FNA revealed papillary carcinoma

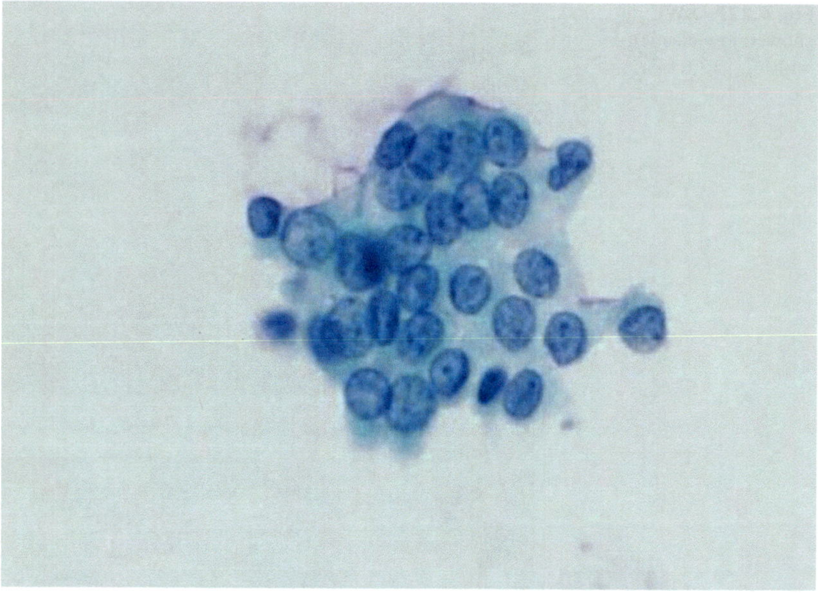

Fig. 4.229 FNA revealed papillary carcinoma showing ground glass appearance nucleus

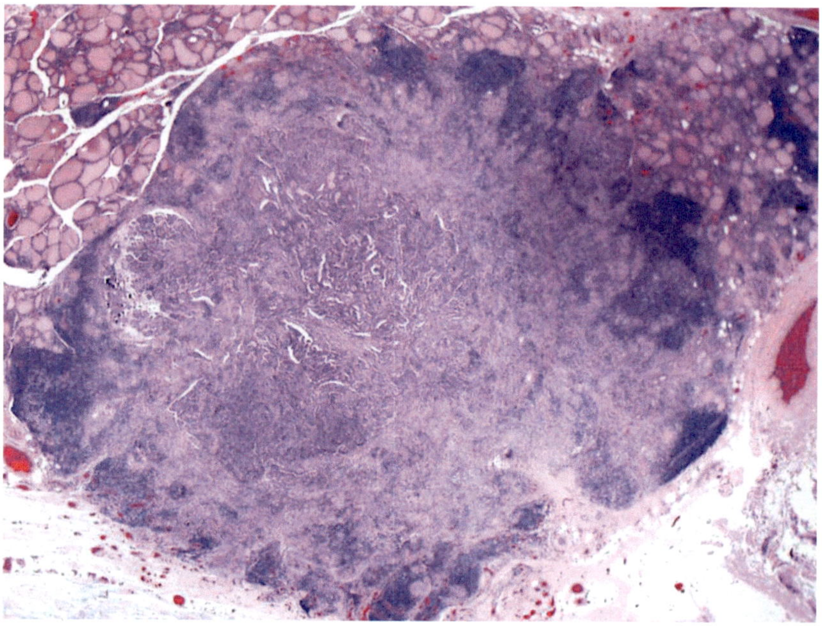

Fig. 4.230 Surgical histopathology showed papillary carcinoma with little fibrotic change which may explain low elasticity on SWE (Fig. 4.227)

Doppler showed increased internal vascularity (Fig. 4.221). Shear wave elastogram showed increased EI areas in the medial and lateral borders of the nodule (E_{Max} 127.7 kPa, Fig. 4.222). The FNA result was Bethesda category V, suspicious of papillary carcinoma. Thyroidectomy was done and surgical histopathology was papillary carcinoma (Figs. 4.223, 4.224, and 4.225) and, on Masson Trichrome stain, areas of fibrosis were observed in the medial and lateral borders of the nodule (Fig. 4.224), compatible with the 2D shear wave elastography.

4.5.7 Case 7

A 41-year-old woman was referred for the recently found thyroid nodule during follow-up after right lobectomy for papillary carcinoma nine years ago. On B-mode USG, a 0.49 cm

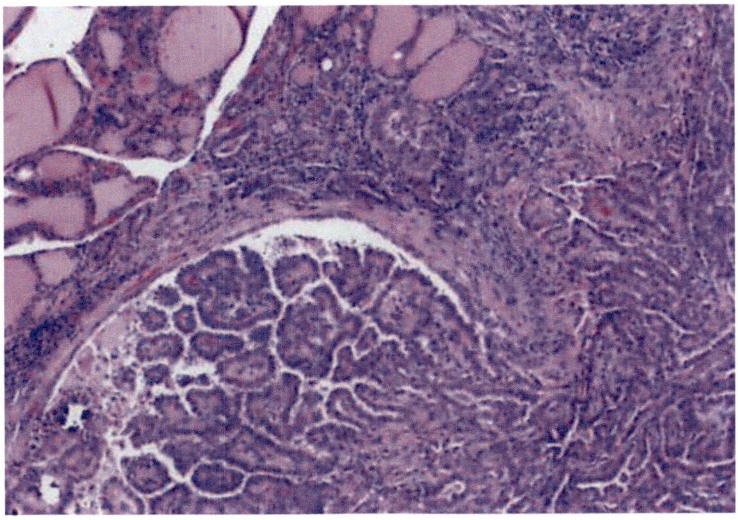

Fig. 4.231 Surgical histopathology showed papillary carcinoma with little fibrotic change which may explain low elasticity on SWE (Fig. 4.227)

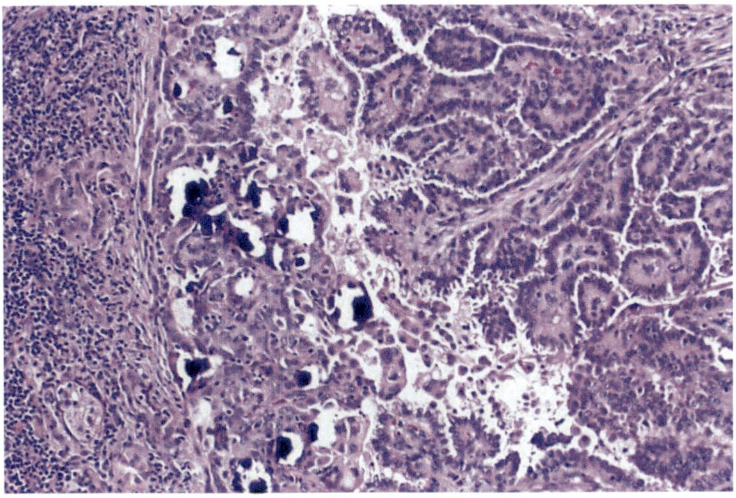

Fig. 4.232 Surgical histopathology showing papillae in papillary carcinoma

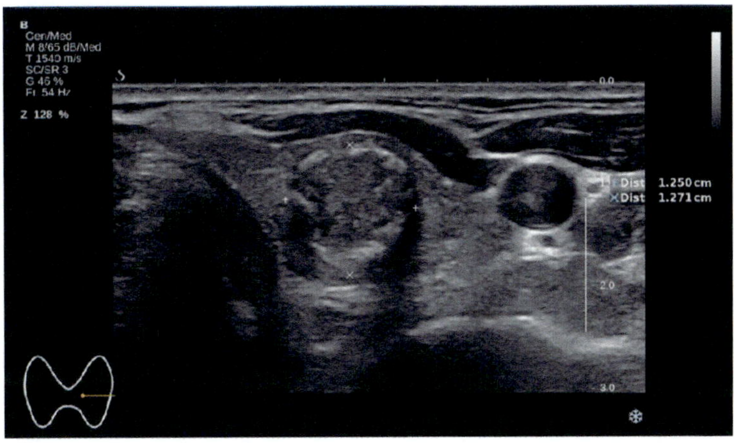

Fig. 4.233 On B mode USG, 1.47 cm rim calcified nodule with internal microcalcification was observed in the left lobe

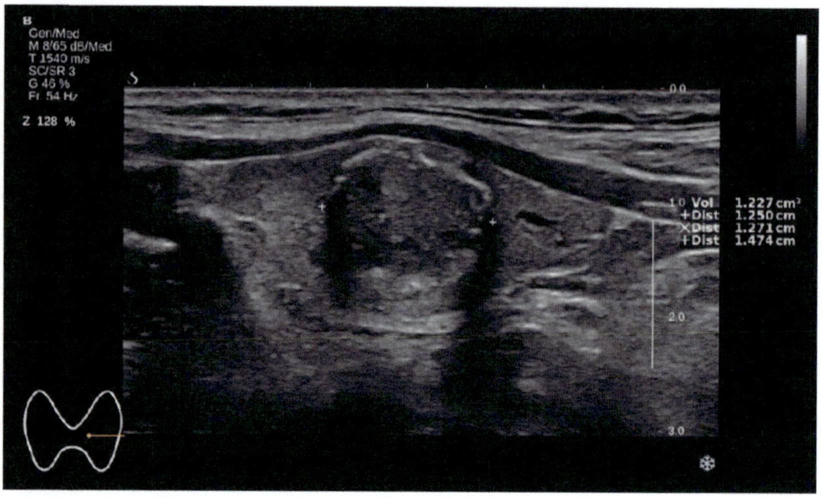

Fig. 4.234 On B mode USG, 1.47 cm rim calcified nodule with internal microcalcification was observed in the left lobe

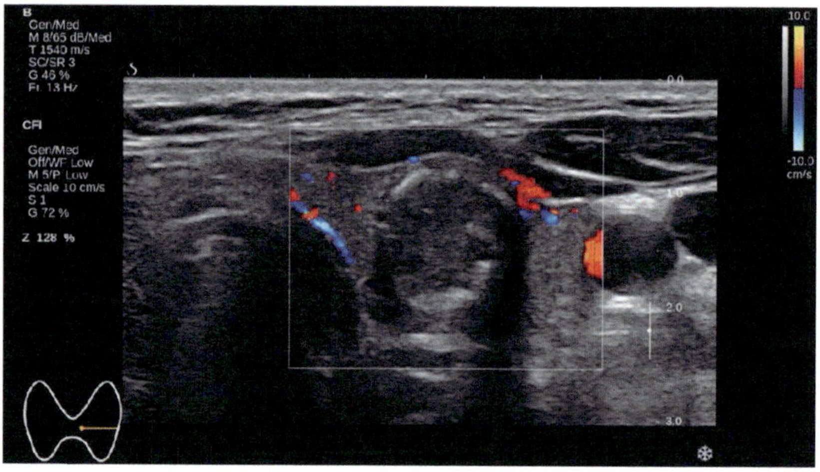

Fig. 4.235 Little internal vascularity was observed on color Doppler

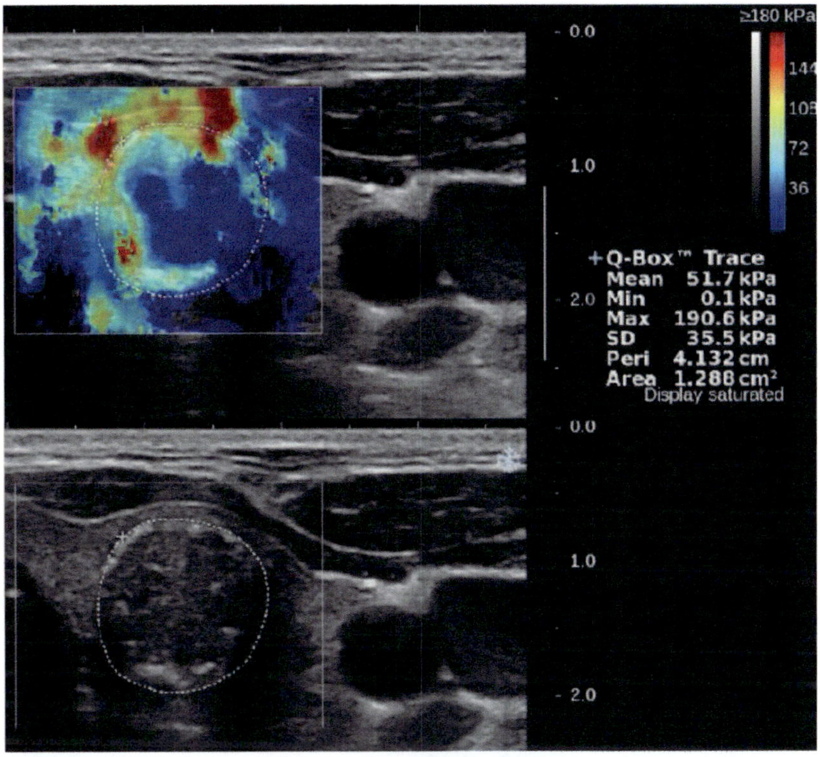

Fig. 4.236 SWE showed increasd elasticity around the margin of the nodule and E_{Max} was 190.6 kPa

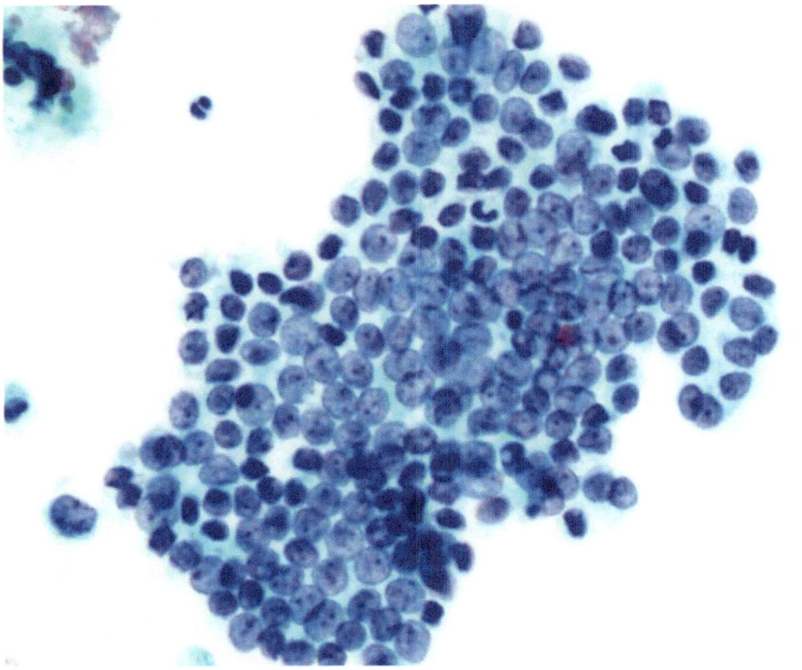

Fig. 4.237 FNAC showed papillary carcinoma cells with nuclear grooves

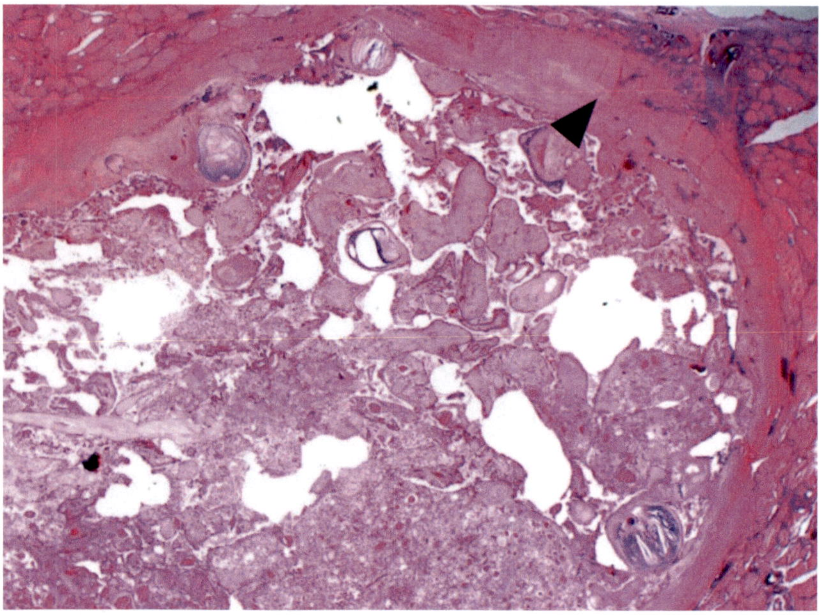

Fig. 4.238 Surgical histopathology was papillary carcinoma showing fibrosis mainly around the margin of the nodule (arrow) similar to high EI region of SWE (Fig. 4.236)

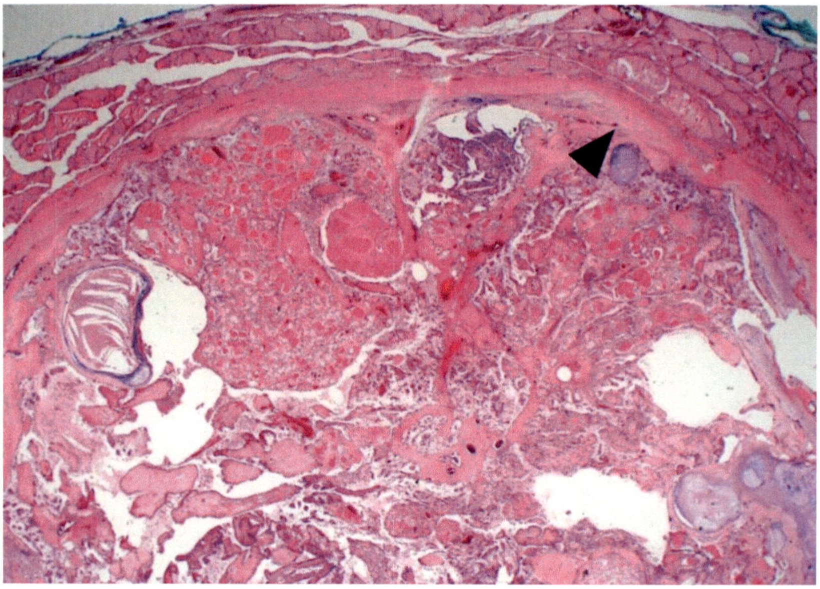

Fig. 4.239 Surgical histopathology was papillary carcinoma showing fibrosis mainly around the margin of the nodule (arrow) similar to high EI region of SWE (Fig. 4.236)

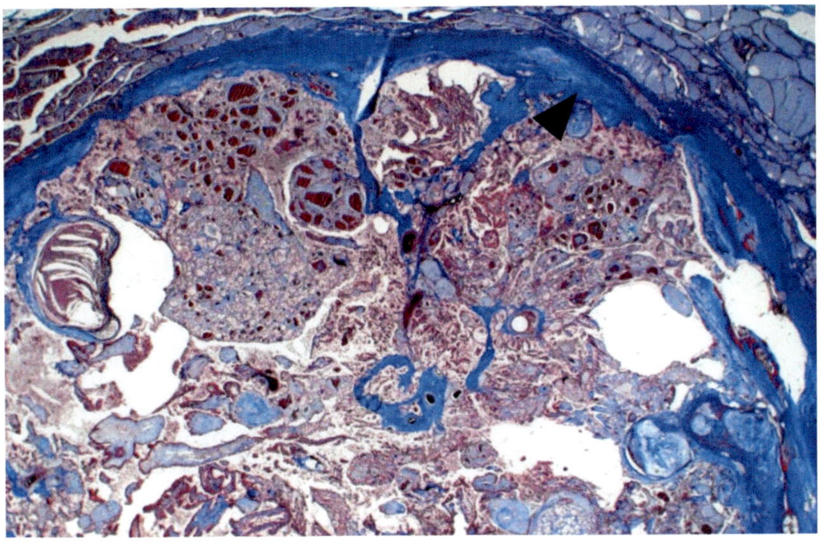

Fig. 4.240 Masson Trichrome stain showing fibrosis mainly around the margin of the nodule (arrow) similar to high EI region of SWE (Fig. 4.236)

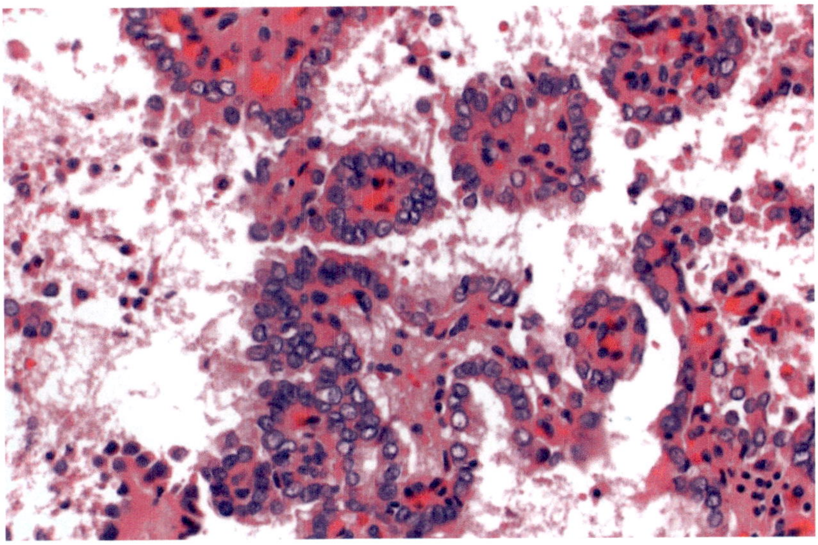

Fig. 4.241 Surgical histopathology showing papillae in papillary carcinoma

hypoechoic nodule was found in the left upper lobe (Figs. 4.225 and 4.226). SWE showed low elasticity with E_{Max} 17.6 kPa (Fig. 4.227). FNA revealed papillary carcinoma, showing a nucleus with ground glass appearance (arrow, Figs. 4.228 and 4.229). Completion thyroidectomy with lymph node dissection was performed and surgical histopathology showed papillary carcinoma with little fibrotic change (Figs. 4.230, 4.231 and 4.232), which may explain low elasticity on SWE (Fig. 4.227 and 4.225).

4.5.8 Case 8

A 51-year-old man was referred for a thyroid nodule found on routine check. On B-mode USG, a 1.47 cm rim calcified nodule with internal microcalcification

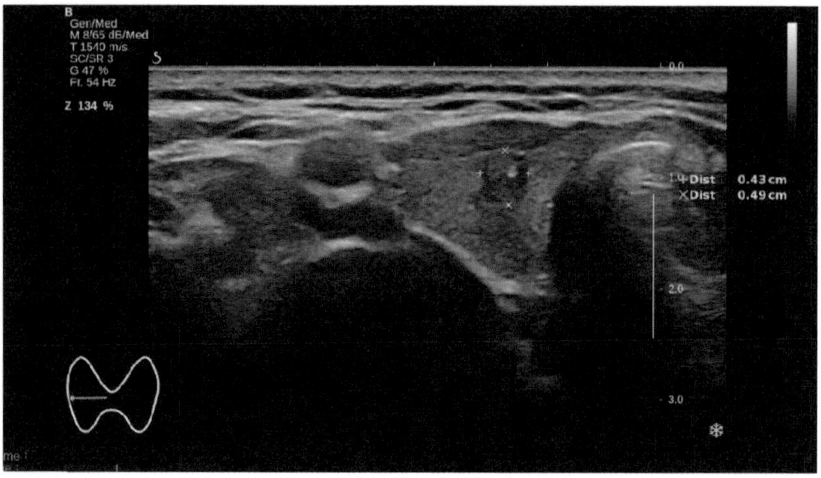

Fig. 4.242 Ultrasonogram revealed 0.52 cm taller than wide nodule in the right middle lobe

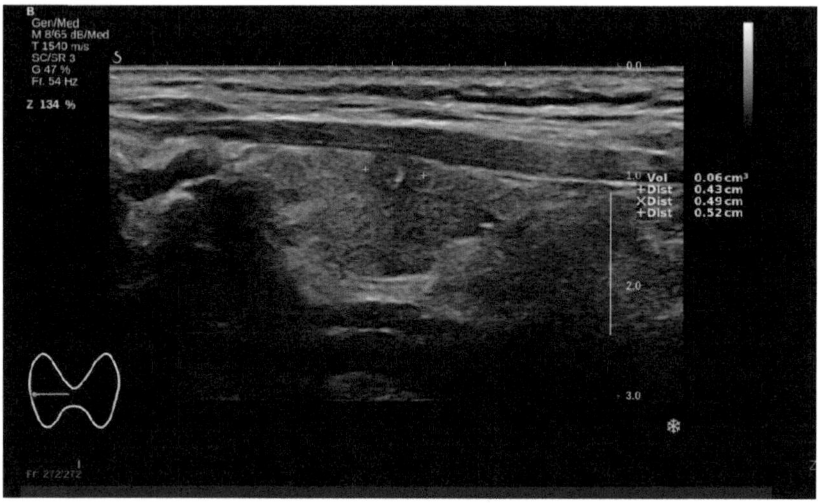

Fig. 4.243 Ultrasonogram revealed 0.52 cm taller than wide nodule in the right middle lobe

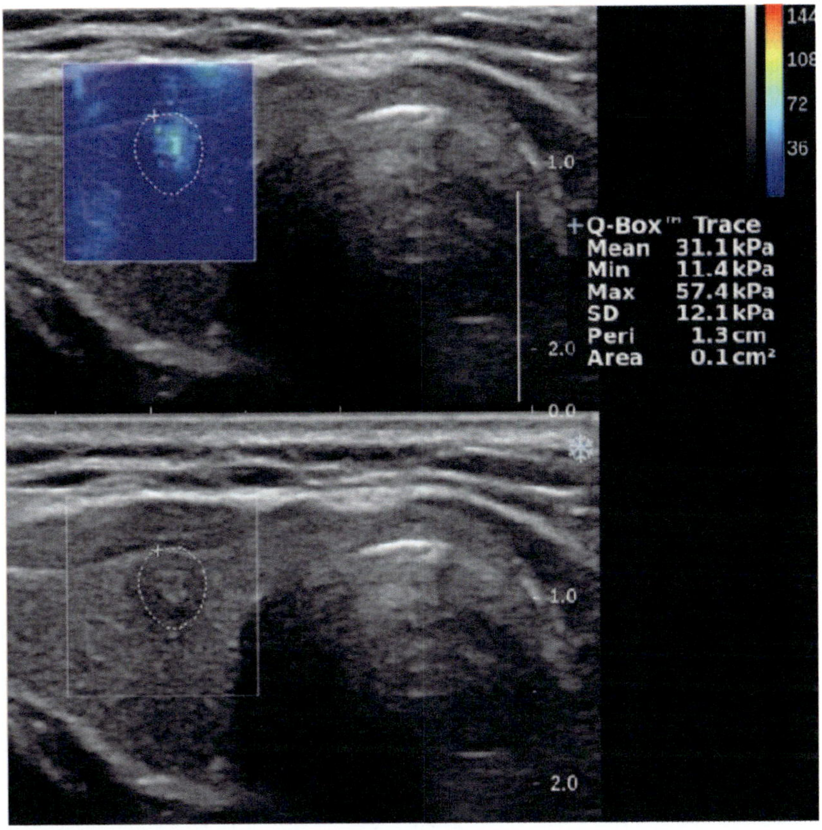

Fig. 4.244 Shear wave elastogram showed increased EI area in the central region of the nodule and E_{Max} was 57.4 kPa

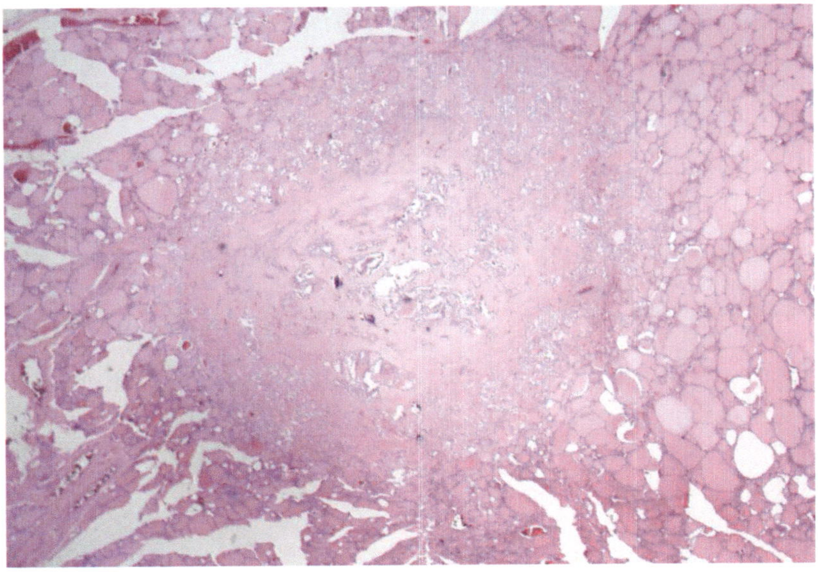

Fig. 4.245 Surgical histopathology was papillary carcinoma and showed fibrosis was observed in the central area of the tumor

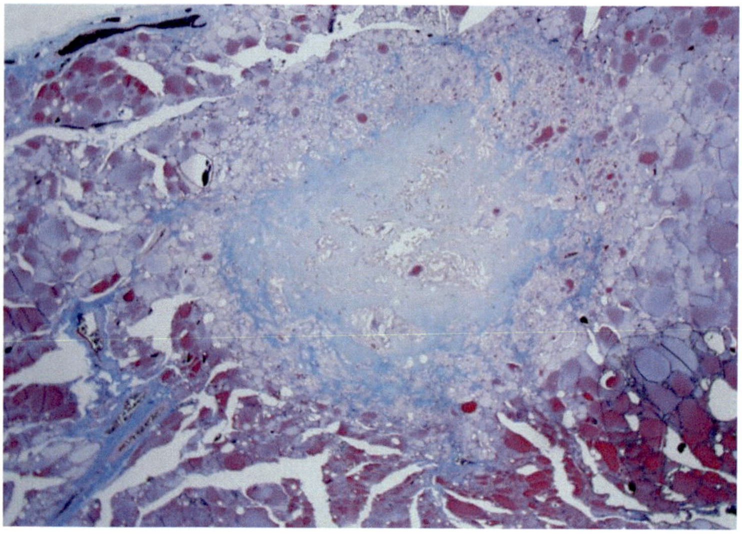

Fig. 4.246 Surgical histopathology was papillary carcinoma and showed fibrosis was observed in the central area of the tumor on Masson Trichrome stain which matched the high elasticity area on the shear wave elastography (Fig. 4.244)

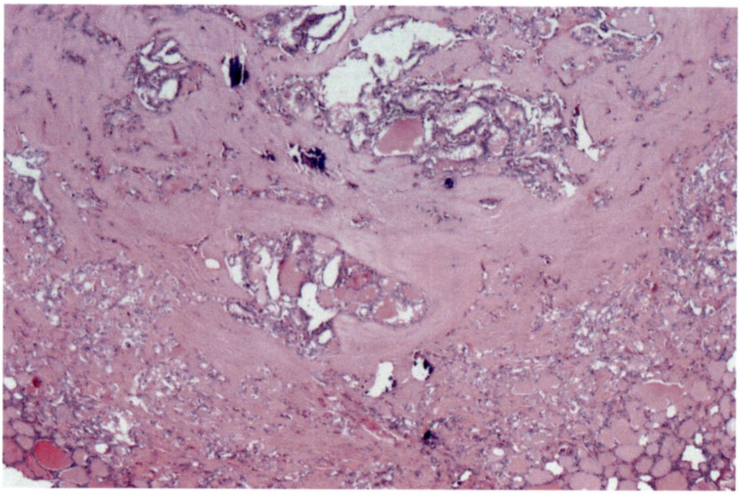

Fig. 4.247 Surgical histopathology was papillary carcinoma showing fibrosis in the central area of the tumor

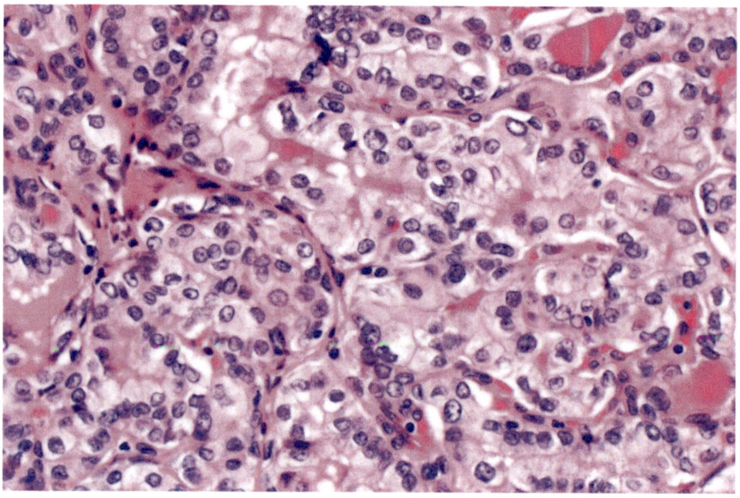

Fig. 4.248 Surgical histopathology showing papillary carcinoma

and little internal vascularity was observed in the left lobe (Figs. 4.233, 4.234, and 4.235). SWE showed increased elasticity around the margin of the nodule (E_{Max} 190.6 kPa, Fig. 4.236). FNAC showed papillary carcinoma cells with nuclear grooves (Fig. 4.237). Total thyroidectomy was performed and histopathology was papillary carcinoma, showing fibrosis mainly around the margin of the nodule (arrow, Figs. 4.238, 4.239, 4.240, and 4.241) similar to high EI region of SWE (Fig. 4.236).

4.5.9 Case 9

A 43-year-old woman was found to have a right thyroid nodule on routine check and was referred for evaluation. Ultrasonogram revealed a 0.52 cm taller-than-wide nodule in the right middle lobe (Figs. 4.242 and 4.243). Shear wave elastogram showed increased EI area in the central region of the nodule and E_{Max} was 57.4 kPa (Fig. 4.244). The FNA result was atypia, Bethesda category III. Thyroidectomy was performed and surgical histopathology was papillary carcinoma (Figs. 4.245, 4.246, 4.247,

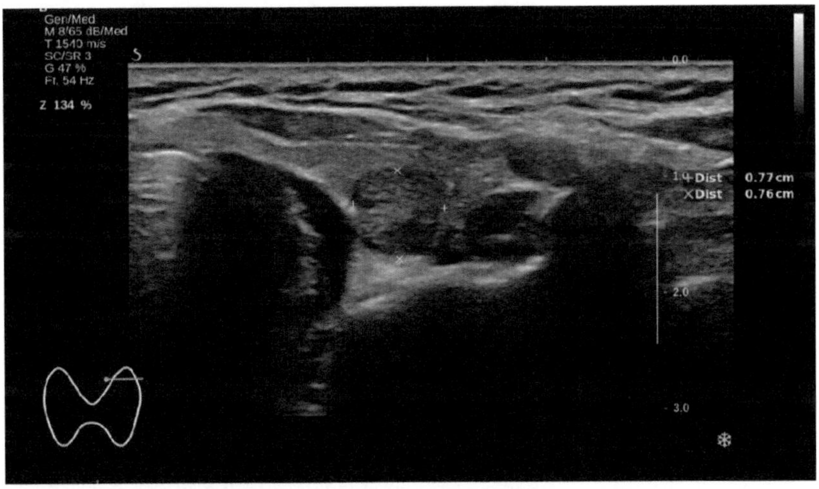

Fig. 4.249 On ultrasonogram 0.87 cm partly hypoechoic irregularly bordered nodule was found in the left upper lobe.

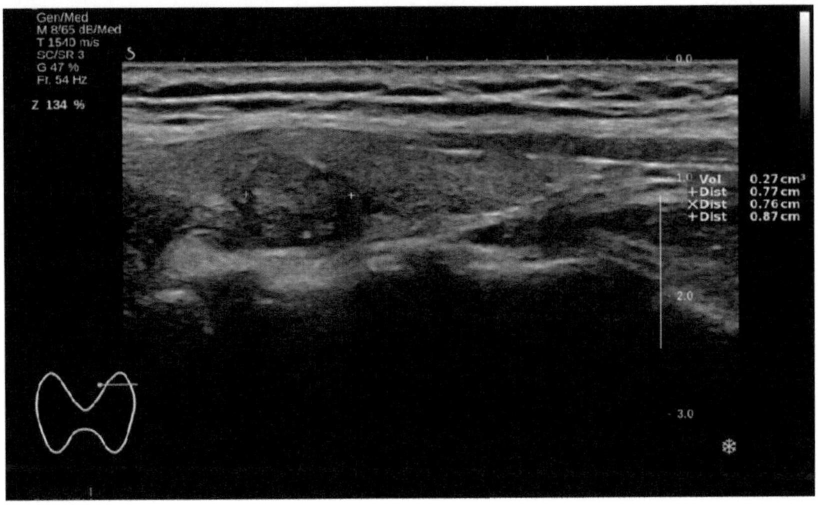

Fig. 4.250 On ultrasonogram 0.87 cm partly hypoechoic irregulalyr bordered nodule was found in the left upper lobe

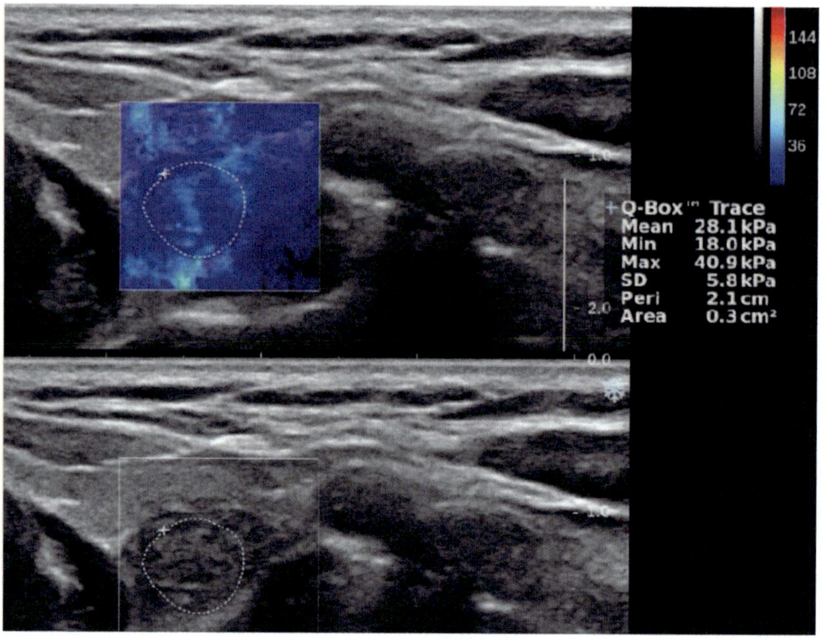

Fig. 4.251 Shear wave elastogram showed low elasticity in the nodule with E_{Max} 40.9 kPa

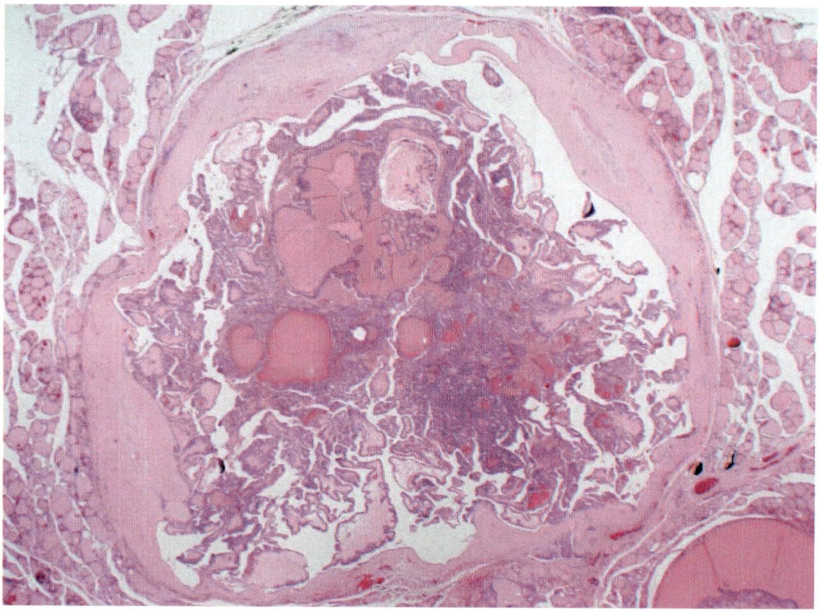

Fig. 4.252 Surgical histopathology revealed papillary carcinoma

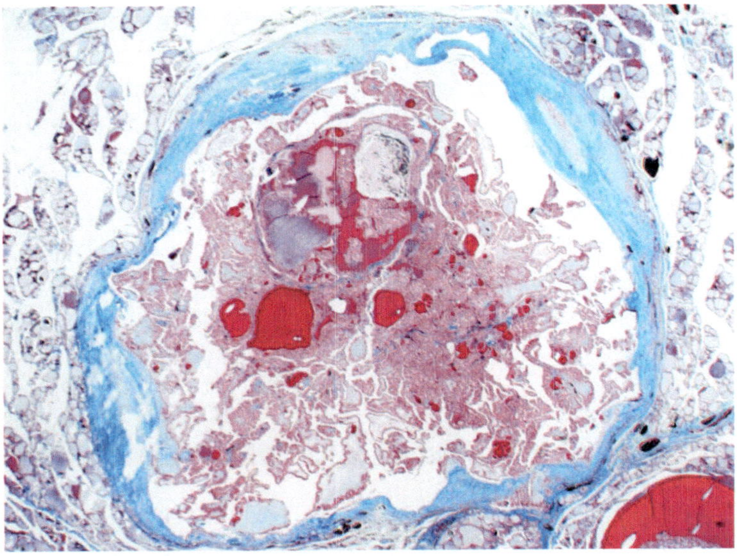

Fig. 4.253 Surgical histopathology revealed papillary carcinoma and Masson Trichrome stain showed no fibrosis in the internal region of the nodule which was compatible with low EI on SWE (Fig. 4.253)

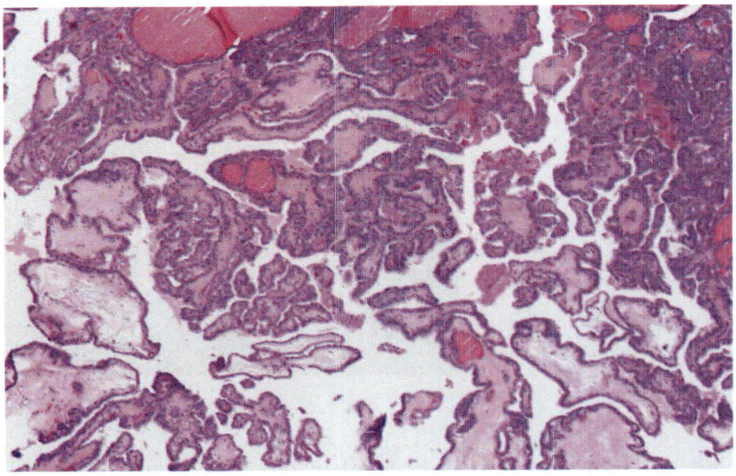

Fig. 4.254 Surgical histopathology showing papillae in papillary carcinoma

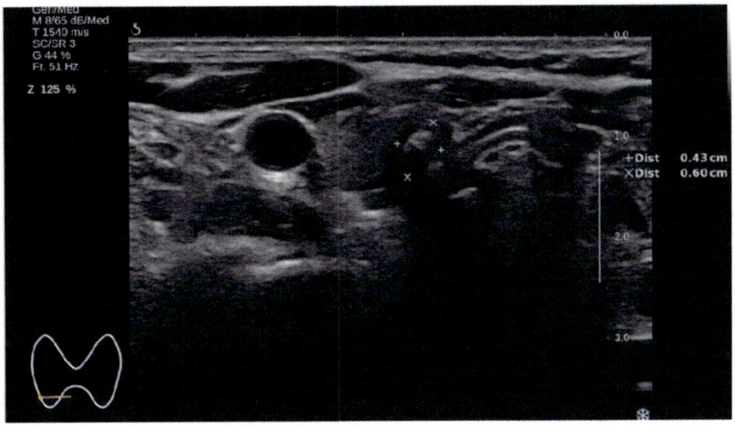

Fig. 4.255 On ultrasonogram 0.60 cm hypoechoeic suspicious malignant nodule with irregular border was found in the right lower isthmic region

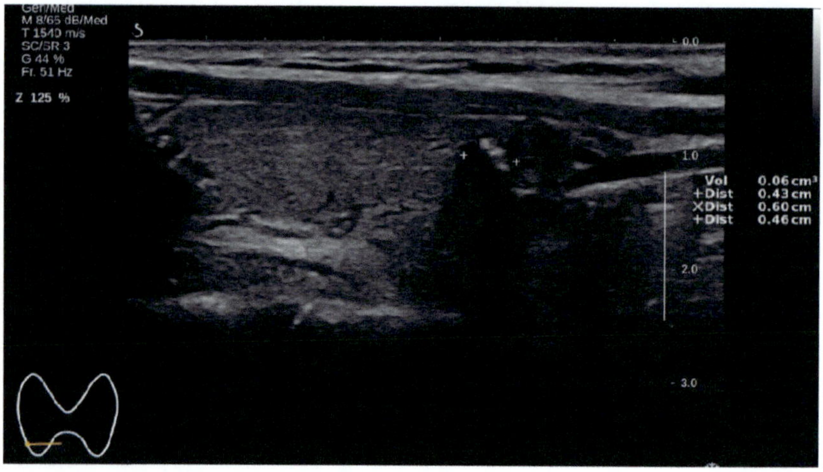

Fig. 4.256 On ultrasonogram 0.60 cm hypoechoic suspicious malignant nodule with irregular border was found in the right lower isthmic region

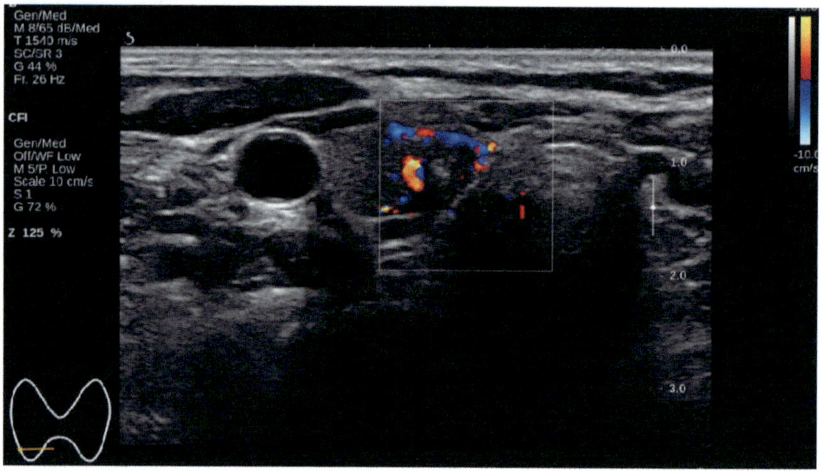

Fig. 4.257 Color Doppler showed moderately increased internal vascularity within the nodule

and 4.248). Fibrosis was observed in the central area of the tumor on the Masson Trichrome stain (Fig. 4.246), which matched the high elasticity area on the shear wave elastography (Fig. 4.244).

4.5.10 Case 10

A 46-year-old woman was found to have a left thyroid nodule on routine check. On ultrasonogram, a 0.87 cm partly hypoechoic irregularly bordered nodule was found in the left upper lobe (Figs. 4.249 and 4.250). Shear wave elastogram showed low elasticity in the nodule with E_{Max} 40.9 kPa (Fig. 4.251). FNA suggested papillary carcinoma and she underwent total thyroidectomy. Surgical histopathology revealed papillary carcinoma (Figs. 4.252, 4.253, and 4.254), and the Masson Trichrome stain showed no fibrosis in the internal region of the nodule (Fig. 4.253), which was compatible with low EI on SWE (Fig. 4.253).

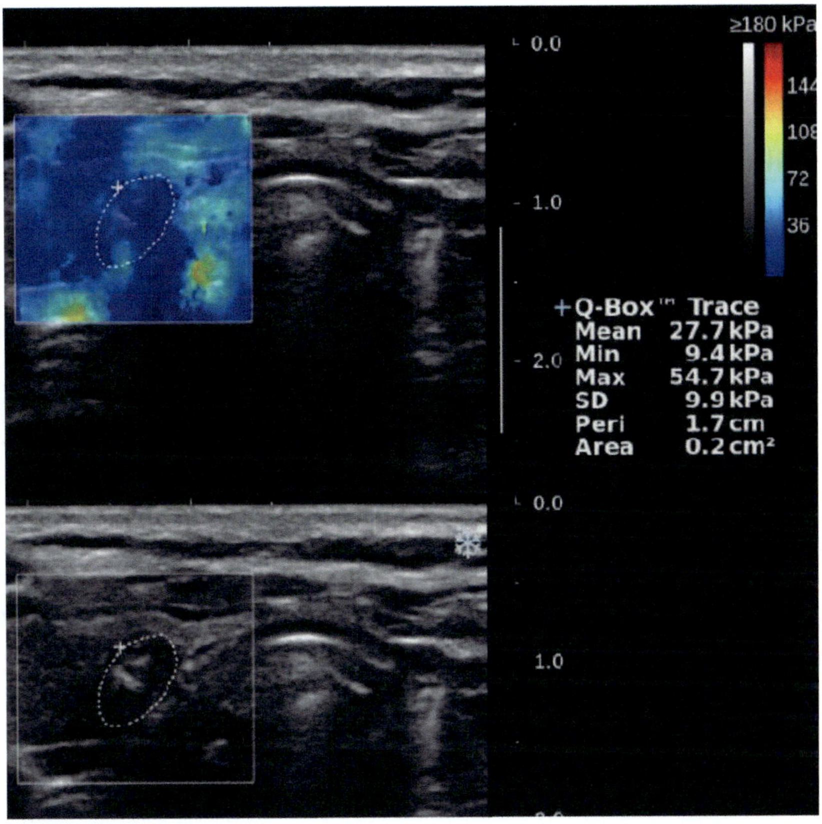

Fig. 4.258 Shear wave elastogram showed increased E1 (E_{Max}; 54.7 kPa) in the central portion of the nodule

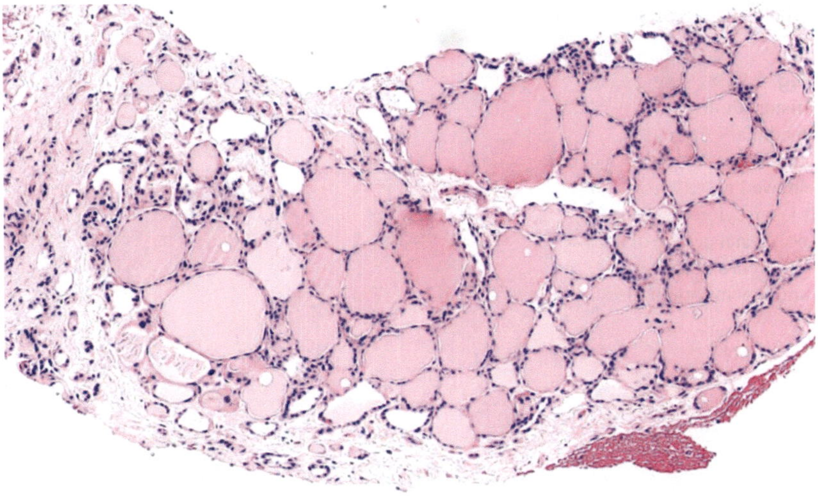

Fig. 4.259 CNB result was nodular hyperplasia

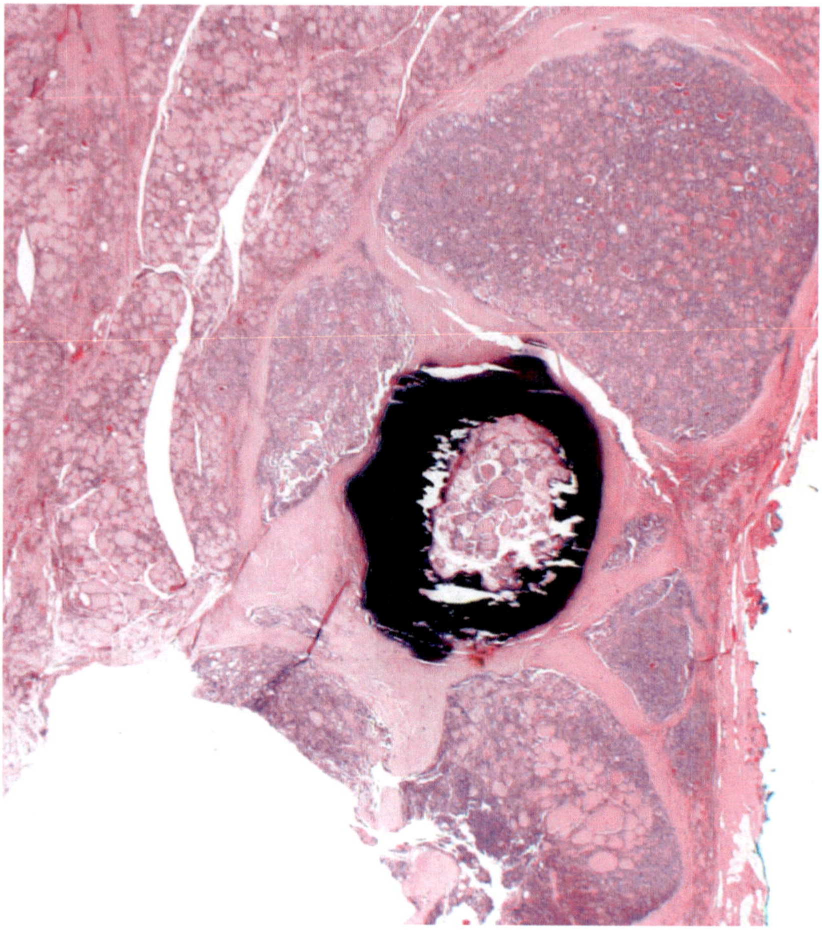

Fig. 4.260 Surgical histopathology was follicular variant papillary carcinoma with fibrosis and calcification in the central region of the tumor

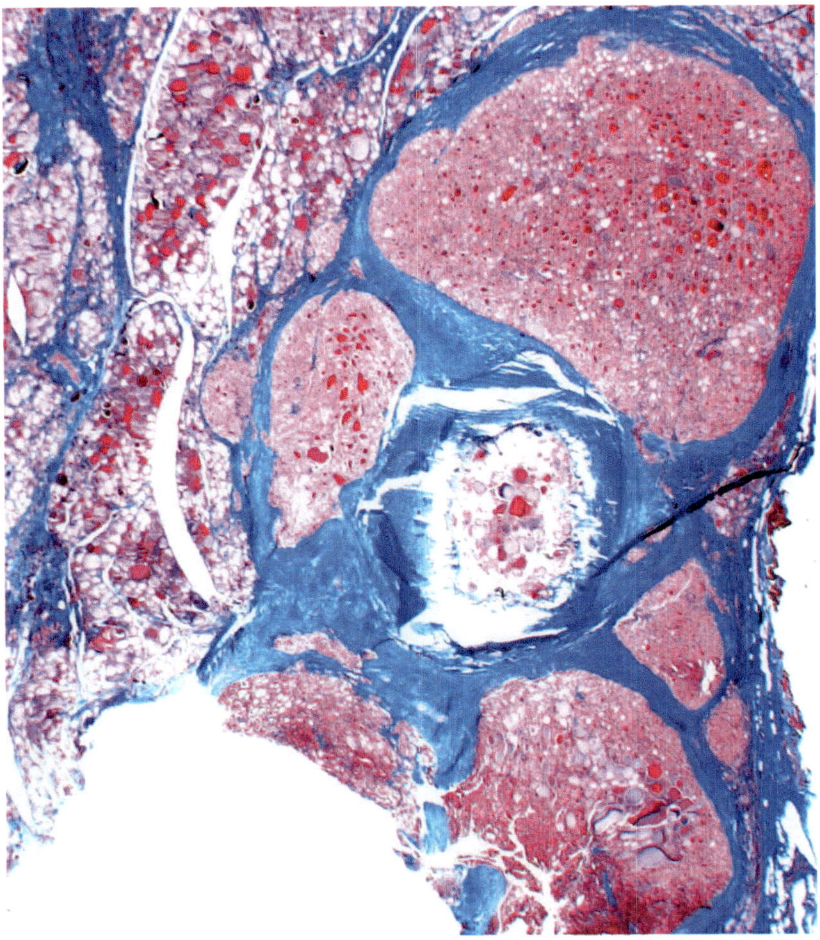

Fig. 4.261 Surgical histopathology was follicular variant papillary carcinoma with lymph node metastasis and showed areas of increased fibrosis with calcification was located in the central portion of the nodule on Masson Trichrome stain which was consistent with the central high EI area on shear wave elastography

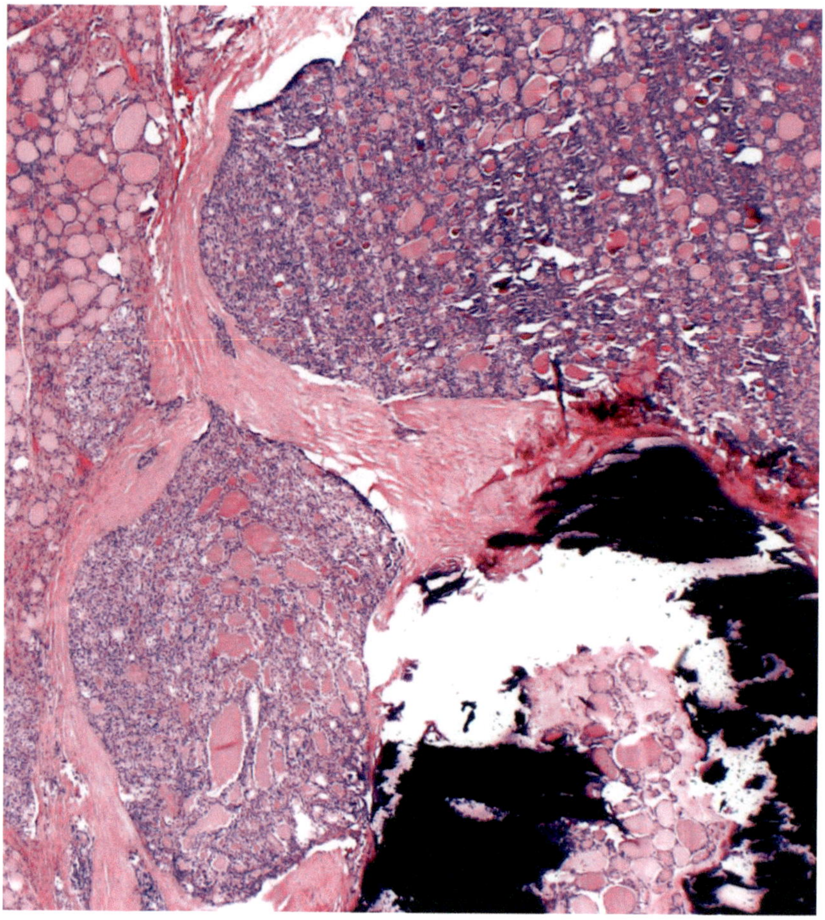

Fig. 4.262 Surgical histopathology showing follicular variant papillary carcinoma

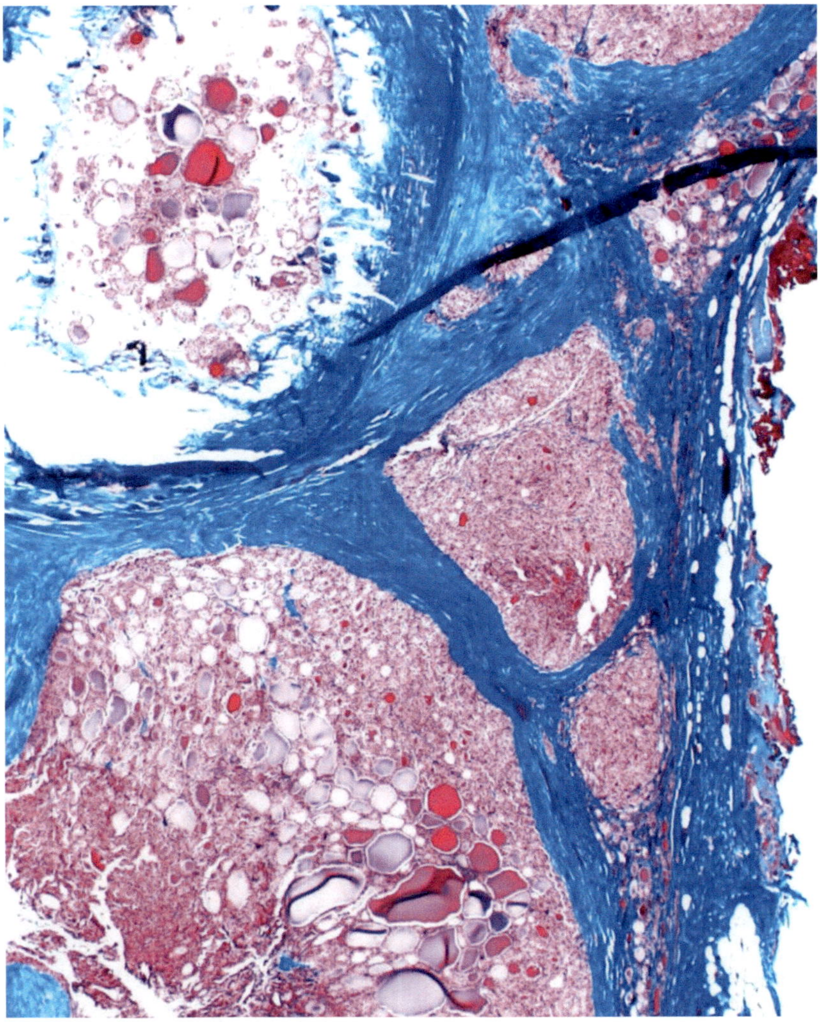

Fig. 4.263 Surgical histopathology showing follicular variant papillary carcinoma with central fibrosis on Masson Trichrome stain

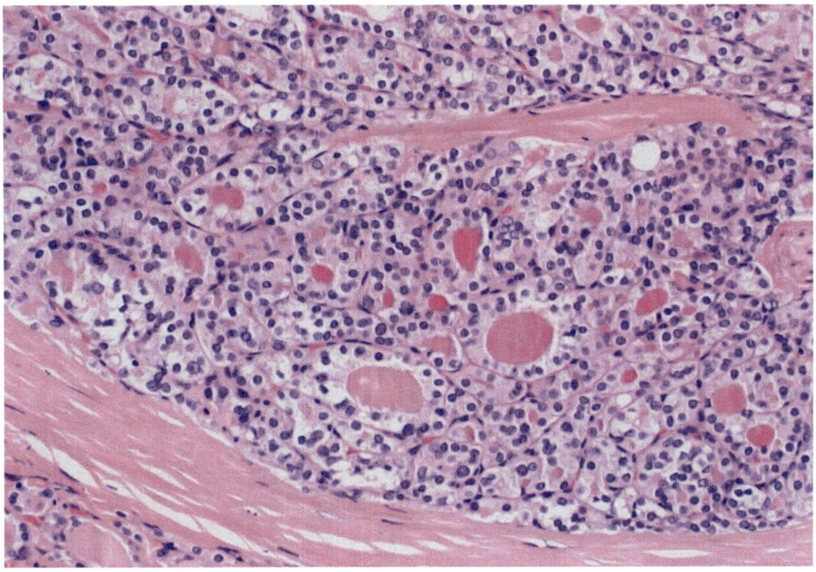

Fig. 4.264 Surgical histopathology showing follicular variant papillary carcinoma

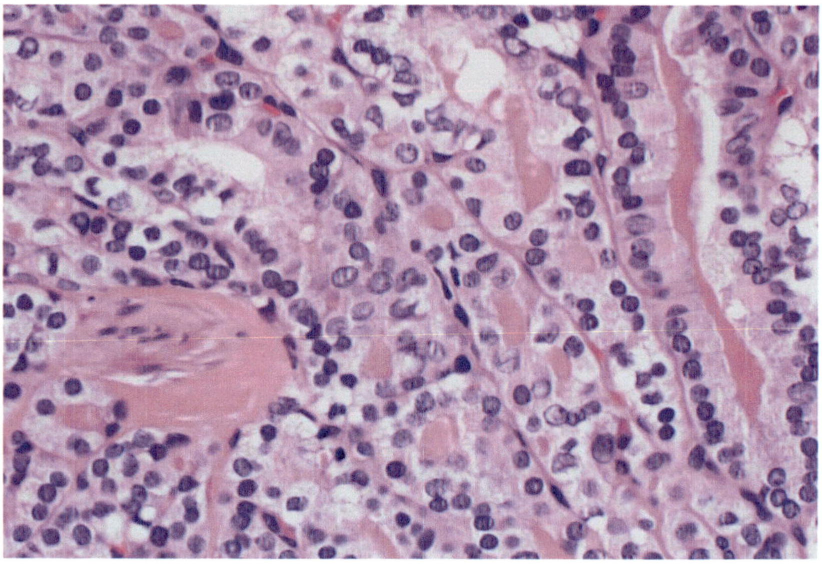

Fig. 4.265 Surgical histopathology showing follicular variant papillary carcinoma

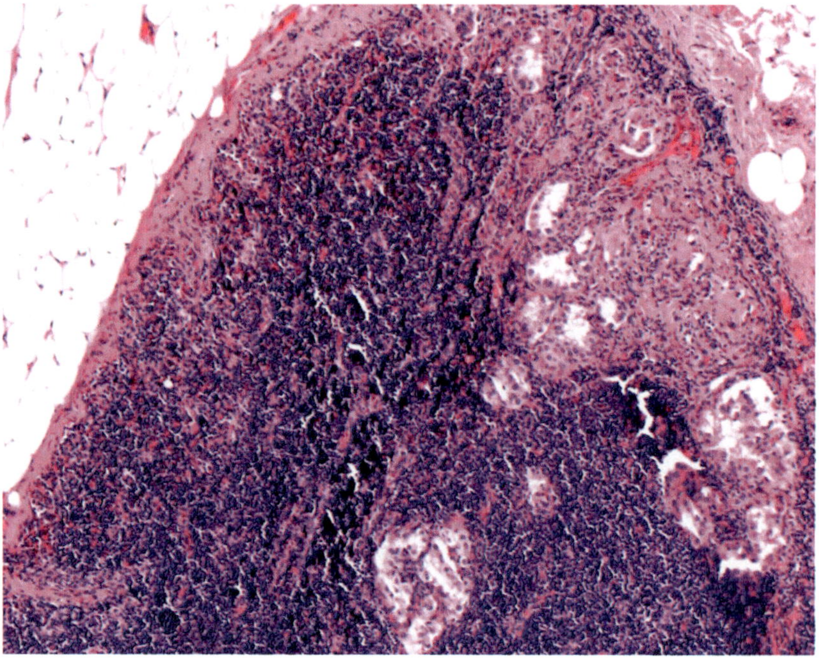

Fig. 4.266 Surgical histopathology showing follicular variant papillary carcinoma with lymph node metastasis

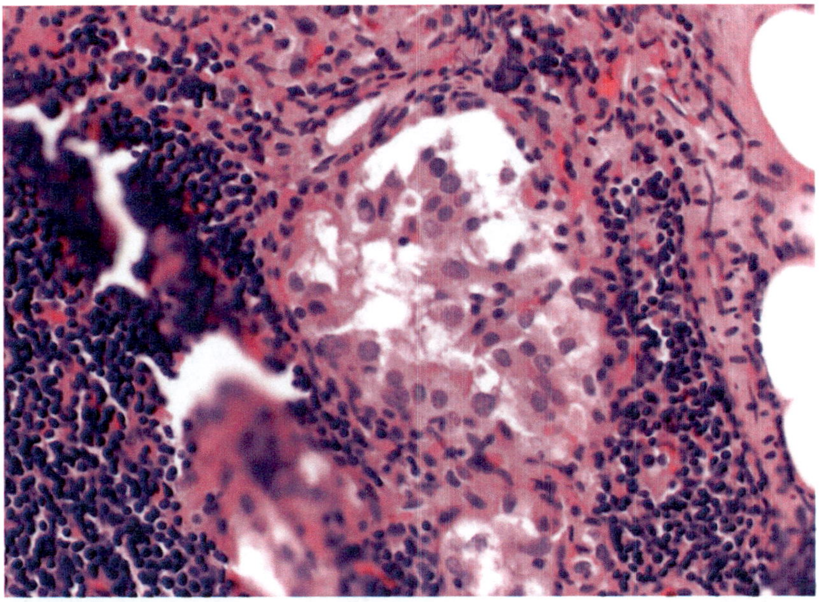

Fig. 4.267 Surgical histopathology was follicular variant papillary carcinoma with lymph node metastasis. Follicular papillary ca cells were seen to invade the lymph node

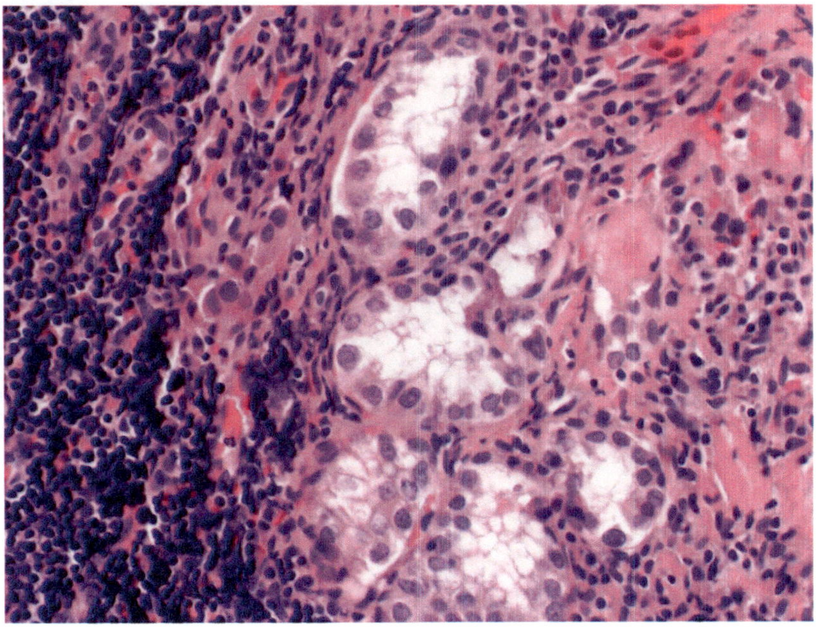

Fig. 4.268 Follicular variant papillary carcinoma cells in the follicular arranngements were seen in the lymph node

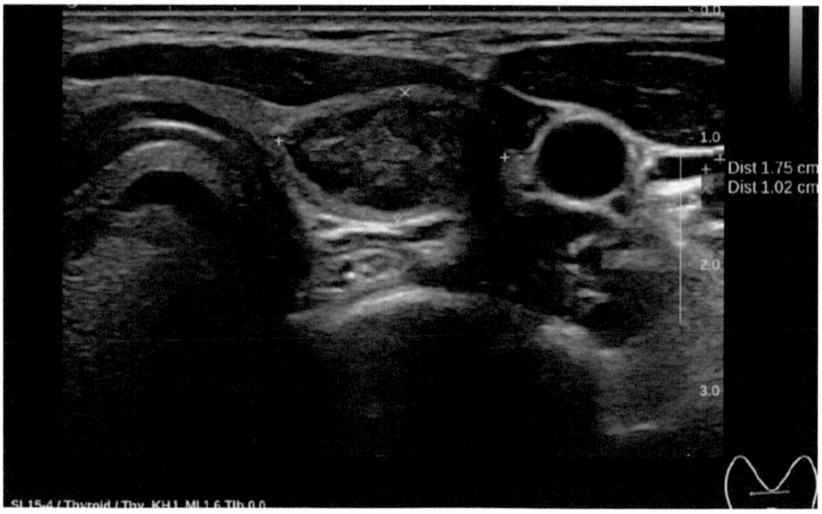

Fig. 4.269 USG showed 2.95 cm round nodule in the left lobe

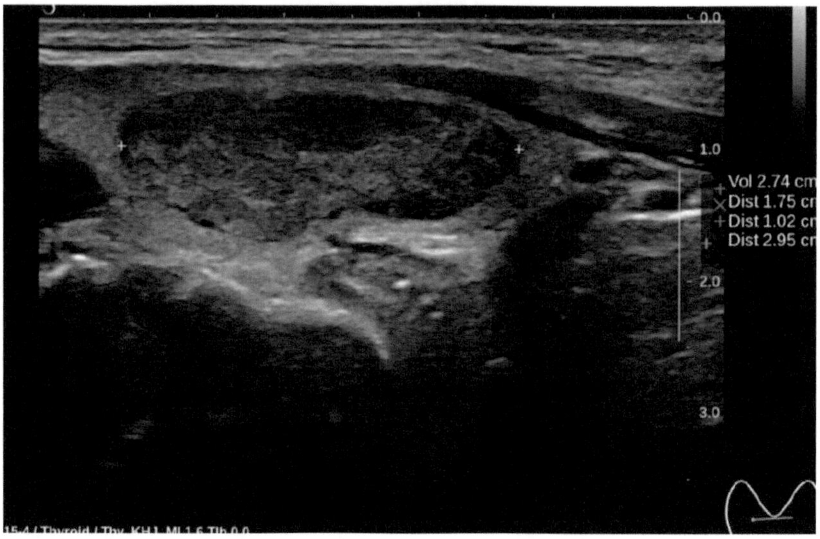

Fig. 4.270 USG showed 2.95 cm round nodule in the left lobe

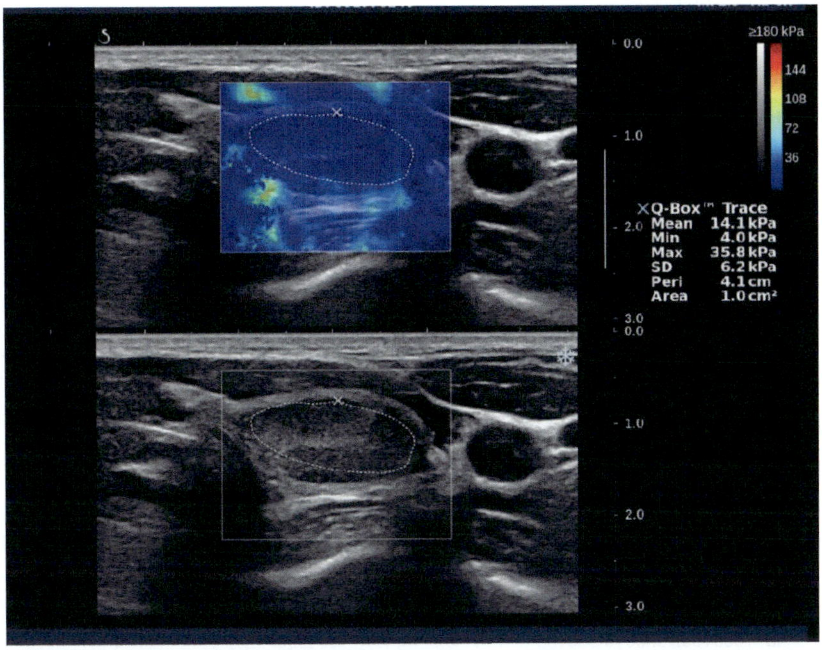

Fig. 4.271 SWE showed low elasticity and E_{Max} was 32.3 kPa and high elasticity was seen only around the margin of the nodule (marginal pattern; E_{Max} 77.6 kPa)

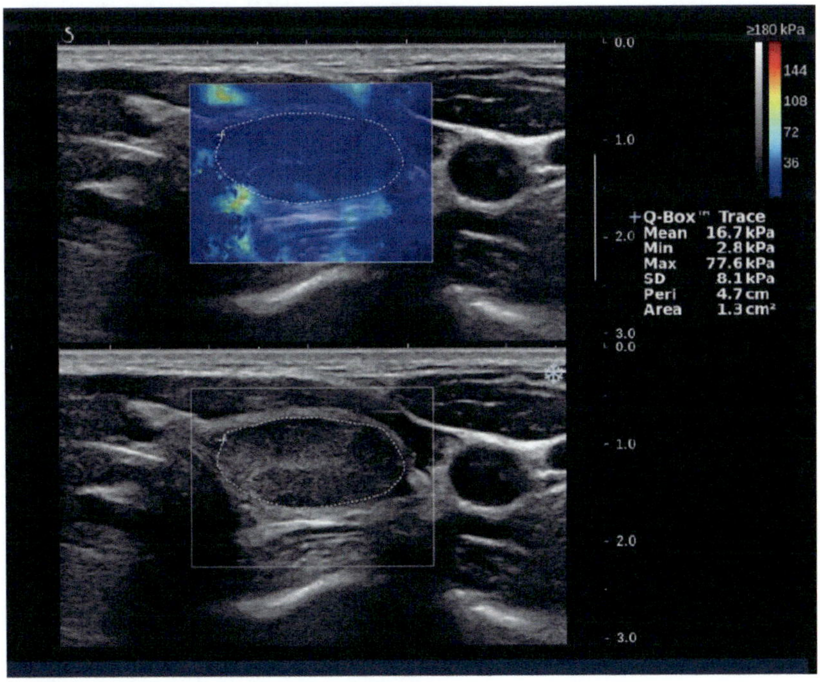

Fig. 4.272 SWE showed low elasticity (E_{Max} 32.3 kPa) and high elasticity only around the margin of the nodule (marginal pattern E_{Max} 77.6 kPa)

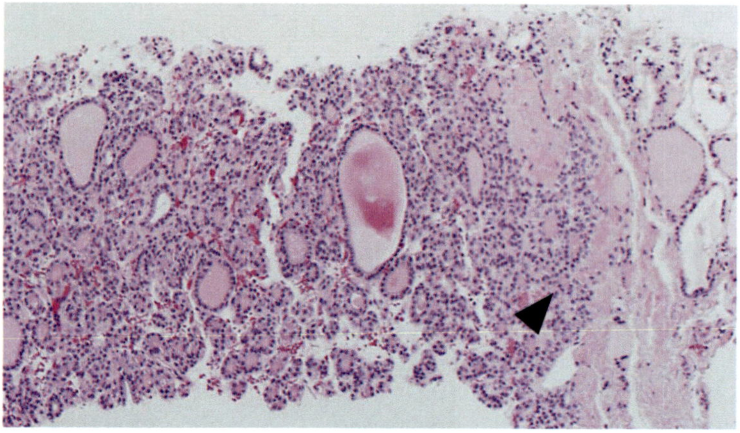

Fig. 4.273 CNB showed microfollicular patterned neoplasm with capsule (arrow)

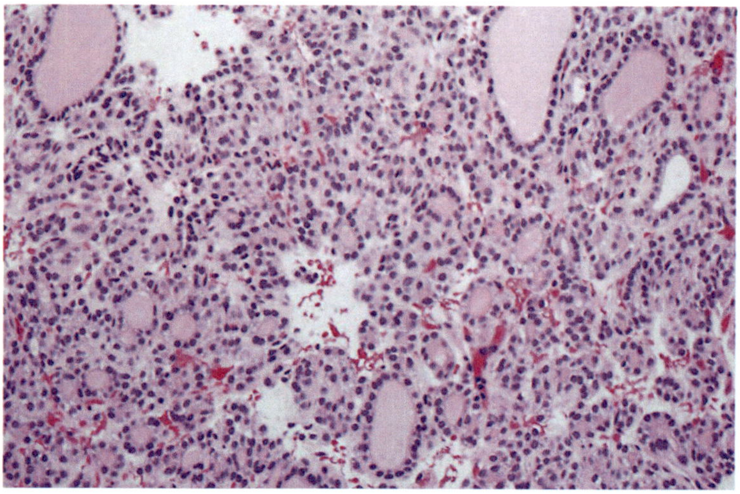

Fig. 4.274 CNB showed microfollicular patterned neoplasm

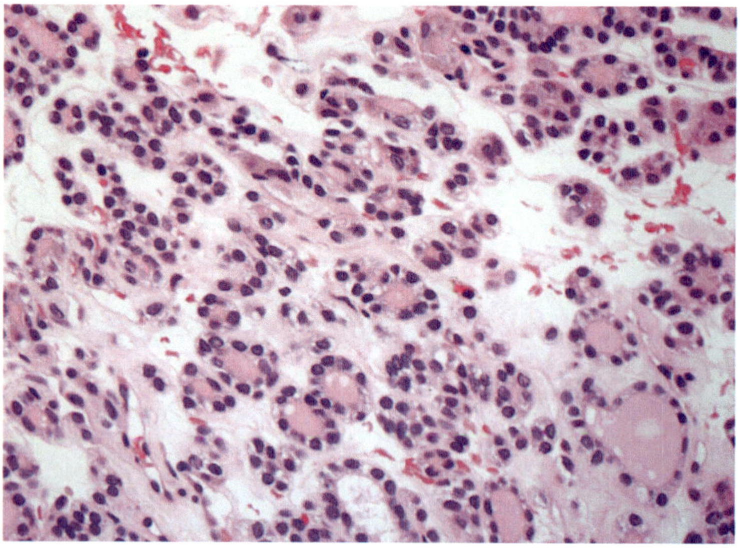

Fig. 4.275 CNB showed microfollicular patterned neoplasm showing microfollicular or abortive follicles

4.5.11 Case 11

A 40-year-old woman was found to have a thyroid nodule on routine check. On ultrasonogram, a 0.60 cm hypoechoic suspicious malignant nodule with irregular border was found in the right lower isthmic region (Figs. 4.255, 4.256, and 4.257). Shear wave elastogram showed increased E1 (E_{Max}; 54.7 kPa) in the central portion of the nodule (Fig. 4.258). The FNA result was atypia

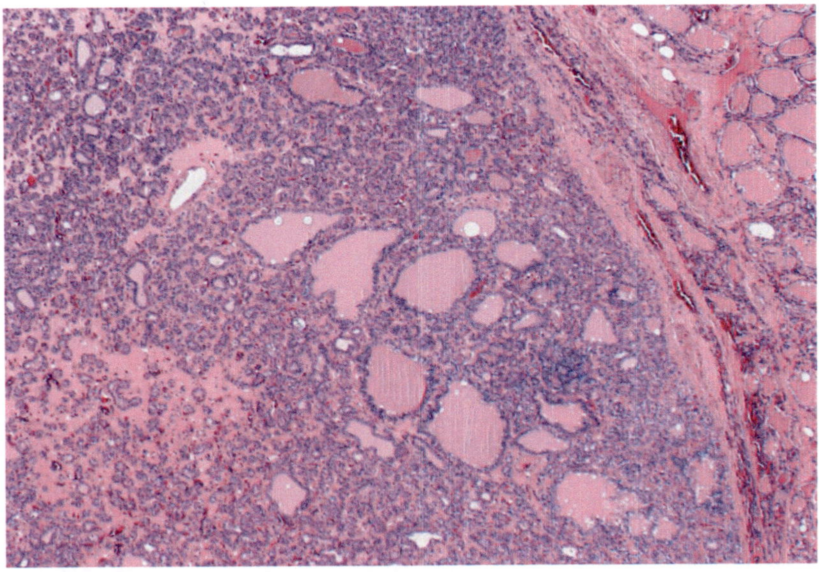

Fig. 4.276 Surgical histopathology was follicular variant papillary carcinoma showing little fibrosis on Masson Trichrome stain (Fig. 4.279) which matches the low elasticity of the nodule (Fig. 4.271)

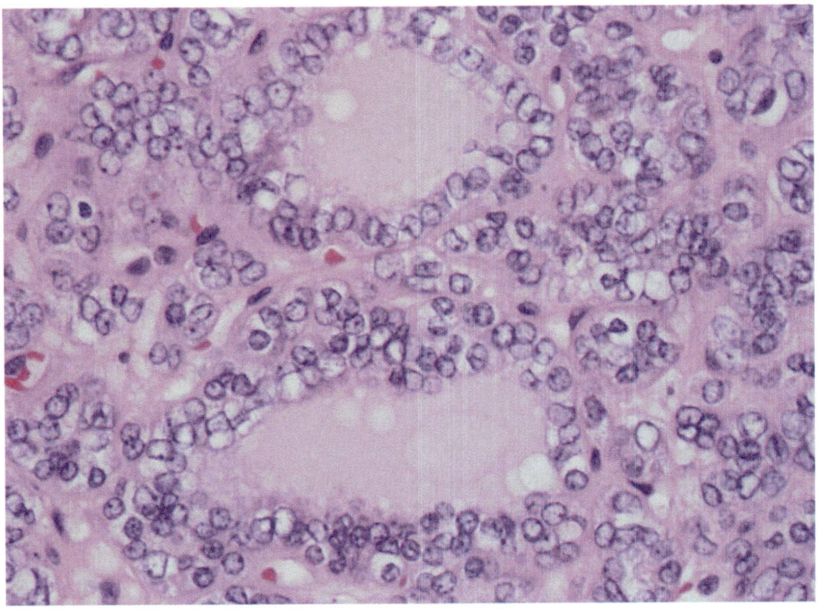

Fig. 4.277 Surgical histopathology showing follicular variant papillary carcinoma

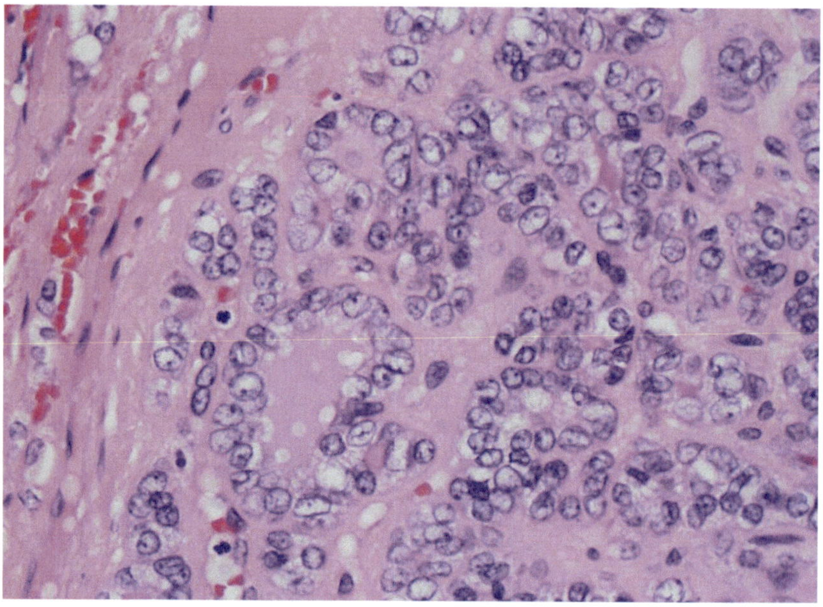

Fig. 4.278 Surgical histopathology showing follicular variant papillary carcinoma

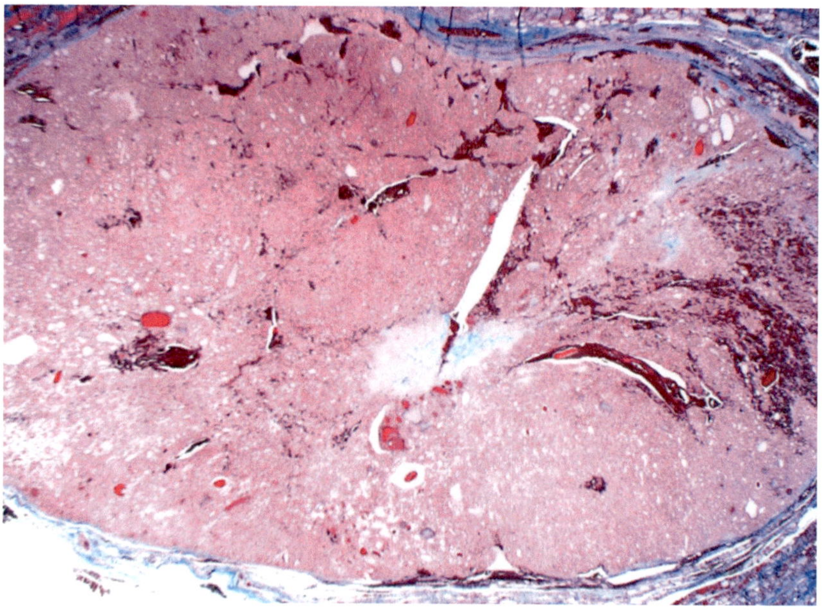

Fig. 4.279 Surgical histopathology was follicular variant papillary carcinoma showing little fibrosis on Masson Trichrome stain (Fig. 4.279) which matches the low elasticity of the nodule (Fig. 4.271)

(Category III), and the CNB result was nodular hyperplasia (Fig. 4.259). Right lobectomy was performed and surgical histopathology was follicular variant papillary carcinoma (Figs. 4.260, 4.261, 4.262, 4.263, 4.264, and 4.265) with lymph node metastasis (Figs. 4.266, 4.267, and 4.268) and showed areas of increased fibrosis with calcification was located in the central portion of the nodule on the Masson Trichrome stain (Figs. 4.261 and 4.263), which was consistent with the central high EI area on shear wave elastography (Fig. 4.258).

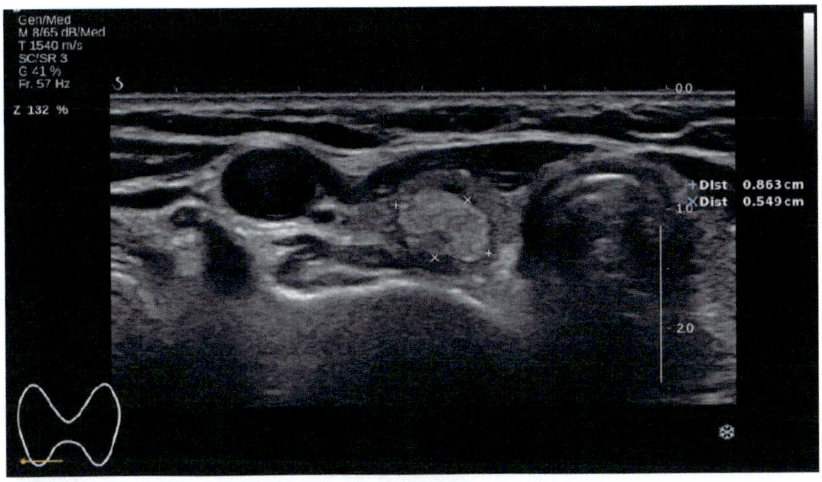

Fig. 4.280 On ultrasonogram 0.97 cm hyperechoic nodule was found in the right lower lobe

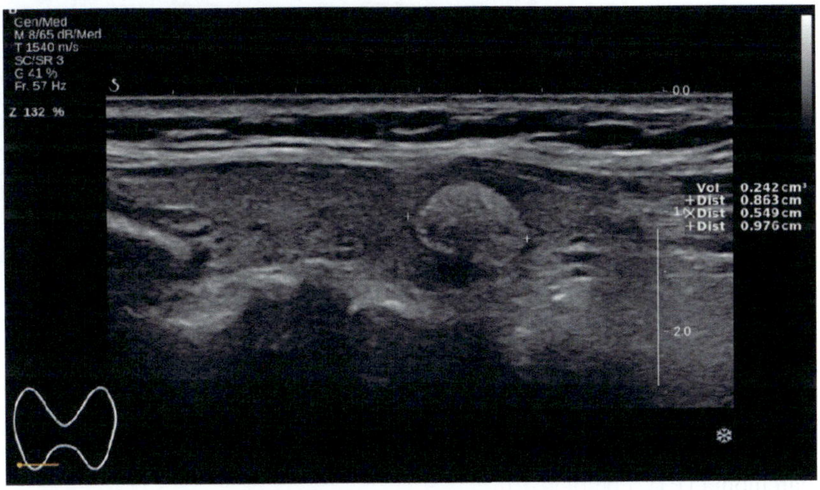

Fig. 4.281 On ultrasonogram 0.97 cm hyperechoic nodule was found in the right lower lobe

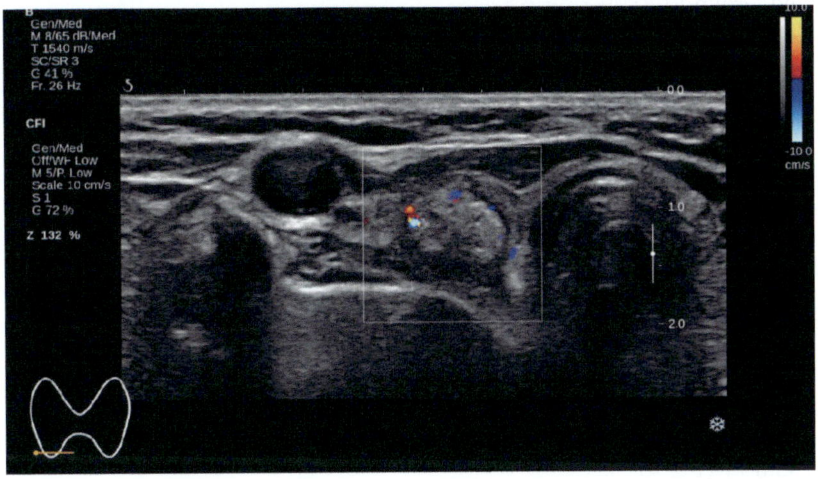

Fig. 4.282 Little internal vascularity was observed on color Doppler

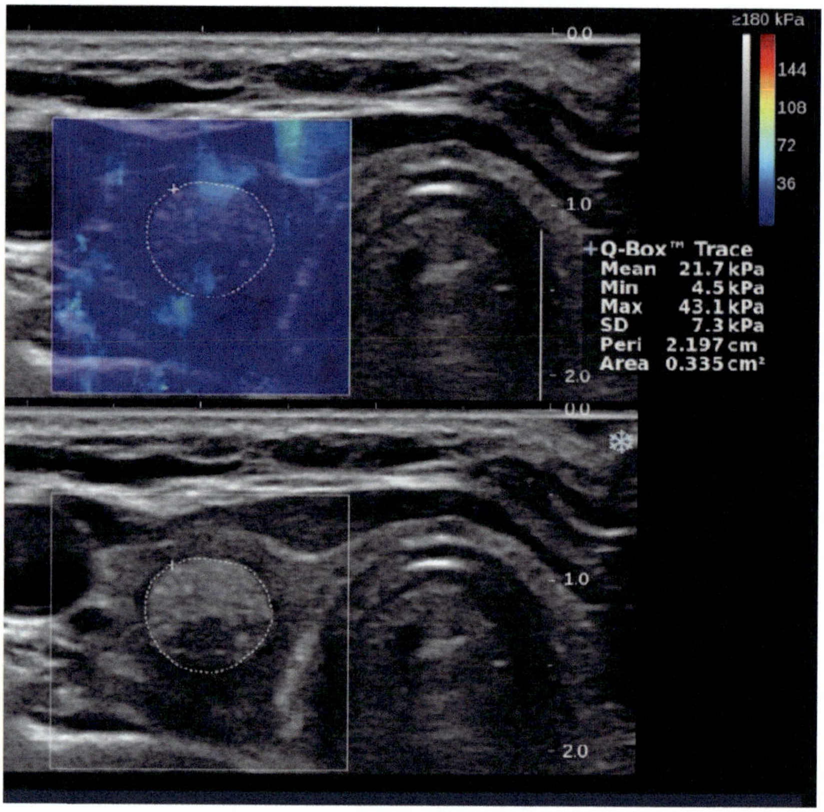

Fig. 4.283 Shear wave elastogram showed low elasticity (E_{Max} 43.1 kPa) in the entire nodule

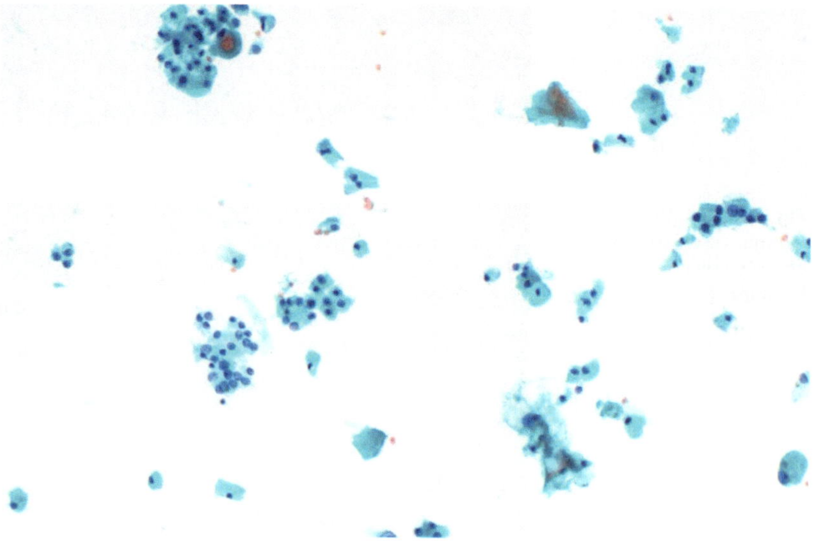

Fig. 4.284 FNA showed many oncocytic cells

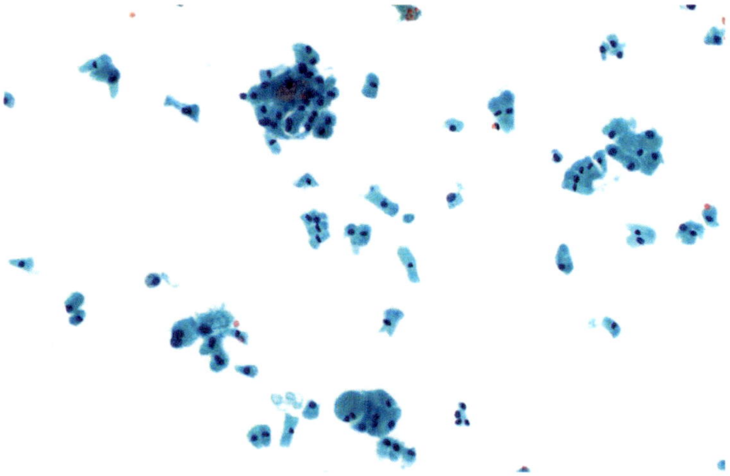

Fig. 4.285 FNA showed many oncocytic cells

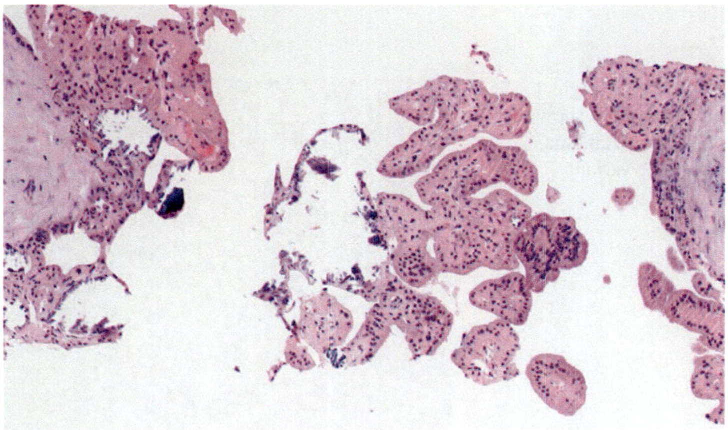

Fig. 4.286 CNB result was oncocytic variant papillary carcinoma showing Hurthle cell proliferative lesion

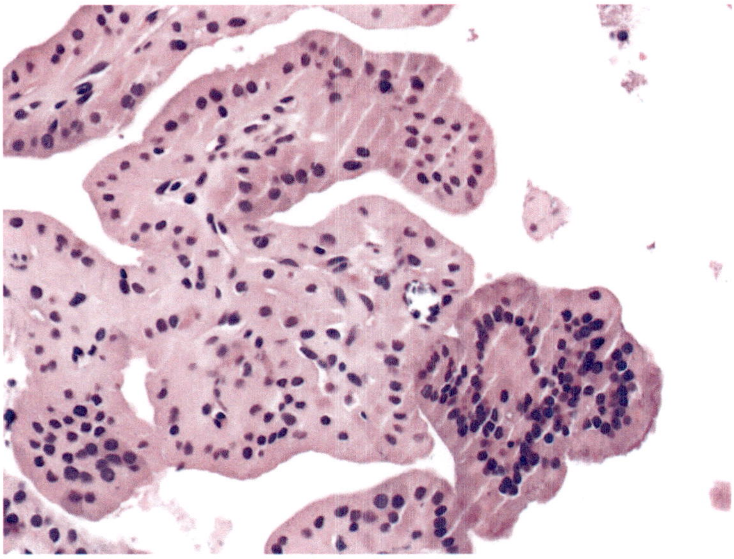

Fig. 4.287 CNB result was oncocytic variant papillary carcinoma. Tumor consists of large cells with abundant eosinophilic cytoplasm and round nuclei with prominent nucleoli

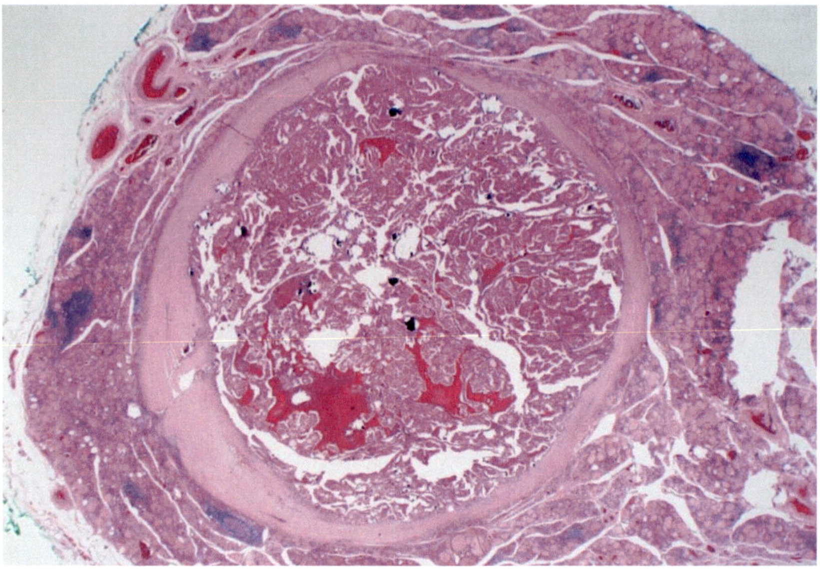

Fig. 4.288 Surgical histopathology was papillary carcinoma, oncocytic variant and showed scanty amount of fibrosis in the tumor which was compatible with the 2D shear wave elastography (Fig. 4.283)

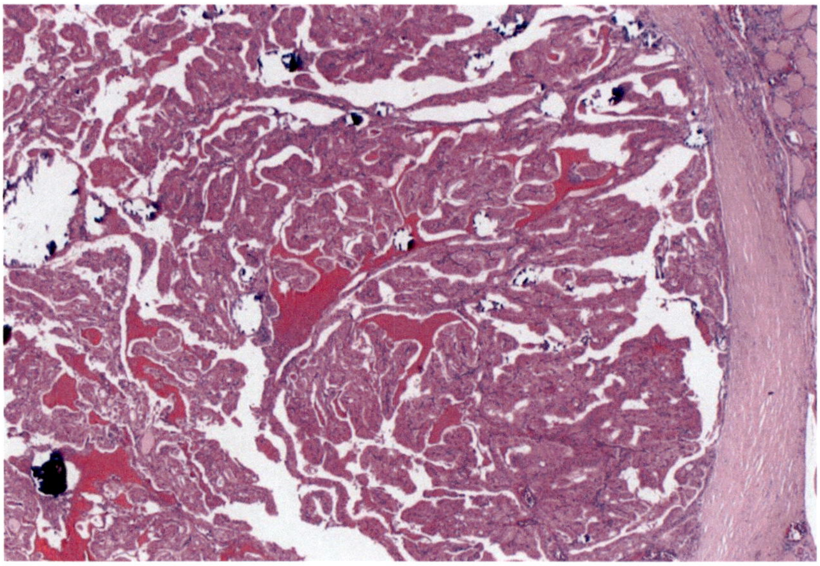

Fig. 4.288 Surgical histopathology showing papillary carcinoma, oncocytic variant

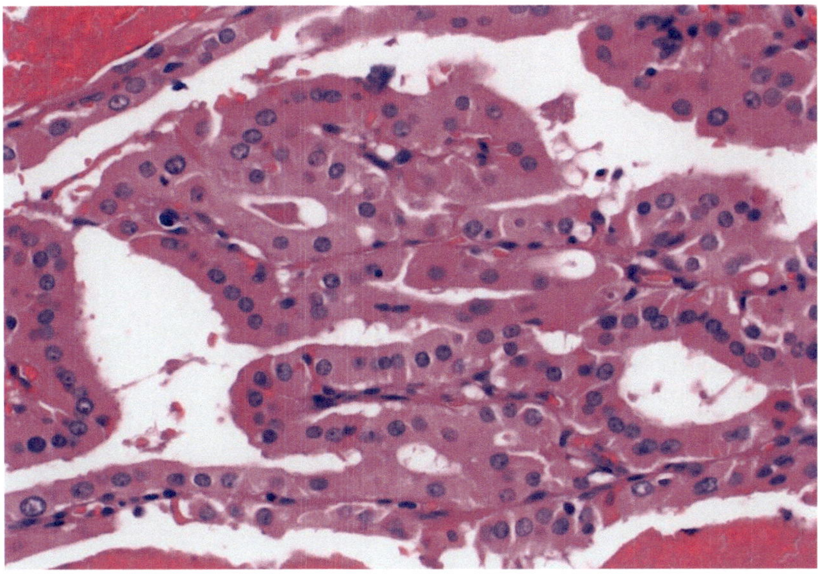

Fig. 4.290 Papillary thyroid carcinoma, oncocytic variant showing tumor cells with abundant eosinophilic cytoplasm and characteristic nuclear features of conventional papillary thyroid carcinoma

4.5.12 Case 12

A 39-year-old man was referred for a thyroid nodule found on routine check. USG showed a 2.54 cm round nodule in the left lobe and the FNA result was benign follicular lesion. A follow-up after three years showed 2.95 cm nodule (Figs. 4.269 and 4.270) and SWE showed low elasticity (E_{Max} 32.3 kPa, Fig. 4.271) and high elasticity only around the margin of the nodule (marginal pattern E_{Max} 77.6 kPa, Fig. 4.272). CNB showed microfollicular patterned neoplasm (Figs. 4.273, 4.274, and 4.275) with capsule (arrow, Fig. 4.273). He underwent total thyroidectomy and histopathology was follicular variant papillary carcinoma (Figs. 4.276, 4.277, and 4.278), showing little fibrosis on the Masson Trichrome stain (Fig. 4.279) which matches the low elasticity of the nodule (Fig. 4.271).

4.5.13 Case 13

A 69-year-old woman presented a thyroid nodule found incidentally. On ultrasonogram, a 0.97 cm hyperechoic nodule was found in the right lower lobe with little internal vascularity (Figs. 4.280, 4.281, and 4.282). Shear wave elastogram showed low elasticity (E_{Max} 43.1 kPa) in the entire nodule (Fig. 4.283). FNA showed many oncocytic cells (Figs. 4.284 and 4.285) and the CNB result was oncocytic variant papillary carcinoma (Figs. 4.286 and 4.287). Total thyroidectomy was done and surgical histopathology was papillary carcinoma, oncocytic variant, and showed scanty amount of fibrosis in the tumor (Figs. 4.288, 4.289, and 4.290), which was compatible with the 2D shear wave elastography (Fig. 4.283).

4.6 Follicular Thyroid Carcinoma

Follicular thyroid carcinoma (FTC) accounts for 6–10% of thyroid carcinoma [1] and is more frequent in dietary iodine deficient areas. FTCs are well encapsulated tumor with capsular or angioinvasion. Capsular invasion is minimally invasive or widely invasive. Vascular invasion is invasion into vessels and intravascular tumor cells should be adherent to the vessels within or beyond the tumor capsule [9].

The cytological and architectural features of FTC are similar to follicular adenoma, showing microfollicular, normofollicular, macrofollicular and trabecular patterns [9]. There is no reliable

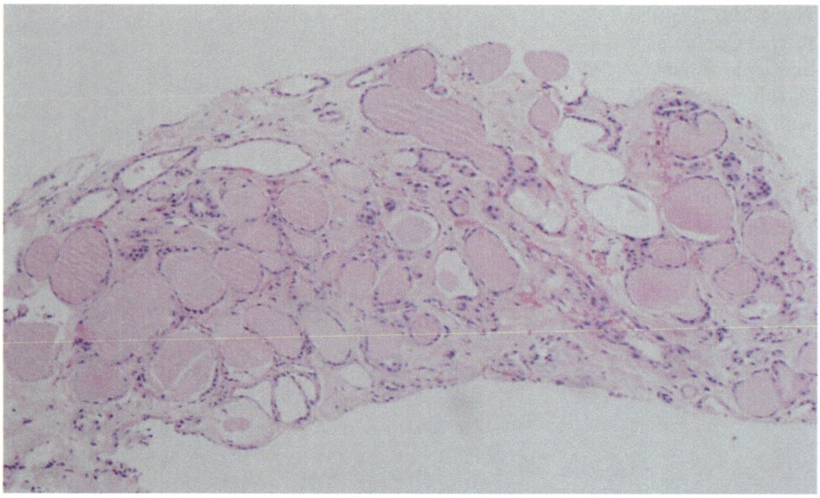

Fig. 4.291 CNB result was follicular lesion

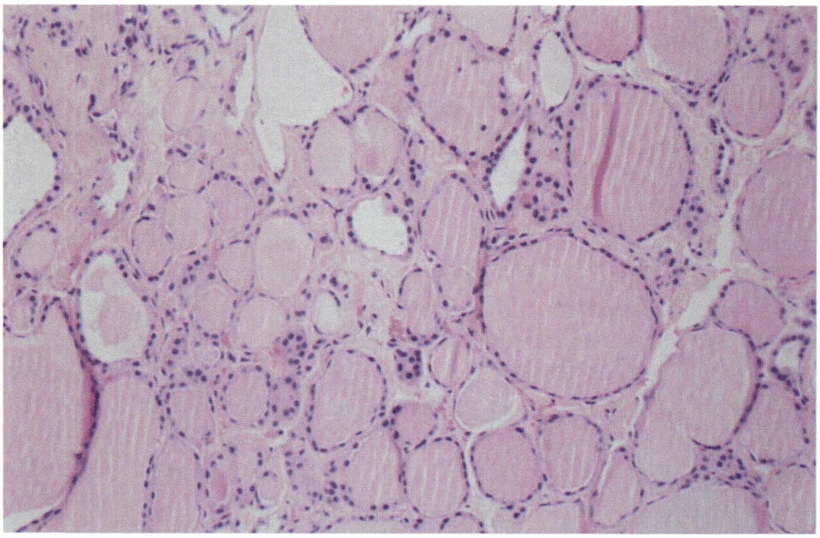

Fig. 4.292 CNB result was follicular lesion

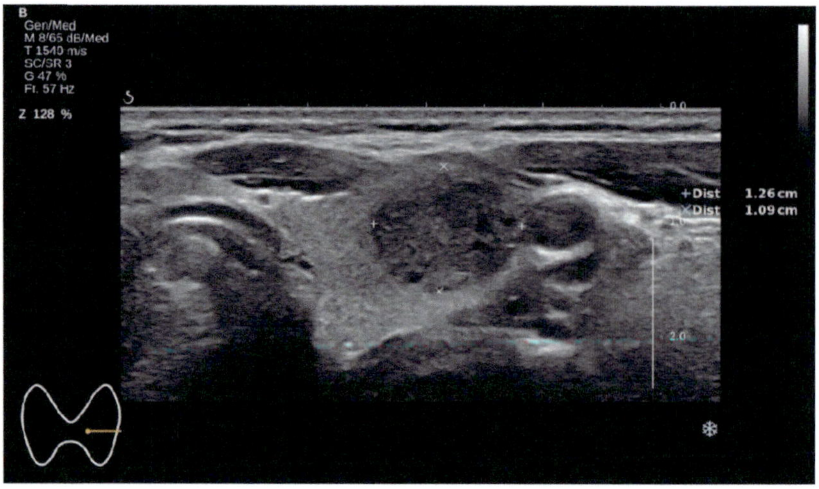

Fig. 4.293 B-mode USG showed a 1.54 cm round nodule in the left lobe

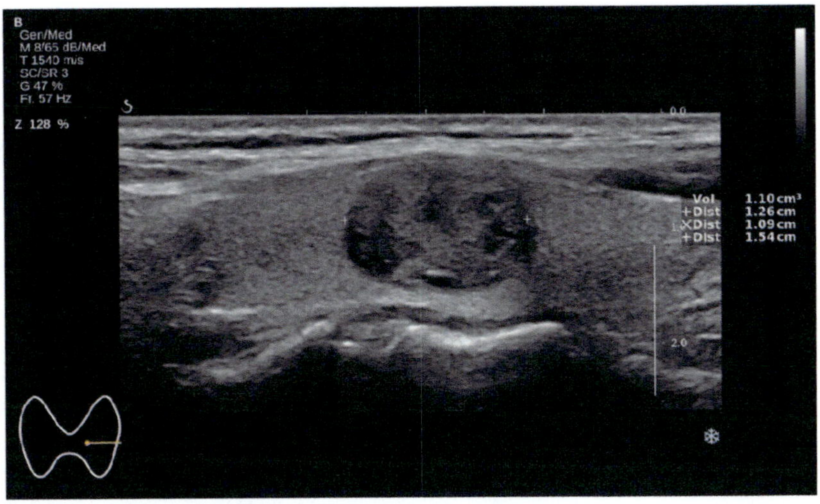

Fig. 4.294 B-mode USG showed a 1.54 cm round nodule in the left lobe

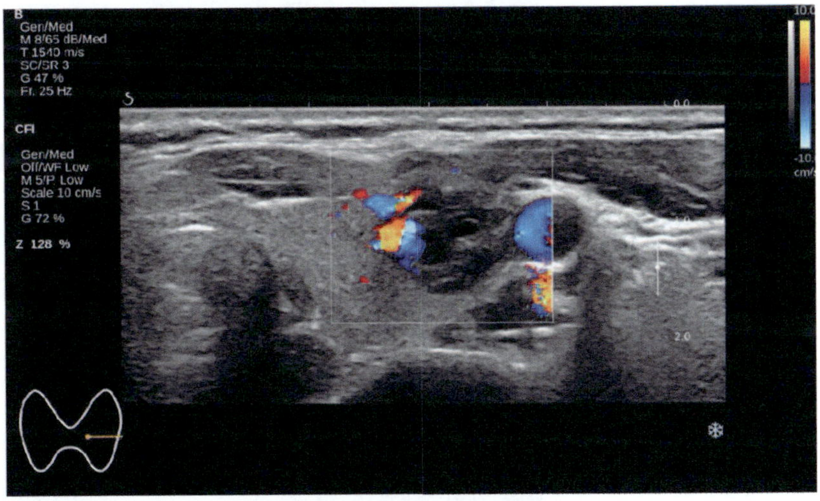

Fig. 4.295 Color Doppler showed moderately increased internal vascularity within the nodule

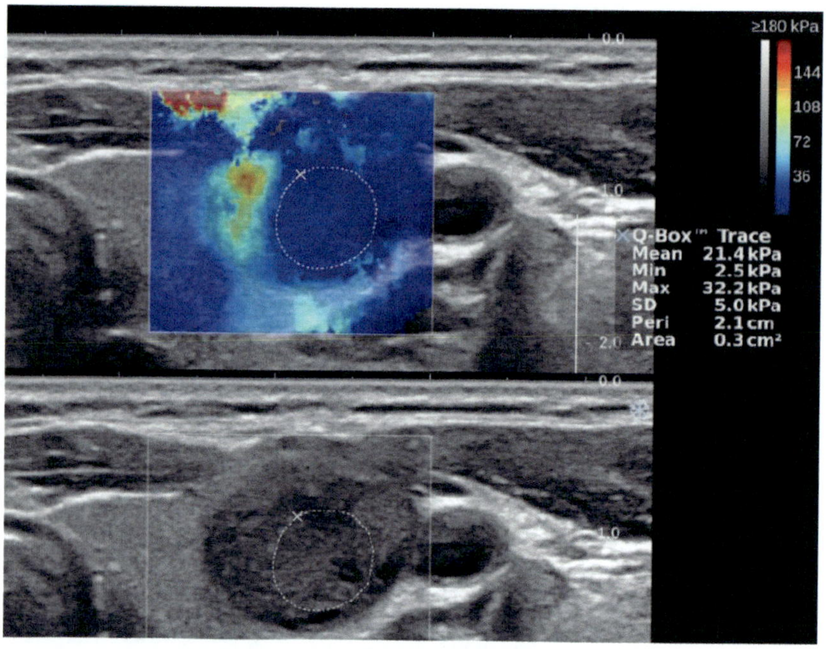

Fig. 4.296 SWE showed low elasticity in the nodule (E_{Max} 32.2 kPa) except medial margin of the nodule (E_{Max} 132.2 kPa)

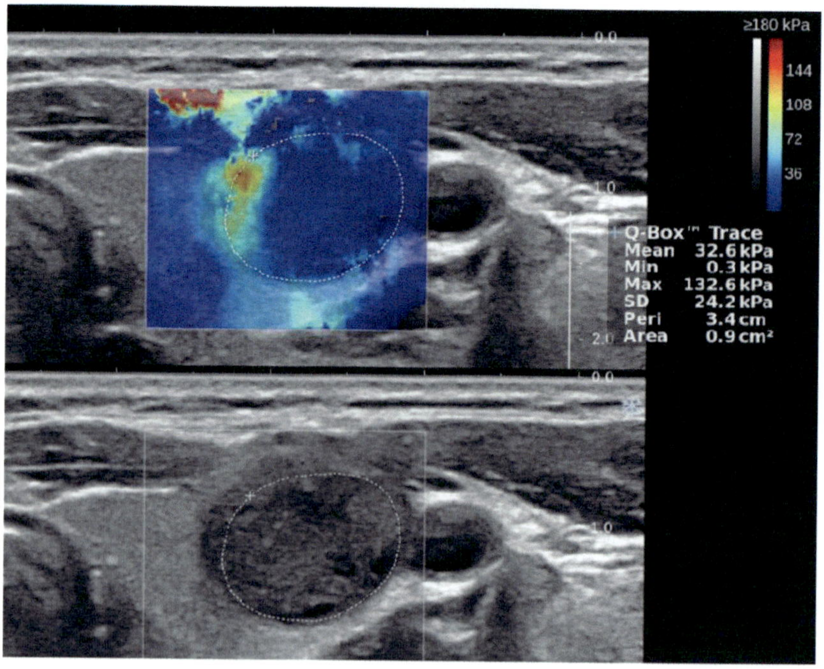

Fig. 4.297 SWE showed low elasticity in the nodule (E_{Max} 32.2 kPa) except medial margin of the nodule (E_{Max} 132.2 kPa)

cytologic difference between follicular adenoma and FTC, and the distinction requires extensive histologic evaluation of the tumor capsule for capsular or vascular invasion [1]. So benign and malignant follicular patterned lesions cannot be distinguished by FNA [9]. Occasionally, follicular tumor cells are dominated by cells with abundant granular, eosinophilic cytoplasm (Hürthle cell or oncocytic cells), and it is called a Hürthle cell tumor if the majority (greater than 75%) of the tumor is composed of Hürthle cells [9]. The cytoplasm of a Hürthle cell is filled with numerous abnormally large mitochondria with loss of cell polarity. Hürthle cell adenomas tend to have thinner capsules than carcinomas and show follicular growth pattern, which is less common in

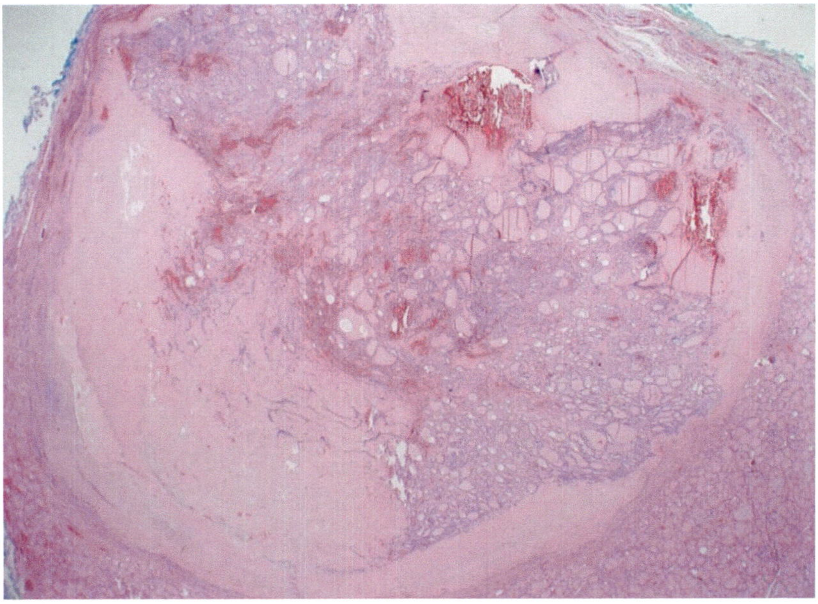

Fig. 4.298 Surgical histopathology was microinvasive follicular carcinoma showing mushroom like capsular invasion showing thick fibrous capsule in the medial margin of the nodule compatible with the finding of the high elasticity on the medial margin on SWE (Fig. 4.297)

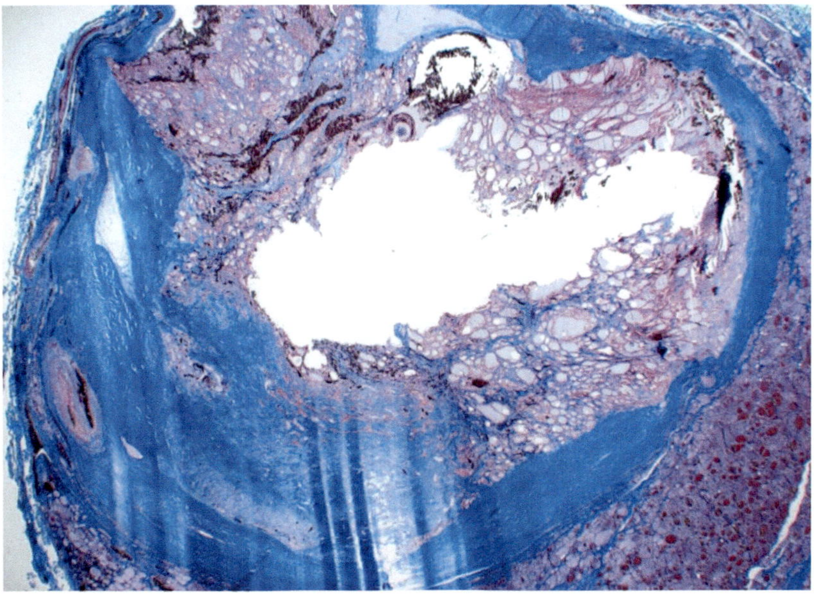

Fig. 4.299 Surgical histopathology was microinvasive follicular carcinoma showing mushroom like capsular invasion showing thick fibrous capsule in the medial margin of the nodule compatible with the finding of the high elasticity on the medial margin on SWE. (Fig. 4.297)

Hürthle cell carcinomas [9]. Malignancy should be defined by the capsular or vascular invasion. Hürthle cell carcinomas are radioiodine resistant and less favorable in prognosis than non-oncocytic FTCs. On B-mode ultrasound, follicular carcinoma showed similar patterns as follicular adenoma. SWE of FTC showed elasticity is not usually elevated in most studies.

4.6.1 Case 1

A 35-year-old woman was referred for the thyroid nodule found on routine check. USG showed a 1.75 cm round nodule in the left lobe, and the CNB result was follicular lesion (Figs. 4.291 and 4.292). Thyroxine suppression therapy was tried for one year without response and discontinued. After five years of follow-up, B-mode USG

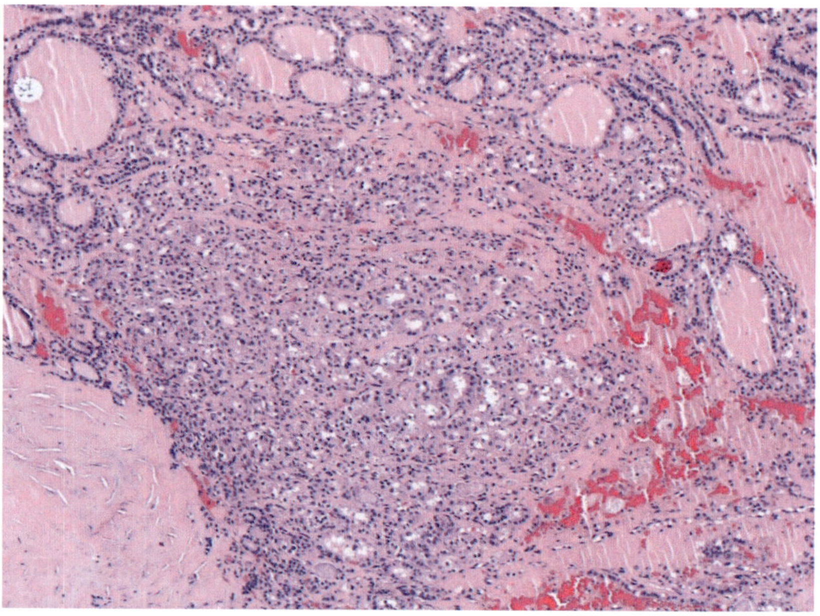

Fig. 4.300 Surgical histopathology was microinvasive follicular carcinoma showing mushroom like capsular invasion

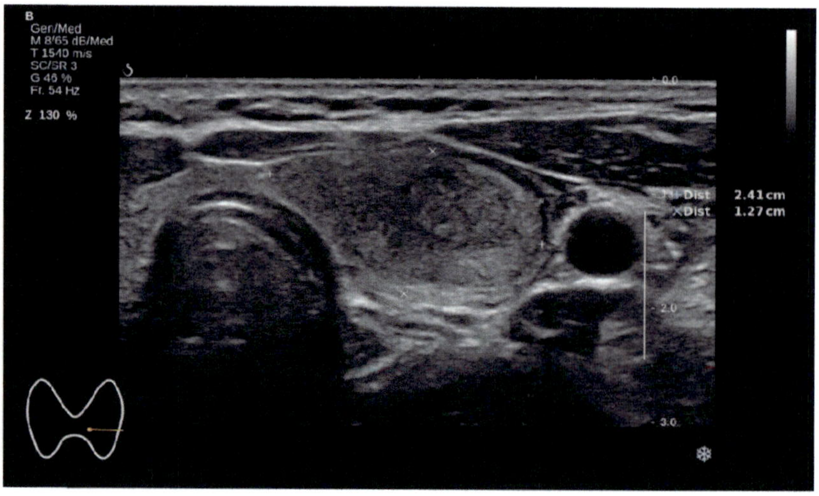

Fig. 4.301 On USG 3.54 cm isoechoic solid nodule was observed in the left lower lobe

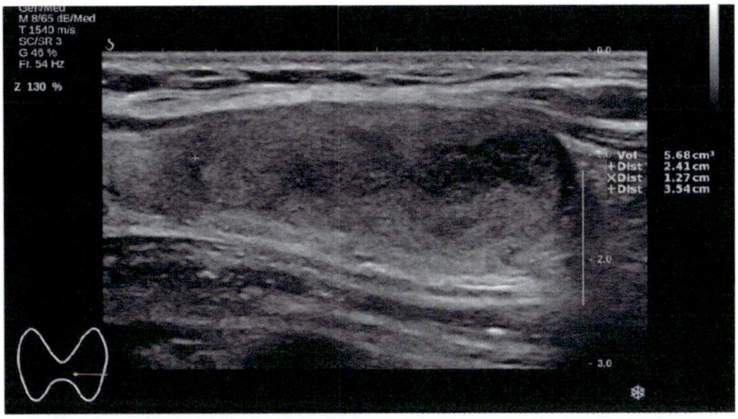

Fig. 4.302 On USG 3.54 cm isoechoic solid nodule was observed in the left lower lobe

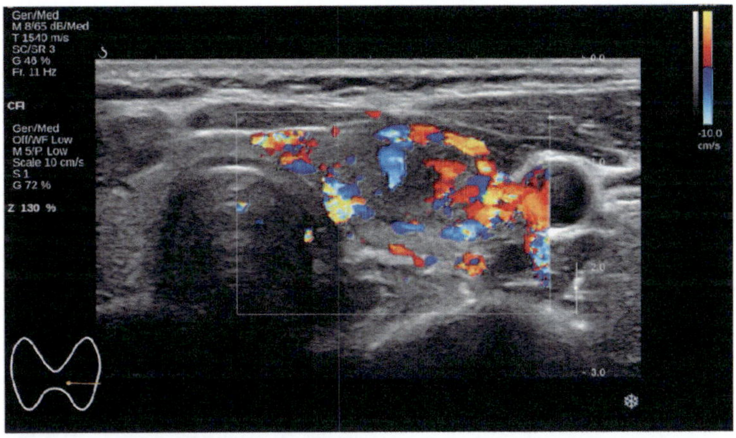

Fig. 4.303 Color Doppler showed increased internal vascularity within the nodule

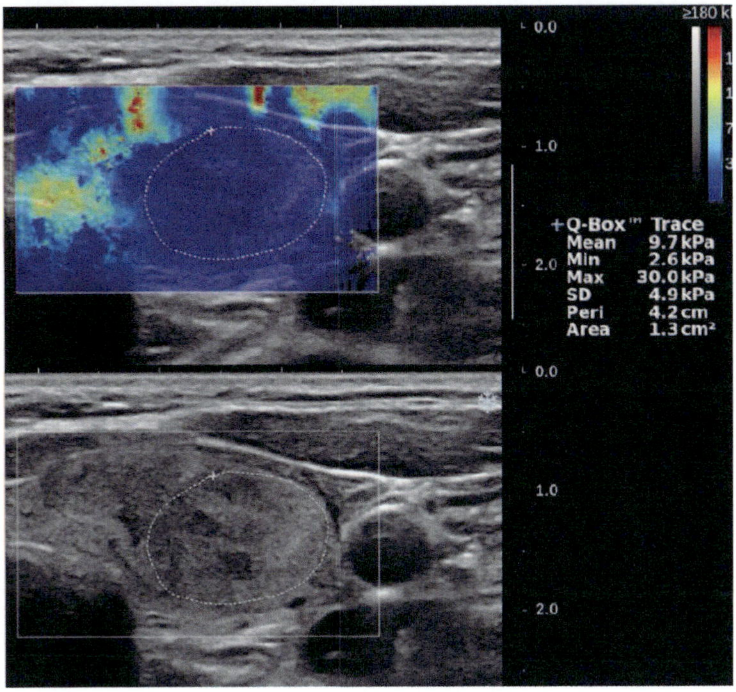

Fig. 4.304 Shear wave elastogram showed low elasticity in the whole nodule which is color coded with deep blue and E_{Max} was 30.0 kPa

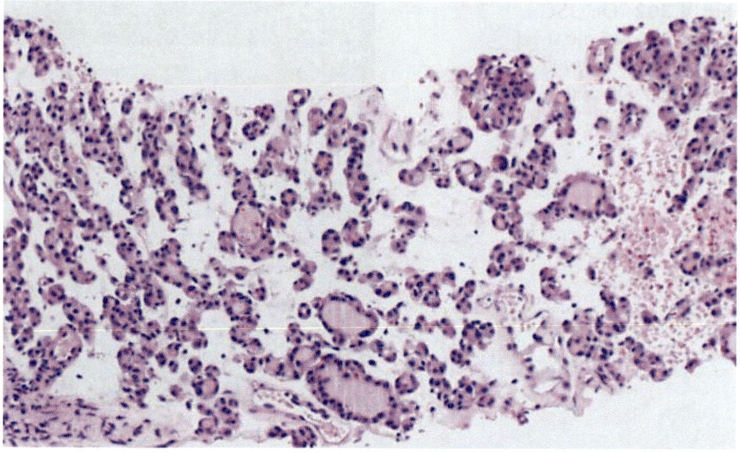

Fig. 4.305 CNB showed abortive oxyphilic microfollicles suggesting oxyphilic follicular neoplasm

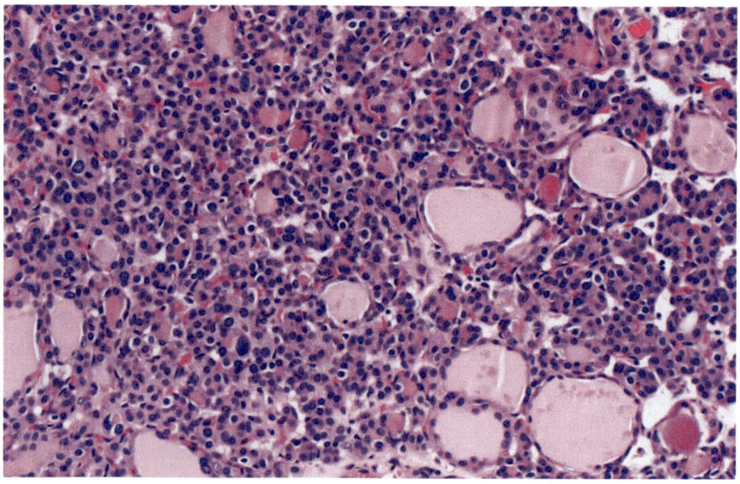

Fig. 4.306 Surgical histopathology revealed hurthle cell carcinoma showing microfollicles and abortive follicles with oxyphilic cells

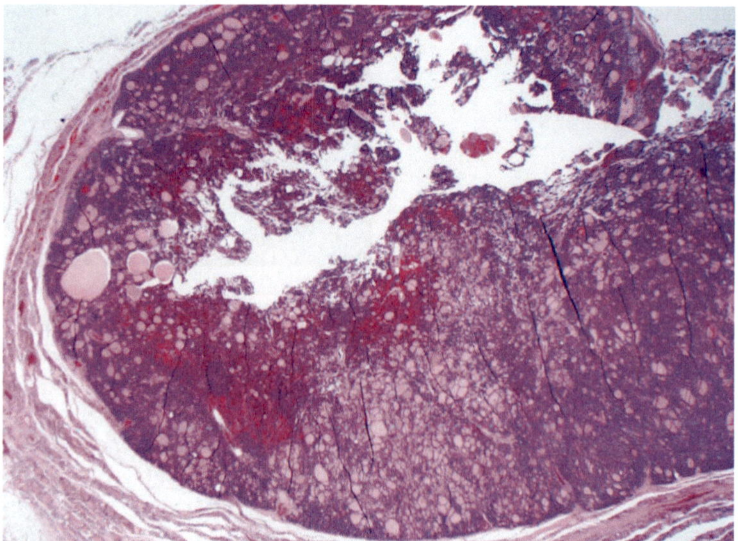

Fig. 4.307 Surgical histopathology revealed hurthle cell carcinoma

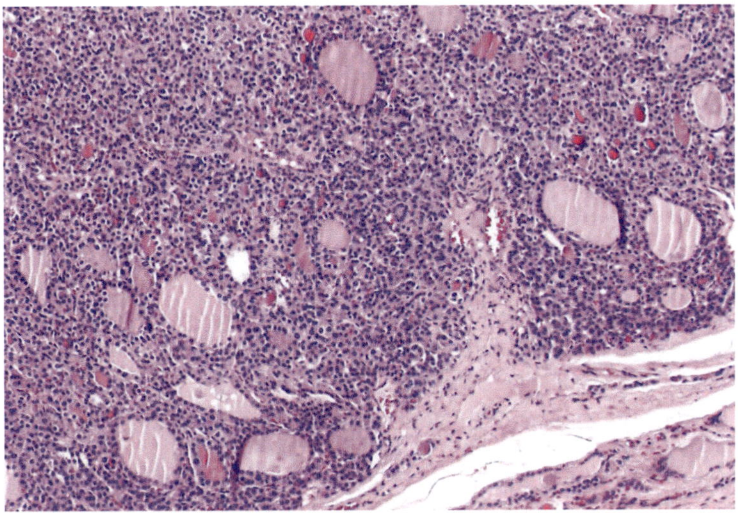

Fig. 4.308 Surgical histopathology revealed hurthle cell carcinoma

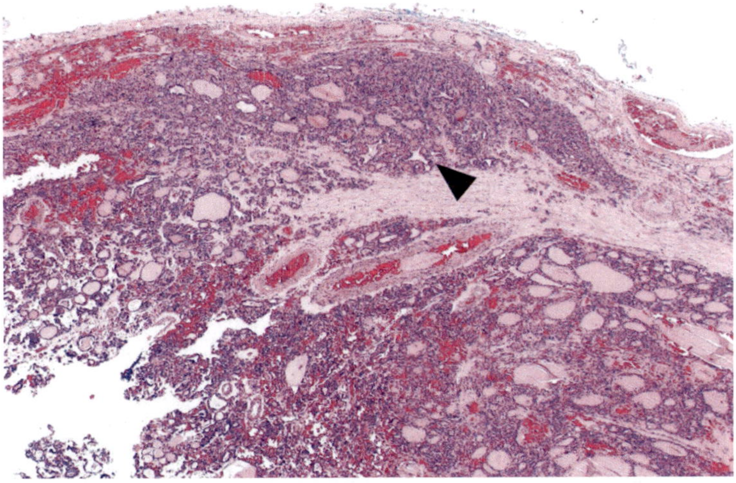

Fig. 4.309 Surgical histopathology revealed hurthle cell carcinoma (Fig. 4.306, Fig. 4.307, Fig. 4.308) showing mushroom like capsular invasion of the tumor (arrow)

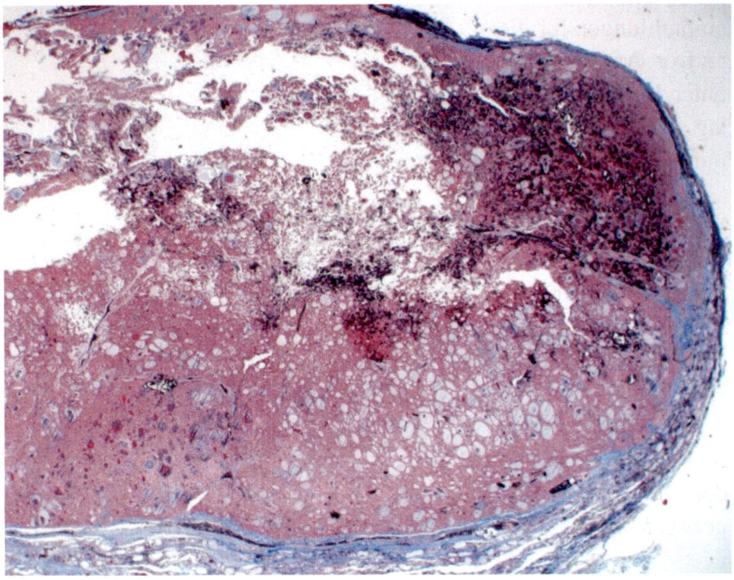

Fig. 4.310 Masson Trichrome stain showed fibrotic area appeared mainly around the margin of the nodule and nearly none in the tumor explaining low elasticity on the stiffeness map, the shear wave elastogram (Fig. 4.304)

showed a 1.54 cm round nodule in the left lobe (Figs. 4.293, 4.294, and 4.295) and SWE showed low elasticity in the nodule (E_{Max} 32.2 kPa, Fig. 4.296) except the medial margin of the nodule (E_{Max} 132.2 kPa, Fig. 4.297), suggesting the probability of follicular neoplasm. After the explanation of the results, she preferred surgery, and total thyroidectomy was performed. Surgical histopathology was microinvasive follicular carcinoma, showing mushroom-like capsular invasion (Figs. 4.298, 4.299, and 4.300) showing a thick fibrous capsule in the medial margin of the nodule (Fig. 4.299), compatible with the finding of the high elasticity on the medial margin on SWE (Fig. 4.297).

4.6.2 Case 2

A 36-year-old woman was found to have a left 3.0 cm thyroid nodule and FNA showed microfollicles, suggesting follicular neoplasm. On USG follow-up three years later, the nodule increased to 3.84 cm and showed an isoechoic solid nodule, with increased internal vascularity on color Doppler (Figs. 4.301, 4.302, and 4.303). Shear wave elastogram showed low elasticity in the whole nodule, which is color coded with deep blue (E_{Max} 30.0 kPa, Fig. 4.304). CNB showed abortive oxyphilic microfollicles, suggesting oxyphilic follicular neoplasm (Fig. 4.305). She underwent total thyroidectomy. Surgical histopathology revealed Hürthle cell carcinoma (Figs. 4.306, 4.307, and 4.308), showing mushroom-like capsular invasion of the tumor (arrow, Fig. 4.309). The Masson Trichrome stain showed that the fibrotic area appeared mainly around the margin of the nodule and nearly none in the tumor (Fig. 4.310), explaining low elasticity on the stiffness map, the shear wave elastogram (Fig. 4.304).

4.7 Medullary Thyroid Carcinoma

Medullary thyroid carcinoma (MTC) is derived from the calcitonin-producing C-cells or parafollicular cells, and accounts for 5% of thyroid malignant neoplasm. About 30% of MTCs are heritable forms; multiple endocrine neoplasia (MEN) type 2A (Sipple's syndrome) including pheochromocytomas and hyperparathyroidism, and MEN type 2B (mucosal neuroma syndrome)

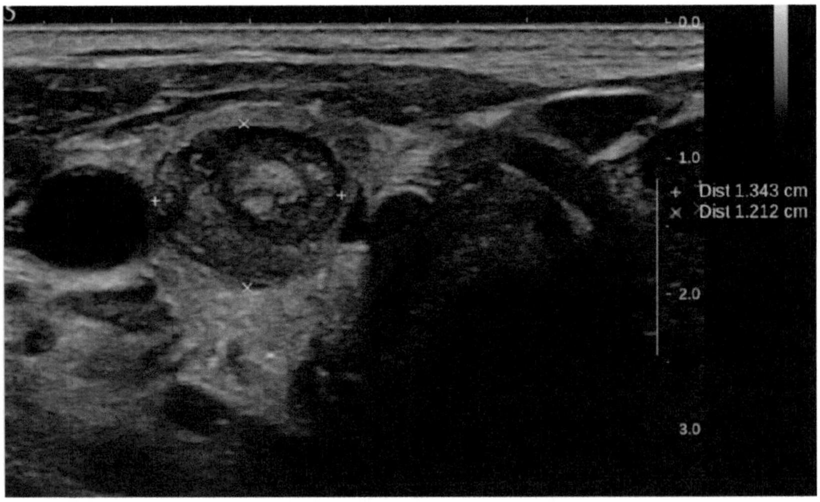

Fig. 4.311 On ultrasonogram, a 1.679 cm isoechoic round nodule mixed with hypoechoic foci was found in the right upper lobe

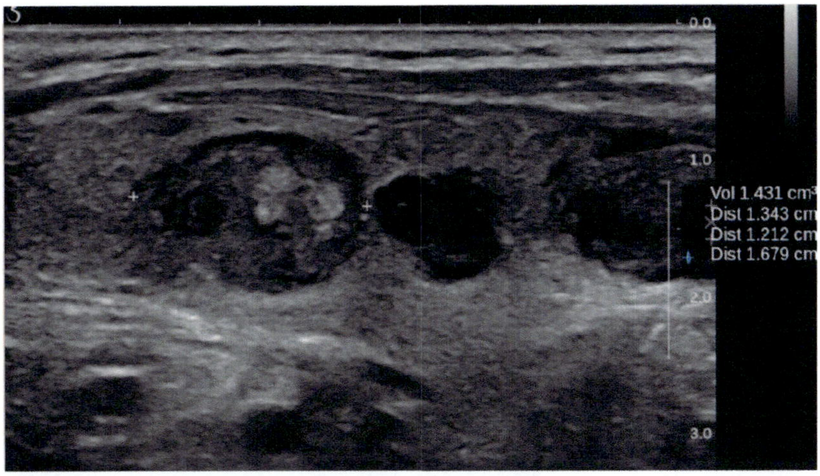

Fig. 4.312 On ultrasonogram, a 1.679 cm isoechoic round nodule mixed with hypoechoic foci was found in the right upper lobe

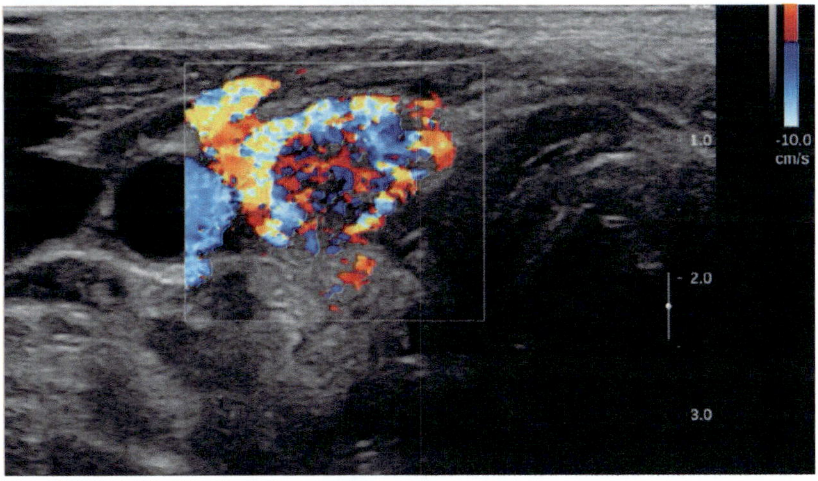

Fig. 4.313 Color Doppler showed increased internal vascularity

and familial MTC (FMTC). The hereditary forms are associated with germ-line mutations in the RET proto-oncogene on chromosome 10 and autosomal dominant mode of inheritance. Sporadic MTC and FMTC are usually found in older age with a peak incidence of 40–50 years. Up to 50–70% of patients with palpable nodules have cervical lymph node metastasis. Serum levels of calcitonin correlate with tumor burden and are helpful for the diagnosis of MTC.

Sporadic MTC presents as a single nodule, but heritable MTCs are usually bilateral and multifocal. MTCs are composed of round, polygonal-to-spindle-shaped cells containing calcitonin secretory granules and form nests, follicles or trabeculae. MTCs exhibit a wide variety of histologic and cytologic appearance including papillary, giant cells, spindle cell, small cells, oncocytic and clear-cell variants. Amyloid depos-

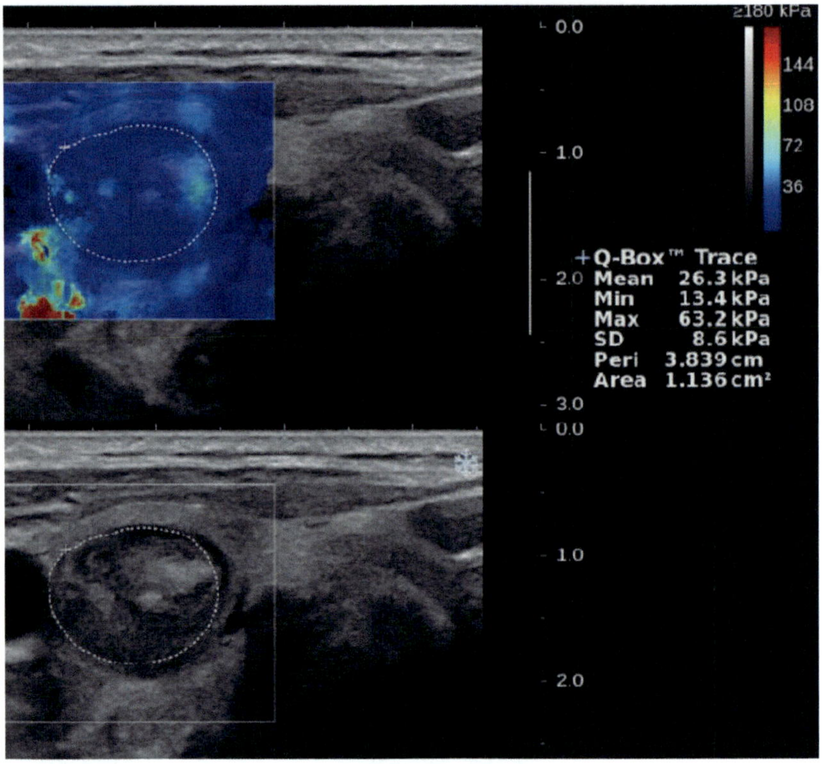

Fig. 4.314 Shear wave elastogram showed focal increased elasticity and E_{Max} was 63.2 kPa

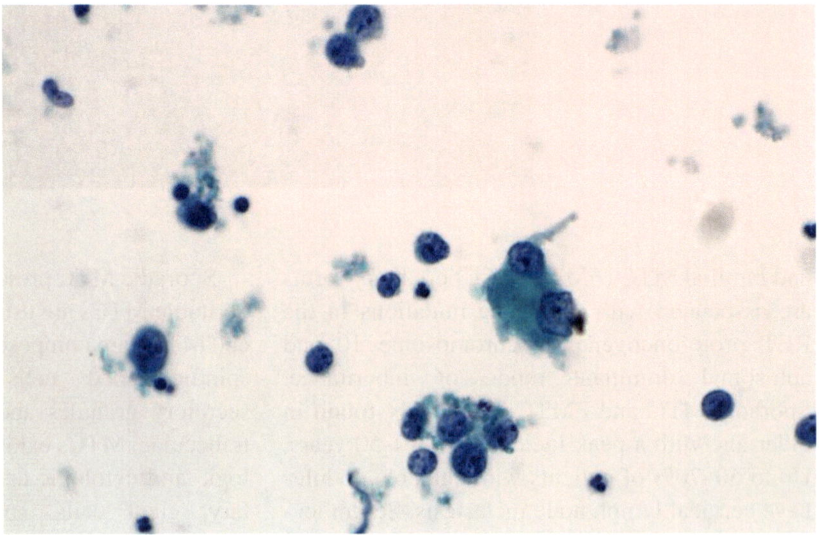

Fig. 4.315 FNA showed ovoid, plasmacytoid cells with abundant cytoplasm and salt and pepper appearance chromatin

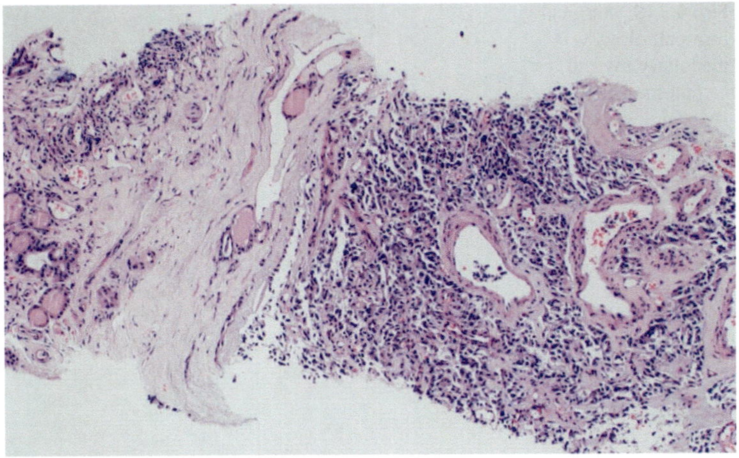

Fig. 4.316 CNB showed sheets of polygonal cells with fibrous capsule-like structure

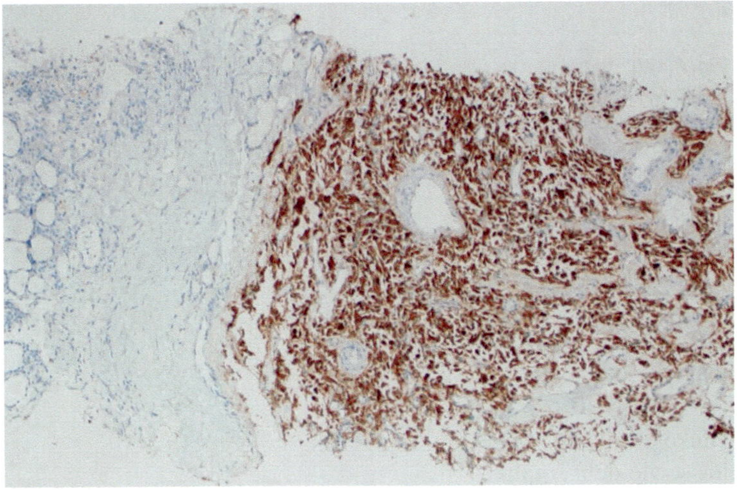

Fig. 4.317 CNB showed sheets of polygonal cells with fibrous capsule-like structure and positivity for calcitonin

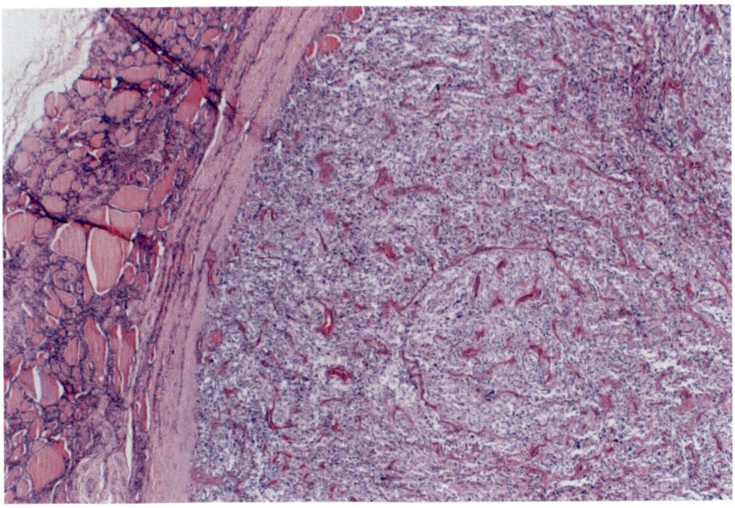

Fig. 4.318 Surgical histopathology was medullary thyroid carcinoma which showed nested growth of plasmacytoid or polygonal cells with hyperchromatic nuclei and low mitotic figures

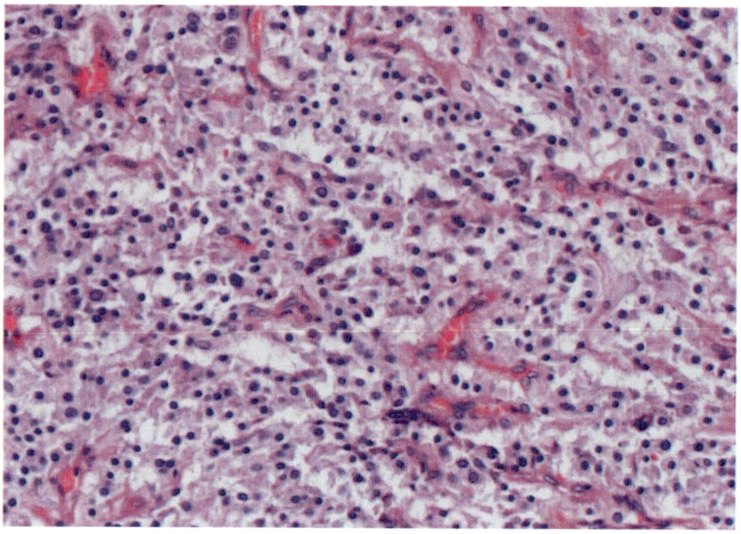

Fig. 4.319 Surgical histopathology was medullary thyroid carcinoma which showed nested growth of plasmacytoid or polygonal cells with hyperchromatic nuclei and low mitotic figures

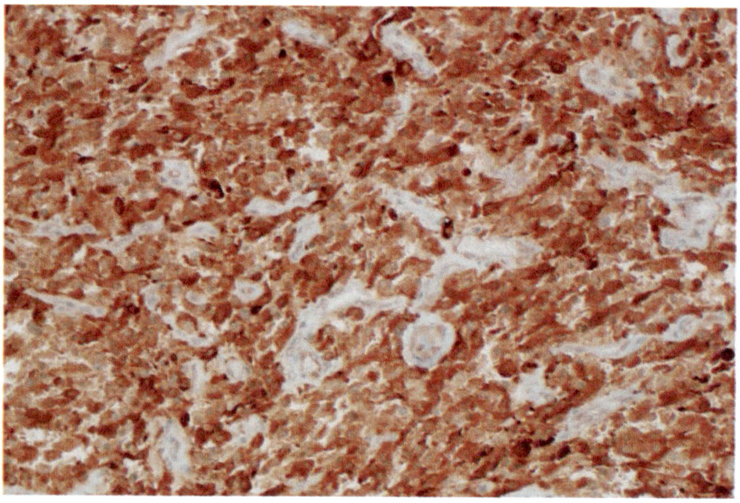

Fig. 4.320 Surgical histopathology was medullary thyroid carcinoma which showed positivity for calcitonin

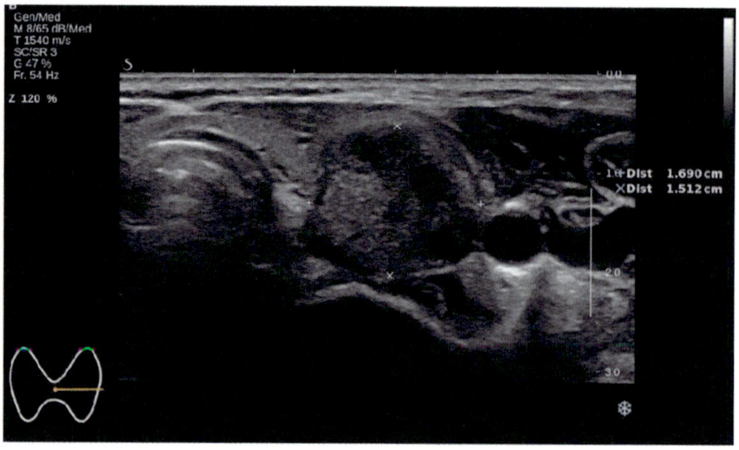

Fig. 4.321 On USG, 2.50 cm suspicious hypoechogenic nodule with echogenic foci was observed in the left middle lobe

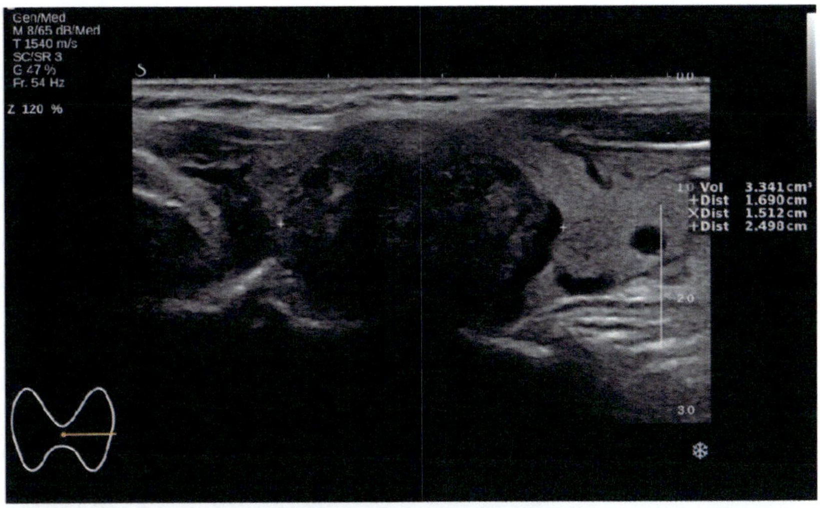

Fig. 4.322 On USG, 2.50 cm suspicious hypoechogenic nodule with echogenic foci was observed in the left lobe

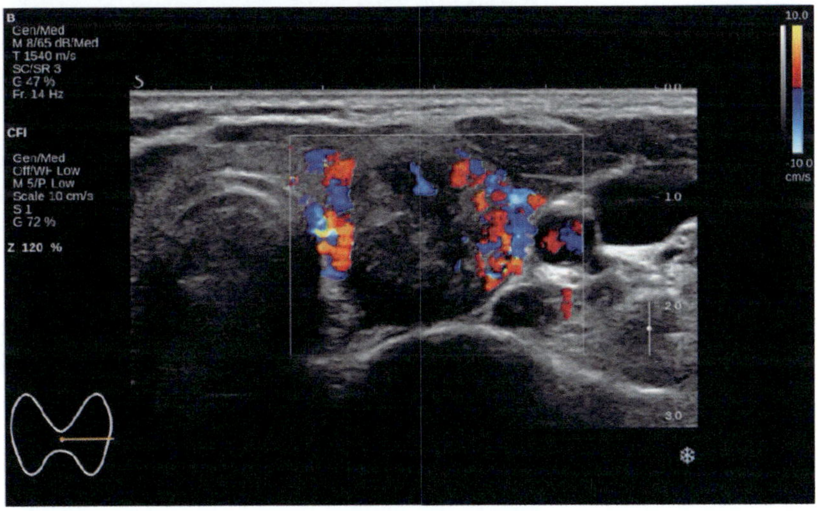

Fig. 4.323 Moderately increased internal vascularity was observed on color Doppler

its derived from calcitonin polypeptides are present in the stroma in 90% of cases [9].

On B-mode ultrasound, MTC showed a solid hypoechoic nodule with echogenic foci in 80–90% due to amyloid deposition or calcification [16]. SWE results have not been reported yet.

4.7.1 Case 1

An 84-year-old woman was found to have a thyroid nodule on routine check and referred for evaluation. On ultrasonogram, a 1.679 cm isoechoic round nodule mixed with hypoechoic foci was found in the right upper lobe (Figs. 4.311 and 4.312) and color Doppler showed increased internal vascularity (Fig. 4.313). Shear wave elastogram showed focal increased elasticity (E_{Max} 63.2 kPa, E_{mean} 26.3 kPa, Fig. 4.314). The preoperative level of serum calcitonin was 248.88 pg/mL. FNA showed ovoid, plasmacytoid cells with abundant cytoplasm, and chromatin with salt and pepper appearance (Fig. 4.315). CNB showed sheets of polygonal cells with fibrous capsule-like structures (Fig. 4.316) and positivity for calcitonin (Fig. 4.317), suggesting medullary thyroid carcinoma. Total thyroidec-

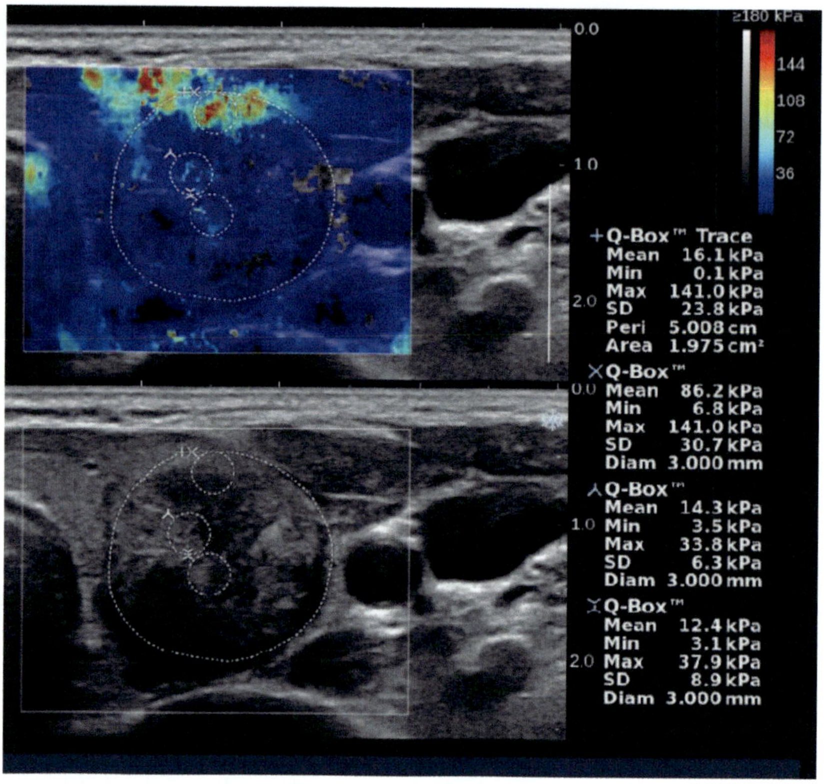

Fig. 4.324 SWE showed low elasticity (E_{Max} 33.8 kPa) except in the upper margin of the nodule (E_{Max} 141.0 kPa)

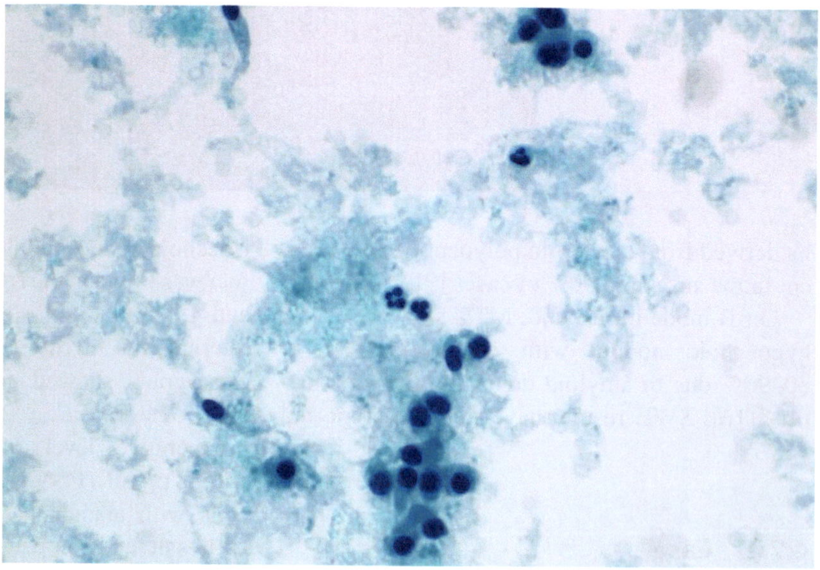

Fig. 4.325 FNA showed clusters of ovoid cells with small to moderate amount of cytoplasm and hyperchromatic nuclei

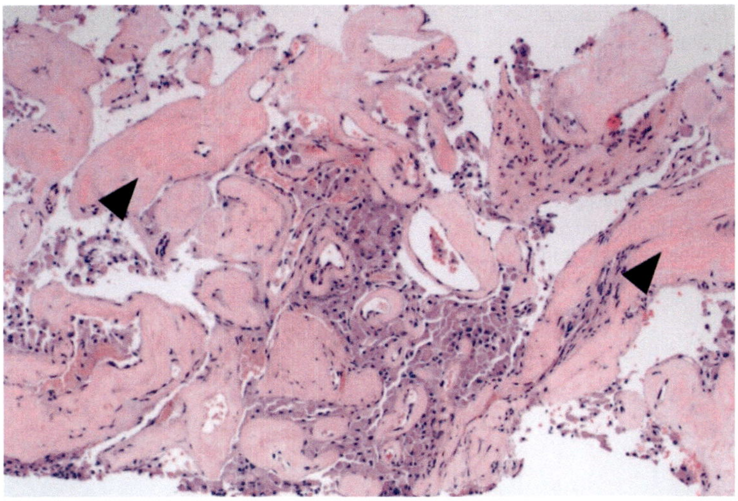

Fig. 4.326 CNB showed proliferation of polygonal cells with amphophilic cytoplasm on the background of hyalinized stroma with amyloid deposition (arrow)

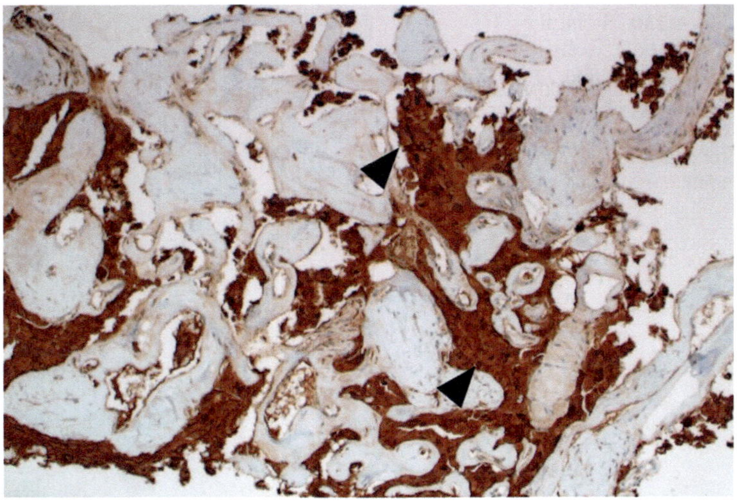

Fig. 4.327 CNB showed tumor cells were positive for calcitonin (arrow).

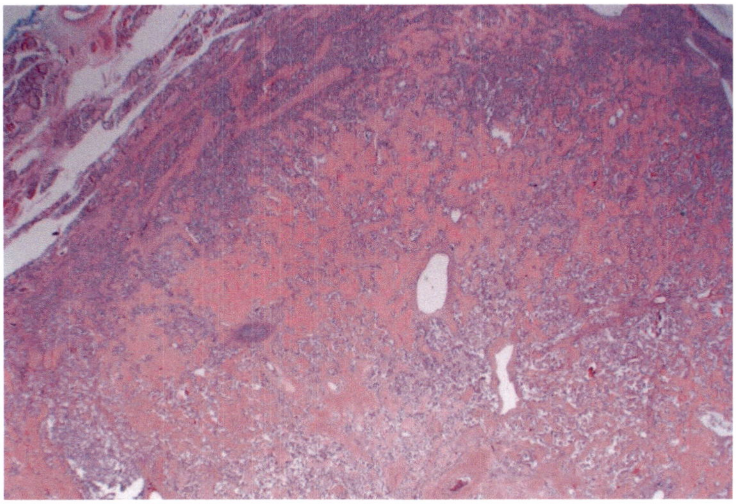

Fig. 4.328 Surgical histopathology was medullary thyroid carcinoma which was consisted of polygonal cells with abundant amphophilic cytoplasm on the markedly hyalinized stroma

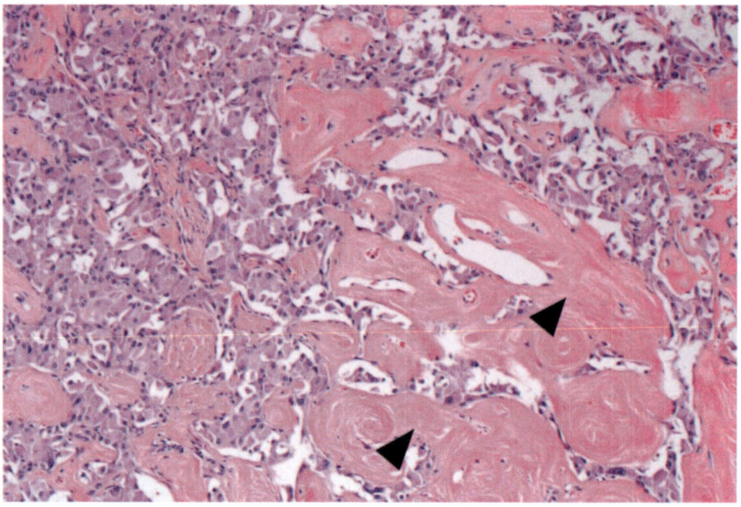

Fig. 4.329 Surgical histopathology was medullary thyroid carcinoma (Fig. 4.328) which was consisted of polygonal cells with abundant amphophilic cytoplasm on the markedly hyalinized stroma with amyloid deposition (arrow).

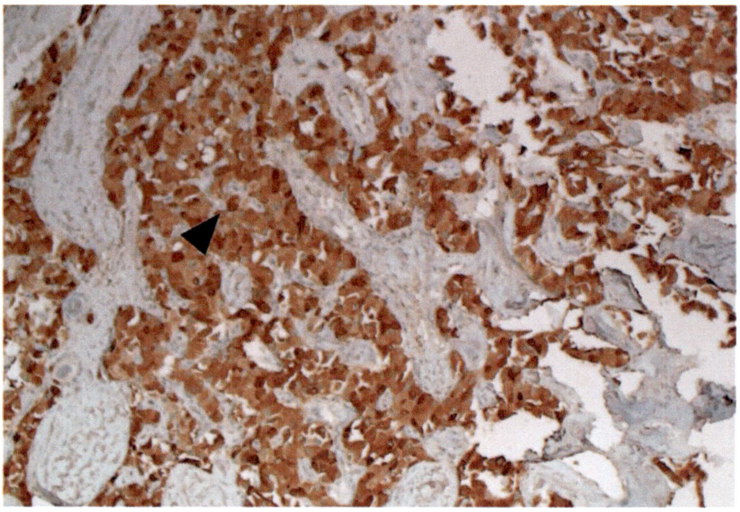

Fig. 4.330 Surgical histopathology was medullary thyroid carcinoma and tumor cells showed positivity for calcitonin immunostaining (arrow)

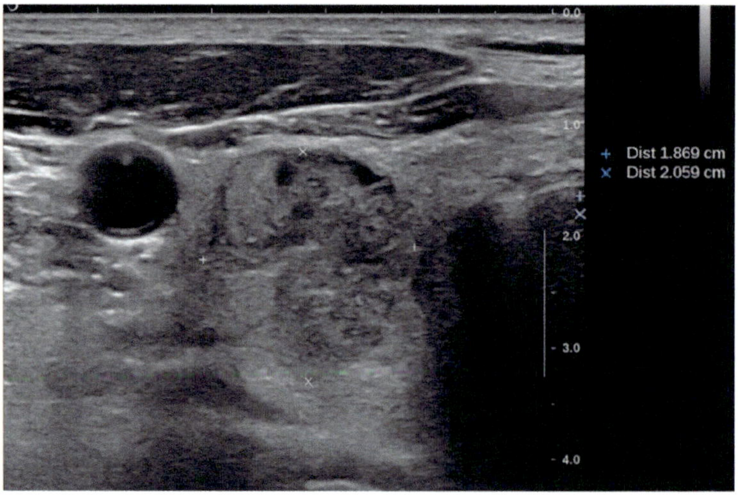

Fig. 4.331 On USG, 2.37 cm isoechogenic nodule was observed in the right middle lobe

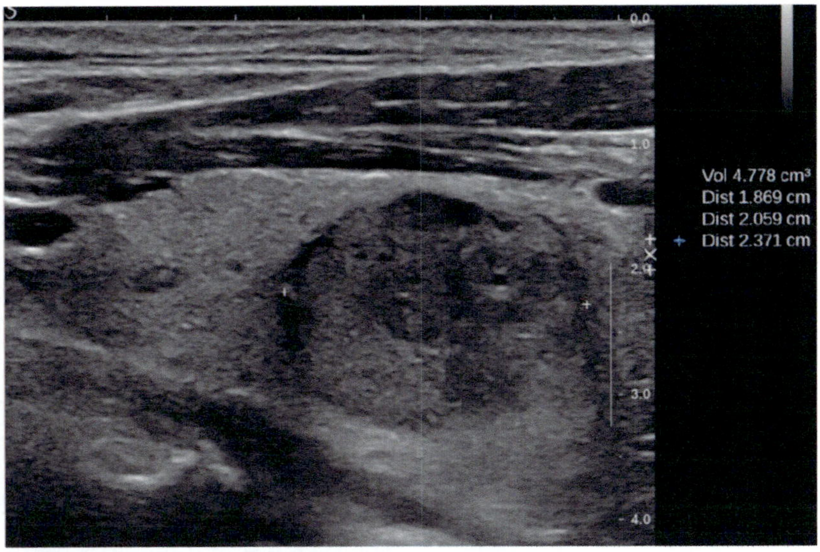

Fig. 4.332 On USG, 2.37 cm isoechogenic nodule was observed in the right middle lobe

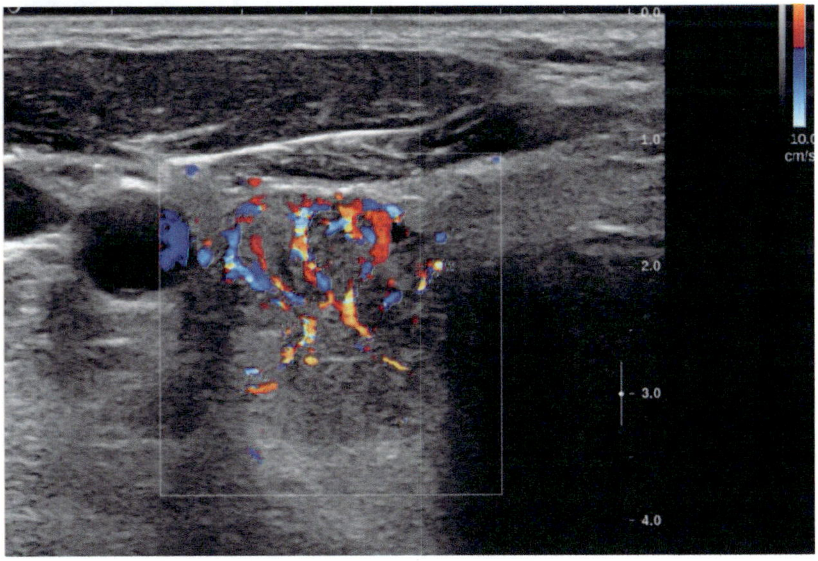

Fig. 4.333 Color Doppler showed increased internal vascularity within the nodule

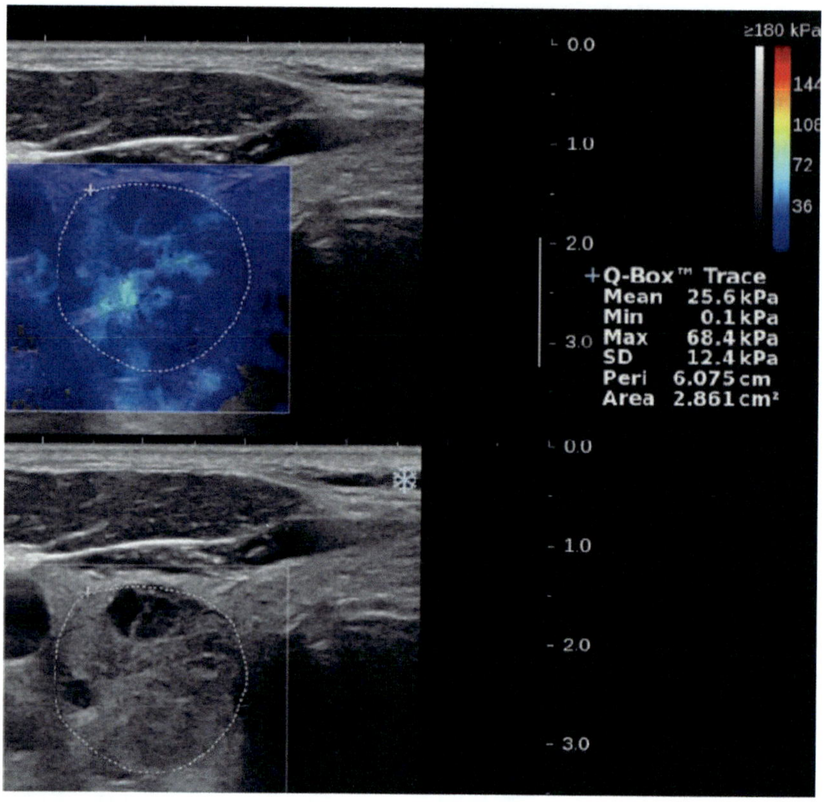

Fig. 4.334 SWE showed uneven distribution of elasticity indices and E_{Max} was 68.4 kPa

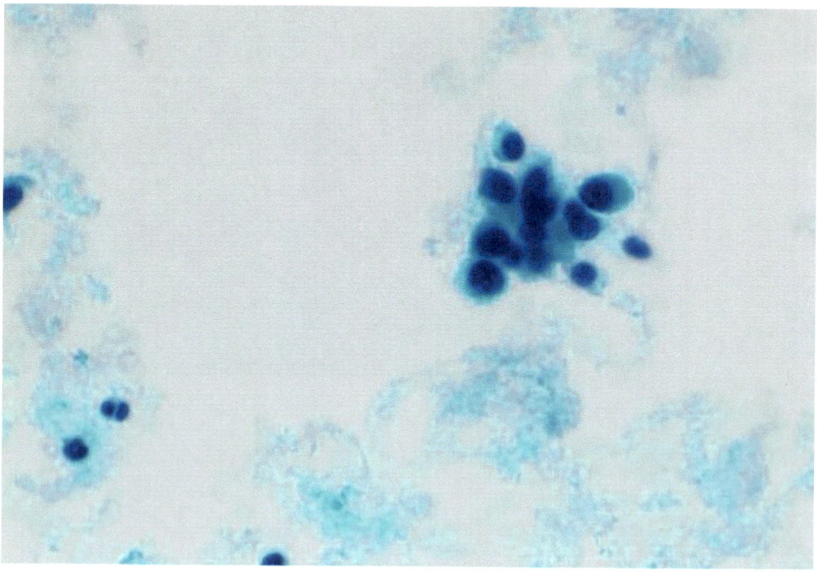

Fig. 4.335 FNA showed a few small clusters of ovoid cells with moderate amount of cytoplasm and hyperchromatic nuclei

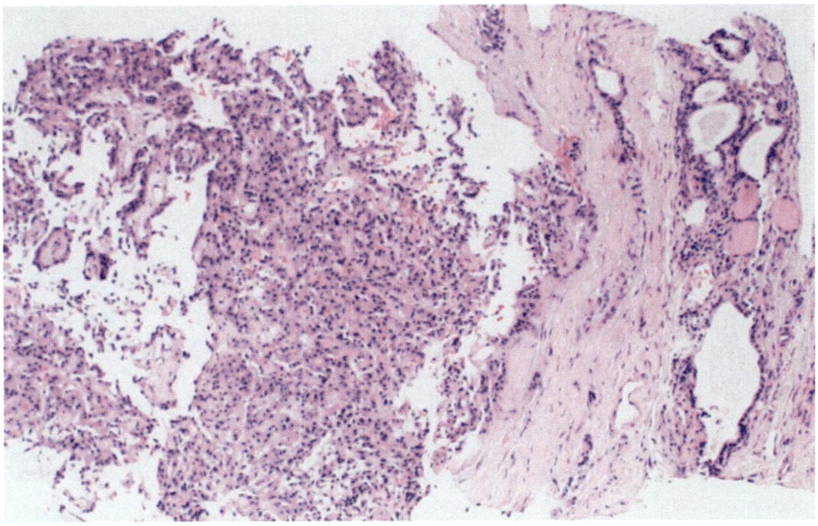

Fig. 4.336 CNB showed ovoid or polygonal cells on the background of hyalinized stroma

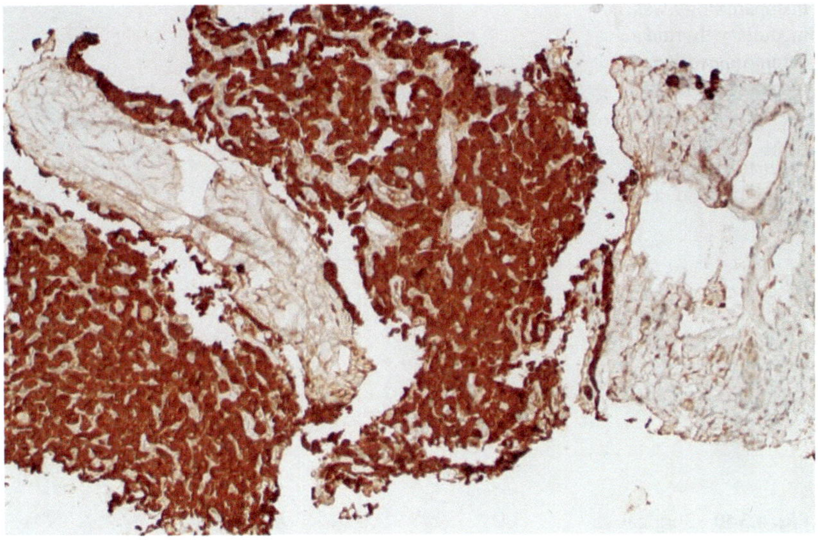

Fig. 4.337 CNB showed ovoid or polygonal cells on the background of hyalinized stroma and positivity in calcitonin immunostaining

tomy was performed and surgical histopathology was medullary thyroid carcinoma, which showed nested growth of plasmacytoid or polygonal cells with hyperchromatic nuclei and low mitotic figures (Figs. 4.318 and 4.319) and positivity for calcitonin (Fig. 4.320).

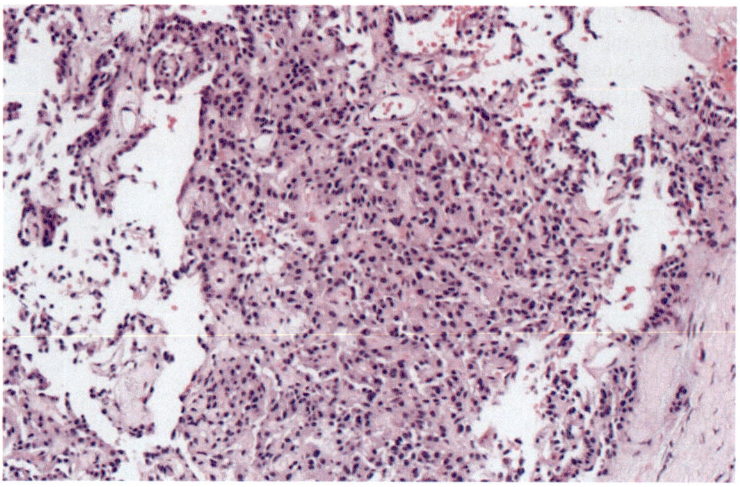

Fig. 4.338 Surgical histopathology was medullary thyroid carcinoma which showed sheet-like growth of round to ovoid cells with hyperchromatic nuclei and abundant amphophilic cytoplasm

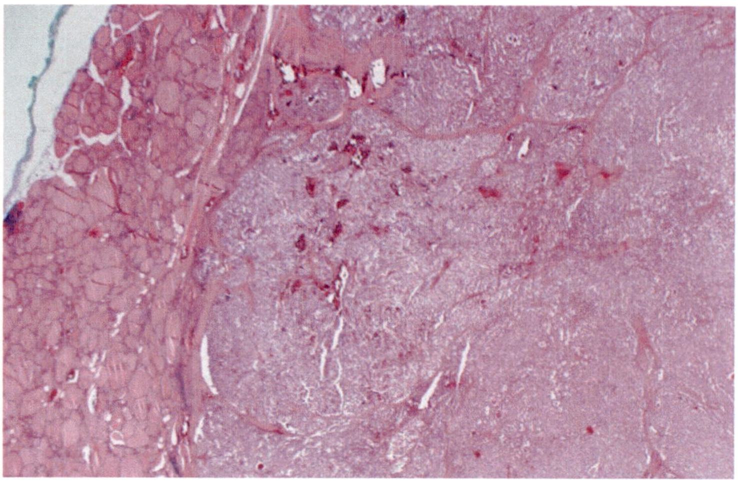

Fig. 4.339 Surgical histopathology was medullary thyroid carcinoma with a relatively well circumscribed, solid mass, which showed sheet-like growth of round to ovoid cells

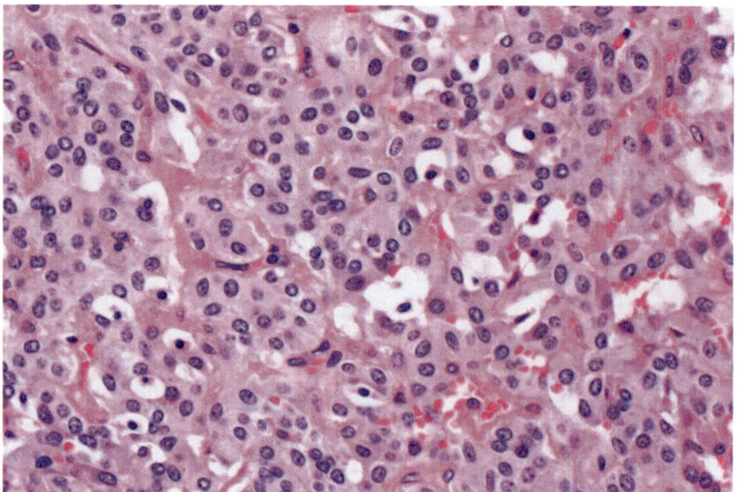

Fig. 4.340 Surgical histopathology was medullary thyroid carcinoma showing sheet-like growth of round to ovoid cells with hyperchromatic nuclei and abundant amphophilic cytoplasm

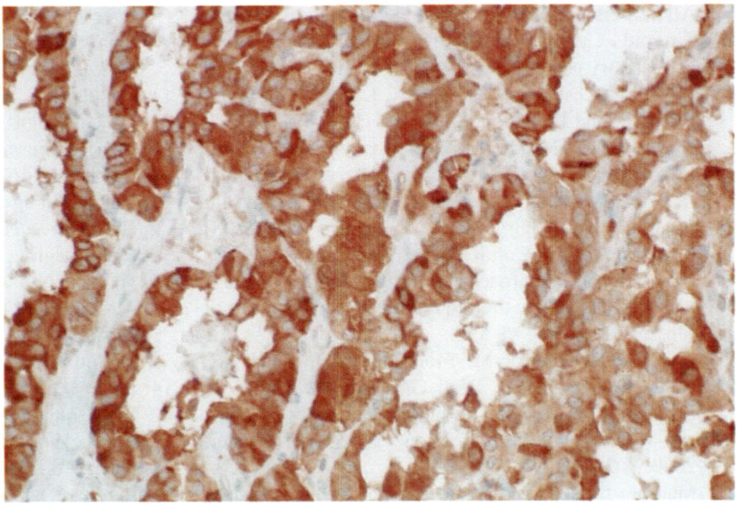

Fig. 4.341 Surgical histopathology was medullary thyroid carcinoma showing positivity for calcitonin

4.7.2 Case 2

A 75-year-old woman presented a thyroid nodule found incidentally. On USG, a 2.50 cm suspicious hypoechogenic nodule with echogenic foci and moderate internal vascularity was observed in the left lobe (Figs. 4.321, 4.322, and 4.323). SWE showed low elasticity (E_{Max} 33.8 kPa, Fig. 4.324) except in the upper margin of the nodule (E_{Max} 141.0 kPa). The serum calcitonin level was 1025.05 pg/mL. FNA showed clusters of ovoid cells with small to moderate amount of cytoplasm and hyperchromatic nuclei (Fig. 4.325). CNB showed proliferation of polygonal cells with amphophilic cytoplasm on the background of hyalinized stroma with amyloid deposition (arrow, Fig. 4.326) and positivity for calcitonin (arrow, Fig. 4.327). Surgical histopathology was medullary thyroid carcinoma (Fig. 4.328), which consisted of polygonal cells with abundant amphophilic cytoplasm on the markedly hyalinized stroma (arrow, Fig. 4.329), and positive for calcitonin immunostaining (arrow. Fig. 4.330).

4.7.3 Case 3

A 72-year-old man was referred for the evaluation of a thyroid nodule incidentally found on a C-spine MRI scan that was taken for shoulder pain. On USG, a 2.37 cm isoechogenic nodule with increased internal vascularity was observed in the right middle lobe (Figs. 4.331, 4.332, and 4.333). SWE showed uneven distribution of elasticity indices (E_{Max} 68.4 kPa, Fig. 4.334). The serum calcitonin level was 2444.95 pg/mL. FNA showed a few small clusters of ovoid cells with moderate amount of cytoplasm and hyperchromatic nuclei (Fig. 4.335). CNB showed ovoid or polygonal cells on the background of hyalinized stroma (Figs. 4.336 and 4.337), and positivity in calcitonin immunostaining (Fig. 4.338). Surgical histopathology was medullary thyroid carcinoma with a relatively well-circumscribed, solid mass (Fig. 4.339), which showed sheet-like growth of round to ovoid cells with hyperchromatic nuclei and abundant amphophilic cytoplasm (Fig. 4.340) and positivity for calcitonin (Fig. 4.341).

References

1. Kumar V, Abbas AK, Aster JC. Robbins and Cotran pathologic basis of disease. 9th ed. Philadelphia, PA: Elsevier; 2015.
2. Baloch ZW, Livolsi VA. Follicular-patterned lesions of the thyroid: the bane of the pathologist. Am J Clin Pathol. 2002;117:143–50.

3. Ali SZ, Cibas ES. The Bethesda System for Reporting Thyroid Cytopathology: definitions, criteria and explanatory notes. New York, NY: Springer; 2010.
4. Grant EG, Tessler FN, Hoang JK, Langer JE, Beland MD, Berland LL, Cronan JJ, Desser TS, Frates MC, Hamper UM, Middleton WD, Reading CC, Scoutt LM, Stavros AT, Teefey SA. Thyroid ultrasound reporting lexicon: White Paper of the ACR Thyroid Imaging, Reporting and Data System (TIRADS) Committee. J Am Coll Radiol. 2015;12:1272–9.
5. Alexander EK. Approach to the patient with a cytologically indeterminate thyroid nodule. J Clin Endocrinol Metab. 2008;93:4175–82.
6. Greaves TS, Olvera M, Florentine BD, Raza AS, Cobb CJ, Tsao-Wei DD, Groshen S, Singer P, Lopresti J, Martin SE. Follicular lesions of thyroid: a 5-year fine-needle aspiration experience. Cancer. 2000;90:335–41.
7. Maruta J, Hashimoto H, Suehisa Y, Yamashita H, Noguchi S, Aratake Y, Ohno E, Kobayashi TK. Improving the diagnostic accuracy of thyroid follicular neoplasms: cytological features in fine-needle aspiration cytology. Diagn Cytopathol. 2011;39:28–34.
8. DeMay RM. Follicular lesions of the thyroid. W(h)ither follicular carcinoma? Am J Clin Pathol. 2000;114:681–3.
9. Lloyd RV, Osamura RY, Kloppel G, Rosai J. WHO classification of tumours of endocrine organs (Medicine). 4th ed. Lyon: International Agency for Research on Cancer; 2017.
10. Barr RG, Ferraioli G, Palmeri ML, Goodman ZD, Garcia-Tsao G, Rubin J, Garra B, Myers RP, Wilson SR, Rubens D, Levine D. Elastography assessment of liver fibrosis: Society of Radiologists in Ultrasound Consensus Conference Statement. Radiology. 2015;276:845–61.
11. Fukuhara T, Matsuda E, Izawa S, Fujiwara K, Kitano H. Utility of shear wave elastography for diagnosing chronic autoimmune thyroiditis. J Thyroid Res. 2015;2015:164548.
12. Liu J, Zhang Y, Ji Y, Wan Q, Dun G. The value of shear wave elastography in diffuse thyroid disease. Clin Imaging. 2018;49:187–92.
13. Kamaya A, Machtaler S, Safari Sanjani S, Nikoozadeh A, Graham Sommer F, Pierre Khuri-Yakub BT, Willmann JK, Desser TS. New technologies in clinical ultrasound. Semin Roentgenol. 2013;48:214–23.
14. Samir AE, Dhyani M, Anvari A, Prescott J, Halpern EF, Faquin WC, Stephen A. Shear-wave elastography for the preoperative risk stratification of follicular-patterned lesions of the thyroid: diagnostic accuracy and optimal measurement plane. Radiology. 2015;277:565–73.
15. Gregory A, Bayat M, Kumar V, Denis M, Kim BH, Webb J, Meixner DD, Ryder M, Knudsen JM, Chen S, Fatemi M, Alizad A. Differentiation of benign and malignant thyroid nodules by using comb-push ultrasound shear elastography: A preliminary two-plane view study. Acad Radiol. 2018;25:1388–97.
16. Dighe M, Barr R, Bojunga J, Cantisani V, Chammas MC, Cosgrove D, Cui XW, Dong Y, Fenner F, Radzina M, Vinayak S, Xu JM, Dietrich CF. Thyroid ultrasound: state of the art Part 1 – Thyroid ultrasound reporting and diffuse thyroid diseases. Med Ultrason. 2017;19:79–93.

5 Summary

We tried to evaluate the efficacy of shear wave elastography (SWE), the map of stiffness in the differential diagnosis of the histopathology of thyroid nodules. We examined the patterns of the elasticity index (EI) of SWE in various histopathology groups of 212 thyroid nodules and assess the distribution patterns of the histopathology groups in the different ranges of EI to evaluate whether SWE is useful in predicting the histopathology of the thyroid nodules.

5.1 Distribution of EI (E_{Max}) in Various Pathology Groups

Thyroid nodules were divided into three groups according to E_{Max}: Group I (E_{Max} < 41.3 kPa), Group II (E_{Max} 41.3~99.9 kPa) and Group III ($E_{Max} \geq 100.0$ kPa). The cutoff values of Group I and Group II were set using receiver-operating-characteristic (ROC) curve analysis to predict follicular neoplasm (FN) from nodular hyperplasia (NH). The cutoff values for Groups II and III were arbitrarily set by the researcher.

E_{Max} of FN belonged nearly entirely to Group I (96.3%),rarely in Group II (3.7%) and none in Group III (0%). E_{Max} of NH belonged mainly to Group II (82.5%), and the rest in Group I (7.5%) and Group III (10.5%) (Fig. 5.1). E_{Max} of chronic lymphocytic thyroiditis (CLT) belonged in majority to Group II (61.1%), and in minority to Group I (22.2%) and Group III (16.7%). E_{Max} of subacute thyroiditis (ST) belonged entirely to Group III (100%), and none to Groups I (0%) or

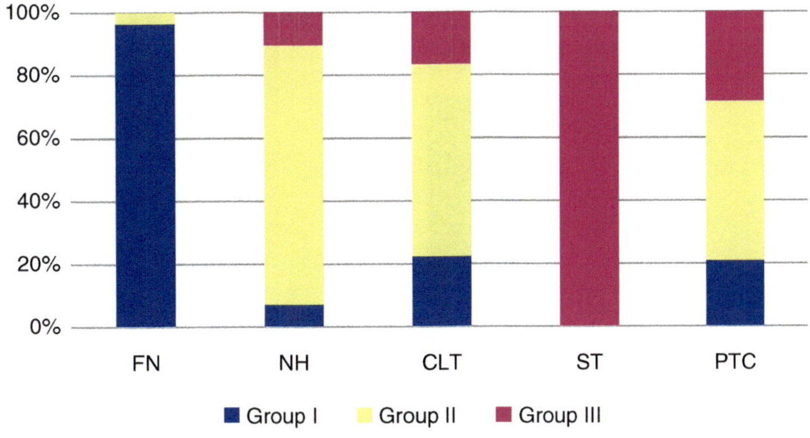

Fig. 5.1 Distribution of elasticity index (E_{Max}) according to pathology groups by fine-needle aspiration or core-needle biopsy. E_{Max}, maximum elasticity; kPa, kilo-Pascal; FN, follicular neoplasm; NH, nodular hyperplasia; CLT, chronic lymphocytic thyroiditis; ST, subacute thyroiditis; PTC, papillary thyroid carcinoma. Data are presented as numbers (percentages)

M. H. Yoo et al., *Shear Wave Elastography of Thyroid Nodules*,
https://doi.org/10.1007/978-981-33-6873-6_5

Group II (0%) (Fig. 5.1). E_{Max} of papillary thyroid carcinoma (PTC) belonged in majority to Group II (50.5%), and followed by Group III (28.6%) and Group I (20.9%) (Fig. 5.1). The distribution of the pathology groups in Group I was significantly different from that in Group II and Group III as per Fisher's exact test (Group I vs II ($p < 0.001$), Group II vs III ($p < 0.001$), and Group I vs III ($p < 0.001$) by Fisher's exact test and bonferroni correction).

5.2 Distribution of Various Pathology Groups According to E_{Max}

Group I was composed of FN (49.1%) and PTC (35.8%) (Fig. 5.2). Group II was composed of NH (44.8%), PTC (43.8%) and CLT (10.5%). Group III was composed of PTC (65.0%), NH (15.0%), ST (12.5%), and CLT (7.5%) (Fig. 5.2). The distribution of the pathology groups in Group I was significantly different from that in Group II and Group III by Fisher's exact test ($p < 0.001$). Also, the distribution of the pathology groups in Group II was significantly different from that in Group III (Group I vs II ($p < 0.001$), Group II vs III ($p < 0.001$), and Group I vs III ($p < 0.001$) by Fisher's exact test and bonferroni correction).

Our data showed that the distribution patterns of pathology groups in Groups I, II, and III were significantly different from each other by Fisher's exact test (Fig. 5.2), suggesting different elasticity might predict different probability of the possible histopathology of the thyroid nodules. All these patterns of each EI group may provide the physician with information about the probability of the histopathology of thyroid nodules over the findings of B-mode USG.

SWE illustrates the map of stiffness of the thyroid nodule and may help predicting the histopathology of the nodule. Especially regarding the follicular patterned lesion, which comprises more than 50% of all thyroid nodules, a differential diagnosis of FN and NH is not easy by B mode USG and also frequently by FNA. CNB is helpful in the differential diagnosis of thyroid nodules with follicular patterned lesion, because it can evaluate the architectural structure including the presence of capsules and the presence of involutional changes such as fibrosis to differentiate between FN and NH. But CNB needs experience and skills to perform and therefore has limitations and cannot be used as routine procedure. Also,

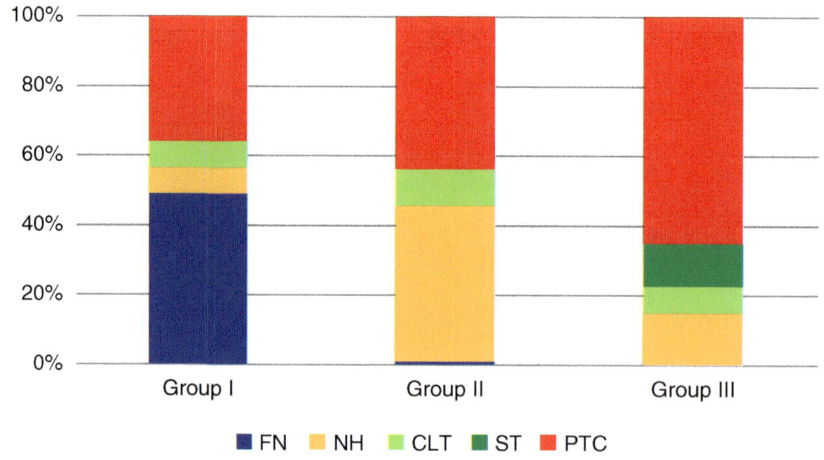

Fig. 5.2 Subgroup analyses of the distribution of the pathology groups by fine-needle aspiration or core-needle biopsy according to the elasticity index (E_{Max}). E_{Max}, maximum elasticity; kPa, kilo-Pascal; FN, follicular neoplasm; NH, nodular hyperplasia; CLT, chronic lymphocytic thyroiditis; ST, subacute thyroiditis; PTC, papillary thyroid carcinoma. Data are presented as numbers (percentages). $p < 0.001$ (Group I vs. II, Group II vs. III, and Group I vs. III by Fisher's exact test)

CNB is invasive and represents the focal tissue rather than the whole area. SWE can provide different stiffness maps because FN and NH show different degrees of fibrosis on histopathology. Our previous study revealed SWE can differentiate between FN and NH with sensitivity, specificity and diagnostic accuracy around 90%. And SWE has an advantage over CNB, like Fibroscan; it is noninvasive and does not need experience and skill like CNB. Also, SWE has the advantage that it can evaluate the whole thyroid nodule rather than small pieces of CNB. SWE will contribute to waiving benign diagnostic surgery of NH, which comprises up to 30–50% of all benign diagnostic surgeries, and to increase the rate of malignancy of thyroid surgery. Also, regarding the differentiation between benign and malignant nodules, SWE will provide additional information about the probability of possible pathology, and help the physician in deciding the candidate nodule of FNA and further management of the nodule.

As Fibroscan (another type of SWE) revolutionized the evaluation of liver cirrhosis and replaced CNB in the diagnosis and management of chronic liver disease, SWE will revolutionize the evaluation of thyroid nodules, especially for the follicular patterned lesion of thyroid with the advantage of noninvasiveness, inexpensiveness and easy appliance (no need of great skill), and will contribute to decrease the benign diagnostic surgery. We hope this book will serve as a beginning reference for that purpose.

GPSR Compliance

The European Union's (EU) General Product Safety Regulation (GPSR) is a set of rules that requires consumer products to be safe and our obligations to ensure this.

If you have any concerns about our products, you can contact us on ProductSafety@springernature.com

In case Publisher is established outside the EU, the EU authorized representative is:

Springer Nature Customer Service Center GmbH
Europaplatz 3
69115 Heidelberg, Germany

Batch number: 10091957

Printed by Printforce, the Netherlands